OXFORD MEDICAL PUBLICATIONS

Oxford Handbook of
**Nephrology and
Hypertension**

Published and forthcoming Oxford Handbooks

Oxford Handbook of
Nephrology and Hypertension

Edited by

Simon Steddon
Consultant Nephrologist
Guy's and St Thomas' Hospitals
London, UK

Neil Ashman
Consultant Nephrologist
St Bartholomew's and the Royal London Hospitals
London, UK

Alistair Chesser
Consultant Nephrologist
St Bartholomew's and the Royal London Hospitals
London, UK

and

John Cunningham
Professor of Nephrology
Royal Free & University College Hospitals
London, UK

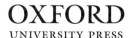

OXFORD
UNIVERSITY PRESS

OM LIBRARY (WEST SMITHFIELD)

OXFORD
UNIVERSITY PRESS

Great Clarendon Street, Oxford OX2 6DP

Oxford University Press is a department of the University of Oxford.
It furthers the University's objective of excellence in research, scholarship,
and education by publishing worldwide in

Oxford New York

Auckland Cape Town Dar es Salaam Hong Kong Karachi
Kuala Lumpur Madrid Melbourne Mexico City Nairobi
New Delhi Shanghai Taipei Toronto

With offices in

Argentina Austria Brazil Chile Czech Republic France Greece
Guatemala Hungary Italy Japan Poland Portugal Singapore
South Korea Switzerland Thailand Turkey Ukraine Vietnam

Oxford is a registered trade mark of Oxford University Press
in the UK and in certain other countries

Published in the United States
by Oxford University Press Inc., New York

© Oxford University Press 2006

The moral rights of the authors have been asserted
Database right Oxford University Press (maker)

First published 2006
Reprinted 2011

All rights reserved. No part of this publication may be reproduced,
stored in a retrieval system, or transmitted, in any form or by any means,
without the prior permission in writing of Oxford University Press,
or as expressly permitted by law, or under terms agreed with the appropriate
reprographics rights organization. Enquiries concerning reproduction
outside the scope of the above should be sent to the Rights Department,
Oxford University Press, at the address above

You must not circulate this book in any other binding or cover
and you must impose the same condition on any acquirer

British Library Cataloguing in Publication Data
Data available

Library of Congress Cataloging in Publication Data
Data available

Typeset by Newgen Imaging Systems (P) Ltd., Chennai, India
Printed in China
on acid-free paper
through Asia Pacific Offset

ISBN 0–19–852069–7 (flexicover: alk.paper)   978–0–19–852069–6 (flexicover: alk. paper)

10 9 8 7 6 5 4 3

QM LIBRARY (WEST SMITHFIELD)

Foreword

The whole of nephrology in your pocket—can this be achieved? Nephrology has the reputation of being a cerebral specialty which requires the practitioner to understand substantial swathes of physiology and have an academic bent if they are to be a successful clinician. The implication might be that a compact pocket-sized text to assist the practicing clinician day-by-day in assessing people with kidney disease and hypertension might be an unrealistic goal.

I am very pleased to say that the authors of this Oxford Handbook have proved the doubters wrong. By balancing their coverage so that clinically common problems deservedly get more space, they have nicely provided the level of information necessary for everyday clinical practice. Importantly there is sufficient pathophysiology to assist in the evaluation of acutely ill people in whom impaired kidney function is contributing to the illness, an increasingly common problem in clinical practice particularly with an aging population. But at the same time there is pithy and well informed coverage of the uncommon, as well as vignettes about the fascinating rarities, which are such an engaging feature of clinical nephrology.

Proper clinical assessment of hypertension, the identification of those with underlying kidney disease, and the extent to which detailed evaluation of the kidneys in such patients should be pursued, are other practical clinical issues often neglected in texts which prefer to consider nephrology and hypertension as separate matters. Here they have been drawn together well with much practical information.

I am sure that this Oxford Handbook, like so many of its stablemates, will find its way into the pockets and bags of many doctors of all ages working not only in renal units but in many other healthcare settings.

Professor John Feehally
President UK Renal Association
Secretary General International
Society of Nephrology
July 2006

Oxford University Press makes no representation, express or implied, that the drug dosages in this book are correct. Readers must therefore always check the product information and clinical procedures with the most up-to-date published product information and data sheets provided by the manufacturers and the most recent codes of conduct and safety regulations. The authors and the publishers do not accept responsibility or legal liability for any errors in the text or for the misuse or misapplication of material in this work.

Preface

The ability to recognize and understand renal disease and hypertension is an important part of practice in almost any area of medicine. Acute renal failure, often preventable, occurs in up to 7% of all hospital admissions and remains responsible for much morbidity and mortality. The recent reclassification of chronic kidney disease (CKD) has exposed the scale of a serious public health issue, relevant to all medical practitioners both in primary and secondary care. Furthermore, irrespective of specialist interest, regular clinical contact with patients who are dialysis-dependent or who have undergone renal transplantation is now the norm, not the exception. Hypertension needs no introduction as the most common indication for prescription drug therapy and the most important cause of premature death in the developed world.

Many doctors are nervous of renal disease—there persists a belief that renal patients suffer exclusively from complex, esoteric conditions that can only be managed in a specialist environment and by specialists who are often more difficult and demanding than their patients. Our intention has been to write a concise but robust handbook that is first and foremost practical: what needs to be done in a busy casualty department or GP surgery several miles from the nearest renal unit. We hope it will be a useful resource not only to doctors, nurses, and other members of the multiprofessional team already engaged in the care of renal patients but also to a broader audience. For those interested in how renal disease evolves, we've provided a good grounding in the fundamentals of nephrology—hopefully dismantling some myths along the way, and giving readers the confidence to manage the day-to-day associated with kidney disease.

In line with existing Oxford Handbooks we have attempted to strike a balance between practical information, helpful to those working 'at the coal face', and the more detailed knowledge that enables effective ongoing care. The authors are all consultants working in busy renal units where theory and practice are balanced to provide effective and efficient care. The book is as up-to-date as possible and a conscious mix of evidence and reality-based medicine.

The book is laid out in twelve chapters, allowing easy access to information on a particular clinical theme. Clinical importance is measured in space, so diabetic nephropathy is given more attention than, for example, Fanconi's syndrome. The section on renal replacement therapies gives an overview of the essential elements of both dialysis and transplantation. Those looking for more detailed notes on all aspects of dialysis therapy are referred to our sister volume *The Oxford Handbook of Dialysis*, or, for general nephrology and transplant topics, our parent text *The Oxford Textbook of Nephrology*. For completeness, we have included practical procedures but would ask that these pages are used for guidance only—all must be taught by experienced operators and cannot be learnt solely from a book.

We make no apology for emphasizing the importance of clinical assessment. Yes, tubular physiology is here (we are nephrologists after all), but this book is aimed principally at clinicians in training and we still believe that without a detailed history and thorough physical examination it is impossible to order and interpret appropriate laboratory tests or imaging, let alone provide good quality care. This seems more important than ever at a time when many lament a diminished sense of enjoyment in the practice of medicine.

We are grateful to all of our colleagues who helped bring this project to fruition as well as to our families for tolerating so many lost evenings and weekends with such good grace. We hope that we have produced a book with personality, and one that brings its subject matter alive. We would like readers to enjoy the highways and byways of renal medicine and that we have avoided, in the words of Mark Twain, a book that 'everyone wants to have read, but no-one wants to read'.

SS, NA, AC, JC
London, July 2006

Contents

List of contributors

Dr Edward Sharples
Specialist Registrar in Nephrology,
St Bartholomew's and the Royal London Hospitals

Dr Raj Thuraisingham
Consultant Nephrologist,
St Bartholomew's and the Royal London Hospitals

Dr Stanley Fan
Consultant Nephrologist,
St Bartholomew's and the Royal London Hospitals

Professor Magdi Yaqoob
Consultant Nephrologist,
St Bartholomew's and the Royal London Hospitals

Advice on chapter revisions was also provided by:

Dr William Drake
Consultant Endocrinologist,
St Bartholomew's and the Royal London Hospitals

Dr Catherine Nelson-Piercy
Consultant in Obstetric Medicine,
Guys' and St Thomas' Hospitals

Mr Islam Junaid
Consultant Urologist,
St Bartholomew's and the Royal London Hospitals

Dr Marlies Ostermann
Consultant in Nephrology and Intensive Care,
Guys' and St Thomas' Hospitals

Symbols and abbreviations

⚠	warning
▶	important
♂	male
♀	female
∴	therefore
~	approx
↑	increased
↓	decreased
→	leading to
1°	primary
2°	secondary
📖	page reference
α	alpha
β	beta
⬧	controversial topic
AAA	ACE-inhibitor after anthracycline (study)
AAA	abdominal aortic aneurysum
ABPM	ambulatory blood pressure monitoring
ACEI	angiotensin converting enzyme inhibitors
ACR	albumin/creatine ratio
ACS	acute coronary syndrome
ADMA	asymmetric dimethyl arginine
ADQI	Acute Dialysis Quality Initiative
AG	anion gap
AGE	advanced glycation end-products
ANA	anti-nuclear antibodies
ANCA	anti-neutrophil cytoplasmic antibodies
ANP	atrial natriuretic peptide
APD	automated peritoneal dialysis
ARB	angiotensin-receptor blocker
ARF	acute renal failure
ASOT	anti-streptolysin O titres
ATN	acute tubular necrosis
AVF	arteriovenous fistula
BCG	Bacillus Calmette–Guérin
BMD	bone mineral density

BOO	bladder outflow obstruction
BP	blood pressure
BPH	benign prostatic hypertrophy
CAH	congenital adrenal hyperplasia
CAN	chronic allograft nephropathy
CAPD	continuous ambulatory peritoneal dialysis
CCPD	continuous cycling peritoneal dialysis
CD	collecting duct
CDC	complement-dependent crossmatch
CEPD	continuous equilibrium peritoneal dialysis
cfu	colony forming units
CKD	chronic kidney disease
CMV	cytomegalovirus
CO	cardiac output
COX	cyclo-oxygenase
CT	computerized tomography
CVVHF	continuous venovenous haemofiltration
DBP	diastolic blood pressure
DT	distal tubule
DTPA	Diethylenetriamine penta-acetic acid
EABV	effective arterial blood volume
ECF	extracellular fluid
EDD	extended duration dialysis
EG	ethylene glycol
ENaC	epithelial sodium channel
EPO	erythropoietin
ESRD	end-stage renal disease
FSGS	focal and segmental glomerulosclerosis
GBM	glomerular basement membrane
GDP	glucose degradation products
GRA	glucocorticoid remediable aldosterone
Hct	haematocrit
HD	haemodialysis
HF	haemofiltration
HIT	heparin induced thombocytopenia
HRS	hepato-renal syndrome
ICAM	intercellular adhesion molecule
IE	infective endocarditis
IMI	intramuscular injection
IV	intravenous(ly)
IVI	intravenous infusion

IVU	intravenous urogram
KDIGO	Kidney Disease Improving Global Outcomes
KDOQI	Kidney Disease Outcomes Quality Initiative
LUTS	lower urinary tract symptoms
MAG3	mercaptoacetylglycine
MARS	molecular adsorbed recirculating system
MCN	minimal change nephropathy
MCUG	micturating cysto-urethrogram
MI	myocardial infarction
MMF	mycophenolate mofetil
MRI	magnetic resonance imaging
MSA	membrane stabilizing activity
MSH	melanocyte-stimulating hormone
MW	molecular weight
NBM	nil by mouth
NIPD	night-time intermittent peritoneal dialysis
NO	nitric oxide
nocte	each night
nPCR	normalized protein catabolic rate
NR	normal range
NSAID	non-steroidal anti-flammatory drug
od	once daily
PAF	platelet activating factor
PAWP	pulmonary capillary wedge pressure
PCA	patient-controlled analgesia
PCR	protein/creatinine ratio
PCT	proximal convoluted tubule
PD	peritoneal dialysis
PET	peritoneal equilibrium tests
Plt	platelets
po	by mouth
PP	pulse pressure
PR	per-rectal
PRCA	pure red cell aplasia
PSA	prostate specific antigen
PTC	proximal tubular cells
PTFE	polytetrafluoroethylene
PUJ	pelvi-uretic junction
qds	four times daily
RAS	renin–angiotensin–aldosterone
RBF	renal blood flow

RCC	renal cell carcinoma
RIFLE	risk, injury, failure, loss, and end-stage disease
SBP	systolic blood pressure
SC	sub-cutaneous(ly)
SEP	sclerosing encapsulating peritonitis
SGA	subjective global assessment
SHPT	secondary hyperparathyroidism
SIRS	systemic inflammatory response syndrome
SLED	sustained low efficiency dialysis
SNS	sympathetic nervous system
SVC	superior vena cava
SVR	systemic vascular resistance
T1DM	type I diabetes mellitus
T2DM	type II diabetes mellitus
TBW	total body water
TCC	transitional cell carcinoma
tds	three times daily
TGF	tubulo-glomerular feedback
TIPS	trans-jugular intrahepatic portosystemic shunts
TMP	transmembrane pressure
TNM	tumour node metastates
TOD	target organ damage
TPN	total parenteral nutrition
TRUS	trans-rectal ultrasound
TURBT	transurethral resection of bladder tumour
TURP	transurethral resection of the prostate
UF	ultrafiltration
UO	urine output
USS	ultrasound scan
VHL	von Hippel–Lindau
VUJ	vesico-ureteric junction

Clinical assessment
of the renal patient

History

Introduction

In nephrology, as in all branches of medicine, a competent clinical assessment is crucial. This should endeavour to incorporate symptoms and signs:

- Arising locally from the kidneys and urinary tract.
- Resulting from impaired salt and water handling.
- Caused by failing renal excretory and metabolic function.
- Relating to a systemic disease causing or contributing to renal dysfunction.

Three further factors need to be considered:

- Asymptomatic patients often require assessment following the discovery of an abnormal BP, urinalysis, or Cr.
- Symptoms, signs, and investigation findings are organized into clinically useful clinical syndromes (see box below).
- Biochemistry, radiology, or histopathology are almost always required for accurate diagnosis (although a thorough clinical assessment will lessen over-reliance on expensive and invasive tests).

Past medical history

- Urinary problems in childhood (e.g. infections, nocturnal enuresis).
- Previously documented renal or urinary disease of any kind. Ask specifically about infections, stone disease, and, in ♂, prostatic disease.
- Hypertension. When diagnosed? Who is responsible for follow-up? Treatment? Level of control?
- Relevant systemic disease (e.g. diabetes mellitus, connective tissue disorder, gout, vascular disease).
- Insurance or employment medicals can provide invaluable historical benchmarks. Can they recall a BP check or providing a urine specimen? Have they had blood tests in the past?

Renal clinical syndromes

- Asymptomatic urinary abnormalities
  - Proteinuria (📖 p.46)
  - Microscopic haematuria (📖 p.54)
- Macroscopic haematuria (📖 p.50)
- Nephritic syndrome (📖 p.58)
  - Rapidly progressive glomerulonephritis (RPGN)
- Pulmonary renal syndromes (📖 p.60)
- Nephrotic syndrome (📖 p.48)
- Renal tubular syndromes (📖 p.64)
- Hypertension (📖 Chapter 5)
- Acute renal failure (ARF) (📖 Chapter 2)
- Chronic renal failure (CRF)/chronic kidney disease (CKD) (📖 Chapter 3)

Local symptoms of urinary tract disease

- Pain
  - Loin pain
  - Ureteric colic
  - Suprapubic pain
- Haematuria
- Change in urine appearance
- Changes in urine volume
  - Polyuria
  - Oliguria and anuria
- Lower urinary tract symptoms
  - Obstructive (voiding) symptoms:
    — acute retention of urine
    — impaired size or force of the urinary stream
    — hesitancy or abdominal straining
    — intermittent or interrupted flow
    — a sensation of incomplete emptying
  - Storage (filling) symptoms:
    — nocturia
    — daytime frequency
    — urgency
    — urge incontinence
    — dysuria
- Urethral discharge

Review of systems

May provide clues to an underlying systemic condition such as connective tissue disorder or vasculitis.
- Skin rashes
- Painful, stiff or swollen joints
- Myalgia
- Raynauds phenomenon
- Dry, red, or painful eyes
- Thromboembolic episodes
- Fevers
- Night sweats
- Sinusitis, rhinitis, epistaxis
- Haemoptysis
- Mouth ulcers
- Photosensitivity
- Sicca symptoms
- Hair loss

Drug and treatment history

Often tells its own story. Ask about compliance.
- Antihypertensive therapy—past and present. Side-effects.
- Analgesics—ask specifically about common NSAIDS (by their over-the-counter names if necessary). Then ask again.
- Any 'one-off' courses of therapy that may not be mentioned as part of regular treatment e.g. recent antibiotics (interstitial nephritis).
- Oral contraceptive (↑BP).
- Steroids, immunosuppressives—type and duration.
- Non-prescription, recreational (cocaine, IVDU) and herbal (◻ p.409) medicines.
- Exposure to important nephrotoxic drugs (see Table 1.1).

Sexual, menstrual, and obstetric history

- Decreased libido and impotence are extremely common in both ♂ and ♀ with CKD
- Irregular menses and subfertility are frequently encountered in ♀. Amenorrhea is common in ESRD.
- Previous pregnancies and any complications (UTI, proteinuria, ↑BP, pre-eclampsia). Miscarriages, terminations? Were infants healthy and born at term?
- In CKD, maternal and fetal outcomes are closely related to severity (◻ p.584).
- Cytotoxic drugs used in the treatment of glomerular disease, can → premature menopause. This may influence treatment in a ♀ of child-bearing age.

Dietary history

Changes in appetite and weight. Dietary habits (vegan, ethnic diet, alcohol). Dietetics is an important part of the management of several renal disorders (↑BP, ARF, CKD, the nephrotic syndrome, stone disease, dialysis).

Ethnicity and renal disease

- IgA nephropathy: Caucasians and certain Asian populations (China, Japan, and Singapore)
- Diabetic nephropathy: Blacks, Mexican Americans, Pima Indians (a native American tribe in Southern Arizona, beloved of epidemiologists and geneticists). An increasing problem in the immigrant Asian population in the UK.
- SLE: Asians and Blacks
- Hypertension: Blacks

Table 1.1 Important nephrotoxins

'Pre-renal' renal insufficiency	Acute tubular necrosis
Diuretics	Aminoglycosides
Any hypertensive agent (In particular, ACE-inhibitors and ARBs aggravate other pre-renal states)	Antifungals: • Amphotericin • Ifosfamide • Foscarnet
Haemodynamically mediated	Antivirals:
NSAIDs and COX2 inhibitors	• Adefovir
ACE inhibitors and ARBS	• Cidofovir
Ciclosporin	• Tenofovir
Tacrolimus	Cisplatin
Vasoconstrictors	Heavy metals (arsenic, mercury, and cadmium)
Glomerulopathy	
NSAIDs	Herbal remedies
Penicillamine	Interleukin-2
Gold	Intravenous immunoglobulin
Hydralazine	Paracetamol
Interferon α	Paraquat
Anti-thyroid drugs	Pentamidine
Carbon tetrachloride and other organic solvents (e.g. glue sniffing)	X-ray contrast agents
Silica dust (?Wegener's vasculitis)	**Interstitial nephritis (these and many, many others)**
Thrombotic microangiopathy	Antibiotics:
Chemotherapeutic agents:	• Penicillins
• Mitomicin C	• Cephalosporins
• Cisplatin	• Quinolones
• Bleomycin	• Rifampicin
Immunosuppressive agents:	• Sulphonamides
• Ciclosporin	Allopurinol
• Tacrolimus	Cimetidine (rarely ranitidine)
Clopidogrel	NSAIDS & COX-2 inhibitors
Quinine	Diuretics
Oral contraceptive	5-aminosalicylates (sulfasalazine & mesalazine)
Tubular crystal formation	Analgesics
Aciclovir	Omeprazole
Ethylene glycol (antifreeze)	**Chronic interstitial disease**
Sulfonamide antibiotics	Lead
Methotrexate	Lithium
Indinavir	Analgesics
	Chinese herbs

Social history

- Smoking: general CV risk, renovascular disease, urothelial malignancy (2–5 fold risk), pulmonary haemorrhage in Goodpastures disease, progression of CKD.
- Occupational history: risk factors for urothelial malignancy (p.512). Hydrocarbon exposure has been implicated in glomerular disease, particularly anti-GBM disease.
- Hepatitis and HIV risk factors.
- Physical activity.
- Renal diseases are often chronic disorders incurring appreciable social morbidity. At ESRD, social circumstance will exert an important influence on choice of, and ability to cope with, a particular dialysis modality. Livelihood may also be affected—one of the goals of RRT should be to keep an individual in employment.

Family history

- Essential hypertension: more common if one or both parents affected.
- Diabetes mellitus (I and II): more common if close relative affected.

Inherited kidney diseases

- Cystic kidney diseases:
  - Adult and juvenile polycystic kidney disease
- Alport's syndrome and variants
- Metabolic diseases with renal involvement:
  - Non-glomerular—cystinosis, primary hyperoxaluria, urate nephropathy
  - Glomerular—Fabry's disease
- Non-metabolic diseases:
  - Glomerular—congenital nephrotic syndrome, nail-patella syndrome
  - Non-glomerular—nephronophthisis
- Cystic disease:
  - Tuberous sclerosis (renal angiomyolipoma)
  - Von Hippel–Lindau (renal cell carcinoma)
- Primary glomerulonephritides:
  - IgA nephropathy (occasionally)
  - Others (rarely)
- Tubular disorders:
  - Cystinuria
  - Various inherited tubular defects
- Disorders with a 'genetic influence':
  - Vesicoureteric reflux
  - Haemolytic uraemic syndrome.

Approach to the patient on renal replacement therapy

When faced with a dialysis or transplant patient there are a few direct questions that will help you get to grips with (and reassure the patient that you are familiar with) their treatment. It will also facilitate discussion with the patient's renal unit.

The patient on haemodialysis
- Where does the haemodialysis treatment take place?
- How many times per week do they dialyse and how many hours is each treatment?
- What is the patient's current access for dialysis (e.g. an arteriovenous fistula)?
- What is their usual fluid gain between treatments?
- Do they know their blood pressure at the end of a dialysis session?

The patient on peritoneal dialysis
- How many exchanges do they perform in a day?
- How many litres is each exchange?
- Do they need assistance to perform an exchange?
- Do they measure their own blood pressure at home? What have the readings been recently?
- Is the exit site of their dialysis catheter clean and dry?
- Are the dialysis bags clear or cloudy on drainage?
- When was their last episode of peritonitis?

All dialysis patients
- What is the patients dry (aka flesh or target) weight?
- How much urine do they pass, if any?
- What is their daily fluid allowance?
- Do they adhere to a renal diet?
- Do they know the cause of their end-stage renal disease?
- How long have they been on dialysis?
- Do they take regular injections of erythropoietin? Who does these injections?
- Have they always been on the same modality of dialysis?
- Have they previously received a transplant?
- How are they coping with dialysis?

The transplant patient
- When and where was the transplant performed?
- What immunosuppression is the patient taking?
- Do they know if they had any rejection episodes?
- Who is responsible for their follow-up?
- Do they know their baseline Cr?
- Was the transplant from a living or cadaveric donor?
- Do they use sun block and attend a skin clinic?
- Do they know the cause of their end-stage renal disease?
- What mode of dialysis were they on prior to transplantation?

Physical examination

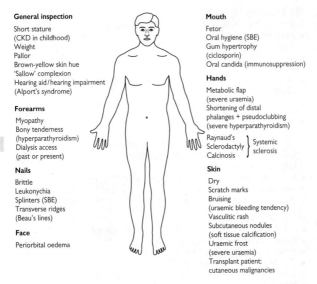

General inspection

Short stature
(CKD in childhood)
Weight
Pallor
Brown-yellow skin hue
'Sallow' complexion
Hearing aid/hearing impairment
(Alport's syndrome)

Forearms

Myopathy
Bony tenderness
(hyperparathyroidism)
Dialysis access
(past or present)

Nails

Brittle
Leukonychia
Splinters (SBE)
Transverse ridges
(Beau's lines)

Face

Periorbital oedema

Mouth

Fetor
Oral hygiene (SBE)
Gum hypertrophy
(ciclosporin)
Oral candida (immunosuppression)

Hands

Metabolic flap
(severe uraemia)
Shortening of distal
phalanges + pseudoclubbing
(severe hyperparathyroidism)
Raynaud's   ⎫
Sclerodactyly ⎬ Systemic
Calcinosis   ⎭ sclerosis

Skin

Dry
Scratch marks
Bruising
(uraemic bleeding tendency)
Vasculitic rash
Subcutaneous nodules
(soft tissue calcification)
Uraemic frost
(severe uraemia)
Transplant patient:
cutaneous malignancies

Fig. 1.1A

Examination by system

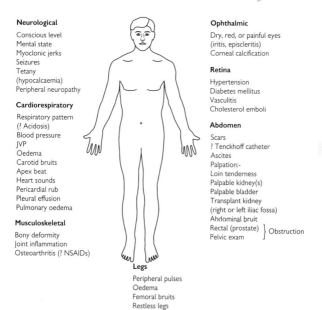

Neurological

Conscious level
Mental state
Myoclonic jerks
Seizures
Tetany
(hypocalcaemia)
Peripheral neuropathy

Cardiorespiratory

Respiratory pattern
(? Acidosis)
Blood pressure
JVP
Oedema
Carotid bruits
Apex beat
Heart sounds
Pericardial rub
Pleural effusion
Pulmonary oedema

Musculoskeletal

Bony deformity
Joint inflammation
Osteoarthritis (? NSAIDs)

Ophthalmic

Dry, red, or painful eyes
(iritis, episcleritis)
Corneal calcification

Retina

Hypertension
Diabetes mellitus
Vasculitis
Cholesterol emboli

Abdomen

Scars
? Tenckhoff catheter
Ascites
Palpation:-
Loin tenderness
Palpable kidney(s)
Palpable bladder
Transplant kidney
(right or left iliac fossa)
Abdominal bruit
Rectal (prostate) } Obstruction
Pelvic exam

Legs

Peripheral pulses
Oedema
Femoral bruits
Restless legs

Fig. 1.1B

Examination: the circulation

▶ The ability to assess the volume status of a patient is critical to the practice of renal medicine. In the vast majority of cases it can be achieved at the bedside without invasive monitoring.

Hypovolaemia

Salt and water or blood loss leads to ↓effective circulating volume and may lead to shock. Signs include:
- ↓BP (and ↓pulse pressure)
- Postural ↓BP (fall in SBP >10mmHg)
- Sinus tachycardia and postural ↑HR (↑ in HR >10 beats/min)
- ↓JVP. Neck veins flat even if supine.
- Cool peripheries and peripheral venoconstriction (⚠ septic patients may be vasodilated and warm)
- Poor urine output.

Less reliable signs include:
- ↓capillary refill
- Poor skin turgor (forehead and anterior triangle of the neck)
- Dry mouth and mucous membranes
- Sunken eyes.

Hypervolaemia

↑ECF volume may be found with ↑intravascular volume, ↑interstitial space volume, or both. ⚠ It is possible to be simultaneously salt and water overloaded and intravascularly depleted (e.g. CCF or nephrotic patient receiving diuretics).

Increased circulating volume
- ↑BP
- Elevation of the JVP

Increased interstitial fluid
- Peripheral or generalized oedema
- Pulmonary oedema (tachypnoea, tachycardia, a third heart sound ± basal crackles)
- Pleural effusion(s)
- Ascites.

The urine

Examination of the urine should be considered a routine extension of the physical examination in all patients.

Appearance

- Depending on concentration, normal urine is clear or given a light yellow hue by urochrome and uro-erythrin pigments.
- Cloudy urine may result from high concentrations of leucocytes, epithelial cells, or bacteria. Precipitation of phosphates can also produce turbidity in urine refrigerated for storage.
- Blood causes a pink to black discolouration depending on the number of RBCs and length of time present.
- Jaundice (conjugated hyperbilirubinaemia) may cause dark yellow or brown urine.
- Haemoglobinuria from intravascular haemolysis (📖 p.131) and myoglobinuria from muscle breakdown (📖 p.128) are both causes of dark urine that tests +ve for blood on dipstick examination. If the sample is centrifuged the supernatant will remain coloured and continue to test +ve. No red cells are seen on microscopy. Specific assays for haemoglobin and myoglobin are available.
- Normal urine tends to darken on standing (urobilinogen oxidizes to coloured urobilin). See box opposite.
- Chyluria is a rare cause of turbid urine. It has a milky appearance (particularly after fatty meals) and settles into layers on standing. Results from a fistulous connection between the lymphatic and urinary systems (usually malignancy, though lymphatic obstruction by *Filaria bancrofti* is more important worldwide).
- Beetroot can produce red urine due to enhanced intestinal absorption of the pigment betalaine in genetically susceptible individuals. Rarely causes diagnostic confusion.

Odour

Offensive urine usually denotes infection (bacterial ammonium production). Sweet urine suggests ketones. Certain rare metabolic diseases confer characteristic smells—one can only hope to encounter maple-syrup urine disease before isovaleric acidaemia ('sweaty feet urine').

Causes of a coloured urine

- Beetroot ingestion (red)
- Blood (pink/red to brown/black)
- Chloroquine (brown)
- Chyluria (milky white)
- Haemoglobin (pink/red to brown/black)
- Hyperbilirubinaemia (yellow/brown)
- Methylene blue (er...blue)
- Myoglobin (pink/red to brown/black)
- Nitrofurantoin (brown)
- Onchronosis (black)
- Phenytoin (red)
- Propofol (green)
- Rifampicin (orange)
- Senna (orange)

Urine that darkens on standing

- Alkaptonuria (homogentisic acid)
- Imipenem-cilastin
- Melanoma (melanogen)
- Methyl dopa
- Metronidazole
- Porphyria (porphobilinogen)

Chemical analysis

Osmolality and specific gravity

Specific gravity refers to the weight of a solution with respect to an equal weight of distilled water (normal range 1.003–1.035 in urine). Can be estimated with a dipstick, but for accurate measurement an osmometer (urinometer) is required.

Osmolality refers to the solute concentration of a solution. It cannot be measured with a dipstick. In the absence of significant glycosuria, the concentrations of Na^+, Cl^-, and urea are the most important determinants in urine. The ability to vary urine osmolality (range 50–1350mosmol/kg) plays a central role in the regulation of plasma osmolality (maintained across a narrow range: 280–305mosm/kg).

Generally speaking, the two measurements correlate. An exception is when relatively large particles such as glucose, proteins, and radiocontrast media are present in the urine. These produce an ↑ in specific gravity with little change in osmolality.

Uses: investigation of polyuria and hypo/hypernatraemic states (📖 p.520). Recurrent stone formers can monitor their own urine specific gravity to maintain a dilute urine.

> #### Isosthenuria
> CKD leads to a progressive ↓ in the range of urinary osmolality that the kidneys can generate. In advanced renal insufficiency the osmolality becomes relatively fixed at ~300mosmol/kg (~1.010 specific gravity) — close to that of glomerular filtrate. In this situation the urine cannot be adequately concentrated or diluted in response to Na^+ and water depletion and overload respectively.

Urinary pH

Urinary pH ranges from 4.5–8.0 (usually 5.0–6.0), depending on systemic acid–base status. Most people (except vegans) pass an acid urine the majority of the time. Isolated urinary pH measurements provide very little useful information. Main clinical use is the investigation of systemic metabolic acidosis. In this situation, a fall in urinary pH (to around 5) is expected as acid is excreted. Failure of this response may indicate renal tubular acidosis (📖 p.556). Most urine dipsticks have an indicator strip for estimation of pH, but if a tubular disorder is suspected a pH meter should be used.

In certain situations the therapeutic manipulation of urinary pH might be useful (see box opposite).

Therapeutic urinary alkalinization

(• see relevant chapters)
- Urinary stone disease (cystine and urate stones)
- Poisoning
  - Salicylates
  - Barbiturates
  - Methotrexate
- Rhabdomyolysis
- ARF 2° myeloma

Further dipstick tests

Leucocyte esterase and nitrites

Increasingly used as indicators of infection. Detection of neutrophil esterase activity identifies pyuria, while the nitrite test exploits the ability of some urinary pathogens (though not all—notably certain Gram +ve organisms including *Strep. faecalis*, *Staph. albus*, *Neisseria gonorrhoeae*, as well as many *Pseudomonas* spp and mycobacteria) to reduce nitrate → nitrite. Positivity requires an adequate dietary nitrate intake, as well as an adequate bladder dwell time (preferably >4h).

When combined, these methods possess good specificity (i.e. take seriously if +ve), though only modest sensitivity (i.e. treat a −ve result with caution if infection is likely clinically). They can serve as a useful screening test in at risk populations, but are not a substitute for microscopy and culture.

Bilirubin and urobilinogen

Conjugated ($\therefore$ water-soluble) bilirubin → biliary excretion → small bowel → converted to urobilinogen → distal reabsorption → partially excreted in the urine. So, (i) unconjugated (water insoluble) bilirubin does not pass into the urine ($\therefore$ dipstick +ve bilirubin indicates hepatic or cholestatic disease); (ii) absence of dipstick urobilinogen in a jaundiced patient suggests biliary obstruction.

Glucose

Glycosuria results when tubular reabsorptive capacity for glucose is exceeded (plasma level >10mmol/L). A valuable screening tool, but less useful for diagnosis and monitoring of DM.

'Renal' glycosuria occurs when proximal tubular injury leads to a failure to reabsorb filtered glucose (🕮 p.64).

Causes of a +ve dipstick for ketones

Dipsticks semi-quantitatively detect acetoacetate (but not β-hydroxybutyrate). A +ve test can be seen in:
- Diabetic ketoacidosis (and occasionally severe intercurrent illness in T2DM)
- Prolonged fasting and starvation diets (e.g. Atkins' diet)
- Alcoholic ketoacidosis
- Severe volume depletion
- Isopropyl alcohol poisoning (hand-rubs, solvents, and de-icers)

Urinary test strips

A variety of test strips for urinanalysis are available. Some have a specific purpose: e.g. Clinistix® (glucose), Hemastix® (blood), and Albustix® (albumin). Others cast a wider net with various combinations of the following:

- Specific gravity
- pH
- Leucocytes
- Nitrites
- Glucose
- Urobilinogen
- Bilirubin
- Ketones
- Albumin or protein*
- Blood

*Dipsticks able to detect microalbuminuria are also available

Proteinuria

Introduction

Urinary protein excretion should not exceed 150mg/day of which less than 20mg is albumin (the remainder consists mainly of non-serum derived tubular mucoprotein such as Tamm–Horsfall/uromodulin). ↑excretion of albumin is a sensitive marker of renal, particularly glomerular, disease (📖 p.46).

> Proteinuria (total protein) and albuminuria (albumin) are not strictly interchangeable terms. When screening for renal disease, specific tests for albumin are preferable.

Protein excretion can be measured in untimed ('spot') or timed (usually 24h) samples.

Dipsticks

Convenient, highly specific, but less sensitive. Contain pH-sensitive indicators that change colour when bound to negatively-charged proteins. Predominantly detect albumin (some are albumin specific; e.g. Albustix®) and may not identify large amounts of other proteins; e.g. Bence–Jones. Have completely superseded sulphosalicylic acid turbidity testing.

A +ve result occurs with protein excretion ≥300mg/L. Lower amounts of proteinuria, particularly in the context of diabetes, are termed microalbuminuria (📖 p.46) (usually defined as 30–300mg/day). This is usually measured by ELISA or radioimmunoassay, although sensitive dipsticks are available.

Dipsticks are semiquantitative. As a *rough* guide:

Trace	~0.15-0.3g/L
+	~0.3g/L
++	~1g/L
+++	~2.5–5g/L
++++	>10g/L

⚠ Changes in urinary concentration affect the result. If volumes are high and the urine dilute, large amounts of protein can go undetected (specific gravity may be a clue). Concentrated morning samples are ∴ preferable.

▶ If a patient has a +ve dipstick test of ≥1+, repeat after 1–2 weeks. If persistent verify with one of the quantitative methods below.

Timed collections

For many clinicians a 24h urine collection remains the gold standard, but there are important drawbacks:
- Inaccurate collection
- Processing is time consuming.

Gradually being supplanted by protein/creatinine ratio (PCR) or albumin/creatinine ratio (ACR). See box.

24h collection: what to tell the patient

- Non acidified, clearly labelled, container
- Pick a convenient day with minimum commitments
- Discard first urine void on that day
- Start collection—all subsequent urine into the container (including overnight)
- First void the following day into the collection
- Since Cr excretion, or creatinine clearance (CrCl) (🕮 p.28), should be similar in two successive samples from the same patient, their measurement in 'back to back' 24h collections may enhance reliability (i.e. disregard the result if CrCl differs greatly between the two)

The albumin/creatinine ratio (ACR)

Untimed ('spot') urine samples can (and many say should[1]) be used to detect and monitor proteinuria. ACR corrects for variations in urinary concentration (caused by changes in hydration) and correlates well with measurements obtained from timed collections.

A first morning urine specimen is preferable. Urinary excretion of creatinine generally remains constant (~10mmol/day).

- Interpretation
  - ACR ≥3mg/mmol: microalbuminuria
  - ACR ≥30mg/mmol: overt proteinuria
  - ACR ≥350mg/mmol: nephrotic range proteinuria
- In the USA and in labs where urinary Cr is measured in mg/dL rather than mmol/L, ACR is expressed as mg/g. (normal: <30mg/g, micro-albuminuria: 30–300mg/g, overt proteinuria: >300mg/g)
- ACR will underestimate proteinuria when Cr excretion is high (Blacks, muscular build) and overestimate proteinuria when Cr excretion is low (elderly, cachectic). However, the ACR remains useful for serial monitoring in individual patients.
- The total PCR is an adequate alternative to ACR in most circumstances. ACR is more sensitive if screening for early disease in high-risk groups (especially diabetes). PCR ≥45mg/mmol indicates significant proteinuria.
- Dipsticks that estimate the PCR (e.g. Multistix Pro®) await further validation.

1K/DOQI Clinical practice guidelines

Red blood cells

Introduction

Haematuria is defined (arbitrarily) as the presence of 2 RBCs per high powered field (hpf) in spun urine. The amount determines whether it is visible to the naked eye (macroscopic haematuria) or requires a dipstick or microscopy for detection (microscopic haematuria). Causes and investigation are considered later (📖 p.50).

Dipstick

Hb induces a colour change (usually green) in a dye linked to organic peroxide. Dipsticks detect as little as 2 RBCs per field and are at least as sensitive as microscopic examination (though appreciable false –ve rate). If dipstick +ve, it is still desirable to perform confirmatory microscopy.

Dipsticks detect Hb and remain +ve even after RBC lysis. Also detect haemoglobinuria from intravascular haemolysis and myoglobin from muscle breakdown, though red cells will be absent on microscopy in both situations.

Urine sediment

Microscopic examination of the urine sediment is still the gold standard.

Urinary RBCs may have variable morphology. Those that have passed through the glomerular basement membrane and suffered osmotic stress in the tubules may have an abnormal appearance, best appreciated under phase-contrast microscopy.

In expert hands, the presence of these 'dysmorphic' red cells can help distinguish glomerular from lower urinary tract bleeding. ⚠ The presence of dysmorphic cells does not rule out a lower tract lesion.

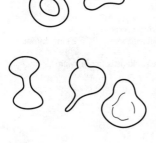

Non-glomerular bleeding:

Red blood cells have normal morphology

Glomerular bleeding:

Red blood cells that pass into the urine through an inflamed or damaged glomerulus may show budding, spiculation. or other surface irregularities.

Fig. 1.2

Examination of the urine sediment

- Tell the patient to discard the first few mL of urine and then collect ~20mL into a universal container.
- Process and analyse the sample within a few hours (red cell lysis).
- Centrifuge a 10mL aliquot at 400g for 10min.
- Remove 9.5mL of supernatant with a pipette.
- Resuspend the pellet in the remaining 0.5mL of urine (gently!).
- Transfer a drop of resuspended urine to a slide.
- Cover the sample (unstained) with a coverslip.
- Examine (preferably) with a phase contrast microscope at 160x and 400x.
- Cellular elements are quantitated as number per high-power field.
- Look also for casts and other elements.
- Use polarized light to identify crystals.
- Clean the microscope and discard all the urine!

In an urgent situation; e.g. for rapid diagnosis of UTI, an unspun sample may be examined. It may be necessary to acidify the urine to prevent precipitation of (view-obscuring) phosphate crystals.

Should we screen for haematuria with urinary dipsticks?

The benefit of screening the general population for haematuria is yet to be established.

Argument for

Dipstick examination is easy, acceptable to patients, and inexpensive. It may assist in the early diagnosis of both urological malignancies (where early intervention may be life-saving) and intrinsic renal disease (where intervention may delay or prevent progression to end-stage renal disease).

Argument against

The basic criteria for general population screening are not fulfilled. Dipstick examination is not a sufficiently specific test and the predictive values for urothelial malignancy and renal disease are quite poor. In both cases the benefits of early detection have not been established.

At present the relevant advisory bodies do not advocate population screening.

QM LIBRARY (WEST SMITHFIELD)

Cells, organisms, and casts

Leucocytes

Neutrophils: leucocytes are a prominent feature of urinary infection, but may be present in inflammatory renal conditions (GN, TIN). Sterile pyuria refers to the situation when leucocytes are seen consistently on microscopy but subsequent culture is sterile.

> **Causes of sterile pyuria**
>
> • Partially treated UTI or fastidious organism (e.g. *Chlamydia*)
> • Calculi
> • Prostatitis
> • Bladder tumour
> • Papillary necrosis
> • TIN
> • TB (send 3x EMUs 🕮 p.488)
> • Appendicitis

Lymphocytes: a feature of chronic tubulointerstitial disease. *Eosinophils:* Hansel's or Wright's stain. Associated with TIN (🕮 p.406), but also possible in several other conditions, including RPGN, prostatitis and atheroemboli. *Renal tubular cells:* large, oval cells. Present in normal urine, but ↑ in tubular damage (ATN or TIN). *Squamous epithelial cells:* large cells with small nuclei. Urethral origin (or skin/vaginal contaminant). *Transitional epithelial (urothelial) cells:* suggest cystitis. *Malignant cells:* special stains, immunocytochemistry, and flow cytometry all aid detection.

Micro-organisms

• **Bacteriuria:** normal urine is sterile. Concomitant presence of leucocytes suggests true infection, rather than contamination. Gram-staining enables initial identification and cell count, while culture and sensitivities are pending.
• **Fungi:** Candida the most frequent. Typical appearance is a small pale green cell, often with visible budding. May result from genital contamination. Risk factors for colonization are: indwelling plastic (ureteric stents, bladder catheter), DM, antibiotic therapy, and immunosuppression.
• **Trichomonas:** oval and flagellate (motile if alive). Usually a genital contaminant.
• **Schistosoma haematobium:** Ova detection an important technique in endemic areas.

Urine culture

M,C+S differentiates contamination from true infection and guides treatment. A pure growth of $>10^5$ colony-forming units (cfu)/mL is the conventional diagnostic criterion for urinary tract infection (🕮 p.424).

OM LIBRARY (WEST SMITHFIELD)

Casts

Casts are plugs of Tamm–Horsfall mucoprotein within the renal tubules, conferring a characteristic cylindrical shape. They are classified according to appearance and the cellular elements embedded in them. Though produced in normal kidneys, they can be valuable clues to the presence of renal disease

Non-cellular casts

- *Hyaline casts:* mucoprotein alone and virtually transparent. A non-specific finding, occurring in concentrated urine.
- *Granular casts:* granular material (aggregates of protein or cellular remnants) is embedded in the cast. Often pathological, but non-specific.
- *Broad or waxy casts:* hyaline material with a waxy appearance under the microscope. Form in dilated, poorly functioning tubules of advanced CKD.

Cellular casts

- *Red cell casts*
  ► Virtually diagnostic of GN.
- *White cell casts:* characteristic of acute pyelonephritis—may help to distinguish upper from lower tract infection. Also occur in TIN.
- *Epithelial cell casts:* sloughed epithelial cells embedded in mucoprotein. A non-specific feature of ATN. Also found in GN.
- *Fatty casts:* contain either lipid filled tubular epithelial cells or free lipid globules. Distinguished from other casts by 'Maltese cross' appearance under polarized light. Occur in the lipid laden urine of the nephrotic syndrome.
  Lipids may also appear as droplets or crystals. When clumped these are referred to as oval fat bodies.
- *Other casts:* under the right conditions any constituent of the urine (micro-organisms, crystals, bilirubin or myoglobin) may become entrapped in a mucoprotein cast.

Crystals

Detected by examining the urine under polarized light. Most crystals are irrelevant.

Uric acid
Usually lozenges with a yellow-brown hue. Precipitate at acid pH. A few may be normal (e.g. high meat intake), but ↑quantities may indicate hyperuricosuria. May be present in acute urate nephropathy (tumour lysis syndrome 📖 p.134).

Calcium oxalate
May be mono-hydrated (ovoid) or bi-hydrated (pyramidal—like the back of an envelope). Prefer an acidic pH, but not always. A few may be normal (spinach and chocolate), but may denote hypercalciuria or hyperoxaluria (see 📖 p.434). A diagnostic clue in ethylene glycol poisoning (📖 p.614).

Calcium phosphate
Heterogeneous in their appearances (needles, prisms, stars). Alkaline pH. Might be a risk factor for calcium stone formation.

Magnesium ammonium phosphate (triple phosphate)
Birefringent prisms ('coffin-lids'). Alkaline pH. If present, check for a proteus UTI.

Amorphous phosphates
Unattractive clumps in (alkaline) urine cooled for storage. No clinical significance.

Cystine
Hexagonal. Cystine is not a constituent of normal urine, so always significant. Prefer an acid urine. A marker of cystinuria (📖 p.432).

Cholesterol
Thin plates with sharp edges. Occur with heavy proteinuria.

Drug induced crystalluria

Many drugs can precipitate in the renal tubule. In severe cases this may → ARF.
- Antibiotics: sulfadiazine, amoxycillin
- Antiviral agents: acyclovir and indinavir
- Methotrexate
- Primidone (a barbiturate)
- Triamterene
- Vitamin C (calcium oxalate deposition)

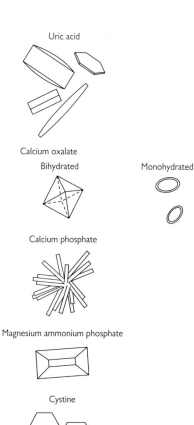

Uric acid

Calcium oxalate

Bihydrated

Monohydrated

Calcium phosphate

Magnesium ammonium phosphate

Cystine

Fig. 1.3 Urinary crystals

Determining renal function

Introduction

Several aspects of renal function can be measured (see opposite). The most important is the glomerular filtration rate (GFR). Glomerular filtrate refers to the ultrafiltrate of plasma that crosses the glomerular barrier into the urinary space. GFR is measured per unit time (usually expressed mL/min) and represents the sum of filtration rates in all functioning nephrons (∴ a surrogate for the amount of functioning renal tissue).

GFR is useful for:
- Providing a consistent measure of kidney function.
- Monitoring progression of CKD (and response to treatment).
- Forecasting the need for RRT.
- Determining appropriate drug dosing in renal impairment.

It provides no information as to the cause of renal insufficiency.

Measurement of GFR
- Measured indirectly by evaluating clearance from plasma of a (renal excreted) marker substance.
- Clearance: the volume of plasma from which this substance is removed per unit time.
- Suitable markers require certain characteristics shown below and may be endogenous (e.g. Cr) or exogenous (e.g. inulin).

Characteristics of an ideal clearance marker
- Safe, economical, and easy to measure
- Freely filtered at the glomerulus
- Not protein bound (able to distribute in the extracellular space)
- Present at a stable plasma concentration
- No extrarenal elimination
- Not reabsorbed, secreted, or metabolized by the kidney

- Inulin, a fructose polysaccharide for which (along with flatulence) we have the Jerusalem artichoke to thank, remains the gold standard. Cost and technical considerations (it requires a continuous infusion) prohibit routine use.

In clinical practice GFR is estimated by one of the following means:
- Serum Cr (and to a lesser extent urea).
- Formulae based on the serum creatinine (estimated or eGFR)
- Creatinine clearance (CrCl) from a 24h urine collection.
- Isotopic clearance (EDTA-GFR or DTPA-GFR).

Aspects of renal function

- Glomerular filtration rate (GFR)
- Tubular function (including Na^+ and K^+ handling and urinary concentrating/ diluting capacity)
- Acid–base balance
- Endocrine function
  - Renin–angiotensin system
  - Erythropoietin production
  - Vitamin D metabolism

Not measured in clinical practice

- Autocrine
  - Production of endothelins, prostaglandins, natriuretic peptides, nitric oxide
- Protein and polypeptide metabolism (e.g. insulin catabolism)

Creatinine

Serum creatinine

Convenient and inexpensive—the most commonly used indirect measure of GFR.

- Generated from non-enzymatic metabolism of creatine in skeletal muscle. Production is proportional to muscle mass (20g muscle → ~1mg Cr). Little short-term variation in an individual.
- ~25% is derived from dietary meat intake (creatine mostly, creatinine in a stew).
- $U_{cr} \times V$ is relatively constant in the formula for CrCl.

  So   CrCl = (UrineCr x V) / PlasmaCr

  Becomes   CrCl = constant / PlasmaCr

Hence, serum Cr varies inversely with GFR: ↓GFR → ↑Cr (until a new steady state is reached).

- ↓muscle mass (elderly, cachectic) → ↓Cr production → overestimates GFR.
- Cr meets many, but not all, of the criteria for a clearance marker. Shortcomings:
  - It is secreted by the proximal tubule (~10–20% when GFR is normal), so the amount excreted in the urine exceeds the amount filtered. As GFR falls, there is a progressive ↑ in tubular secretion until saturation occurs at Cr ~132–176µmol/L. Beyond this Cr rises as expected (see Fig. 1.4).
  - It undergoes extra-renal elimination by secretion and degradation in the GI tract. This becomes more important as GFR falls.
- When ↓GFR is rapid, it takes time for a steady state to be reached and Cr to ↑; i.e. Cr may initially be normal after a catastrophic renal insult.
- Traditionally measured by the Jaffé alkaline pictrate colorimetric assay. Interference by non-creatinine chromogens created a tradition of overestimating Cr. Enzymatic methods on modern auto-analysers are generally more accurate.
- Certain substances interfere with Cr, either through competitive inhibition of tubular secretion (cimetidine, trimethoprim, amiloride, spironolactone, triamterene) or assay interference (in the Jaffé reaction: ketoacids, vitamin C, glucose, and cephalosporins).

Creatinine clearance

CrCl is calculated as: -

$CrCl \times$ plasma creatinine (P_{Cr}) = urine creatinine $(U_{Cr}) \times$ volume (V)

∴ $CrCl = (U_{Cr} \times V) / P_{Cr}$.

Example

- Serum Cr = 106μmol/L
- Urine Cr = 8800μmol/L
- Urine volume = 1.2L
- $CrCl = (U_{Cr} \times V)/P_{Cr}$
- CrCl = (8800 × 1.2)÷106 = 99.6L/day

Conventionally CrCl is shown in mL/min ∴ ×1000/1440

- (99.6 × 1000)/1440 = 69.2 mL/min

Normal range: ♀: 95 ± 20mL/min; ♂: 120 ± 25mL/min

Limitations

- Tubular secretion of Cr means that GFR is overestimated.
- Requires accurate urine collection.
- Heir to all the pitfalls inherent in Cr measurement.
- Even if collections are accurate there is marked serial variation (15–20%).

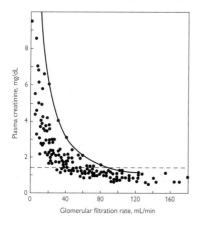

Fig. 1.4 The relationship between Cr concentration and GFR, (measured as inulin clearance) in 171 patients with glomerular disease. The hypothetical relationship between GFR and Cr is shown in the continuous line, assuming that only filtration of Cr takes place. The broken horizontal line represents the upper the upper limit of normal of serum Cr (1.4mg/dL or 115μmol/L). it can be seen that because of Cr secretion, serum Cr consistently overestimates GFR (reproduced from Shemesh O, Golbertz H, Kriss JP, et al. (1985) Limitations of creatinine as a filtration marker in glomerulopathic patients. *Kidney Int* **28**: 830–8.)

eGFR: formulae based on creatinine (see also 📖 p.143)

Introduction

Recent guidelines emphasize the need to diagnose and monitor kidney function using equations based on the serum Cr. These attempt to correct for the confounding effects of body weight, age, sex, race, and muscle mass.

Limitations: still based on Cr and do not take into account tubular secretion, extra-renal elimination, or differences in production between individuals of the same age and sex, or the same individual over time.

Cockcroft–Gault (CG)

$$\text{eGFR (mL/min)} = \frac{1.2 \times \{140 - \text{age(yr)}\} \times \text{weight(kg)}}{\text{Cr } \mu\text{mol/L}}$$

Multiply × 0.85 in ♀ to correct for reduced creatinine production

MDRD

Developed from data in the Modification of Diet in Renal Disease (MDRD) study. Remains unvalidated in children (age <18 years), elderly (age >70 years), pregnancy, ethnic groups other than Caucasians and African Americans, and those without CKD.

eGFR, in mL/min per 1.73 m^2 =

$(170 \times (\text{PCr [mg/dL]})\exp[-0.999]) \times (\text{Age } \exp[-0.176]) \times$
$((\text{S}_{\text{Urea}}[\text{mg/dL}])\exp[-0.170]) \times ((\text{Albumin [g/dL]})\exp[+0.318])$

- Multiply × 0.762 if the patient is female
- Multiply × 1.180 if the patient is black.

Simplified version:

eGFR = $186.3 \times ((\text{serum creatinine}) \exp[-1.154]) \times$
$(\text{Age } \exp[-0.203]) \times (0.742 \text{ if female}) \times (1.21 \text{ if African-American})$

Note: to convert Cr from mg/dL to μmol/L × 88.4. To convert urea from mg/dL to mmol/L × 0.357. Exp=exponential

CG tends to overestimate and MDRD underestimate GFR. Up to 25% of patients will be misclassified if either are used to categorize patients according to the KDOQI CKD classification (📖 p.56).

The formulae are available as web-based and downloadable calculators.
www.nephron.com
www.hdcn.com
www.renal.org
www.nkdep.nih.gov/healthprofessionals/tools/

Reciprocal of plasma creatinine

There is an inverse relationship between GFR and Cr

$$CrCl = constant/Cr$$

Plotting the reciprocal of Cr (1/Cr) against time will often, though not always, produce a straight line, the slope of the curve representing change in GFR with time. A logarithmic plot of Cr can be used in a similar way.

This may be useful in two settings:
- Extrapolation of the line can help predict when CKD is likely to reach ESRD and ∴ assist timely planning of RRT.
- A change in the slope of the curve can be used to monitor treatment: a ↓ in the slope indicates slowed progression; an ↑ may indicate a 2nd insult (acute on chronic renal failure).

Other methods of GFR measurement

Isotopic GFR

Several radiopharmaceuticals (^{51}Cr-EDTA, ^{99m}Tc-DTPA, ^{125}I-Iothalamate) compare favourably to inulin for GFR measurement.

Method: a single IV injection followed by venous sampling at regular intervals (intervals ↑ as expected GFR ↓). Post injection, plasma isotope activity ↓ rapidly as it distributes throughout the ECF. A slower exponential decline (renal elimination) then follows allowing GFR to be determined. Protocols based on urine collection are also described.

With DTPA, renal elimination is often measured with a gamma camera positioned directly over the kidneys. While not as precise as venous sampling, it allows assessment of each kidneys contribution to total GFR ('split function') (📖 p.42).

Note: isotopic techniques are expensive.

Cystatin C

Cysteine protease inhibitor produced by all nucleated cells. Easy to measure, stable production rate, freely filtered at the glomerulus, not influenced by age, sex, muscle mass, diet, or inflammation. Correlates well with GFR. ↑concentration in advance of Cr as GFR falls. Not yet available in routine clinical practice.

β_2 microglobulin

Early ↑ in plasma levels as GFR ↓. Susceptible to 'non-renal' elevation (lymphoid malignancies, inflammatory states). Expensive.

MRI

Gadolinium, a paramagnetic contrast agent, undergoes renal elimination and is well-tolerated in renal insufficiency. MRI could potentially provide both structural and functional information.

Renal function in the elderly

Functioning renal mass declines with age, with progressive glomerulosclerosis from age ~30. This is accompanied by sclerosis of the renal vasculature and altered renal haemodynamics.

The Baltimore longitudinal study (1958–1981) used serial measurements of CrCl to show a ↓GFR of 0.75mL/min/year. Recent studies have used inulin clearances to show that, although GFR is lower in older age groups, it generally stays in the normal range. Associated co-morbidity (↑BP, vascular disease, CCF, etc.) may have more of an impact than age itself.

Clinical relevance
- In the absence of disease, a major age-related ↓ in GFR is uncommon.
- ↓Muscle mass in the elderly → ↓Cr ∴ ↑Cr usually represents a significant ↓GFR.

Urea

- Synthesized in the liver as a means of ammonia excretion
- Rate of production not constant (unlike Cr)
- Inverse relationship with GFR
- Influenced by a number of factors independent of GFR

↑Ur	↓Ur
• High dietary protein intake	• Low protein diet
• GI bleeding	• Liver disease
• Catabolic states	• Pregnancy
• Haemorrhage	
• Trauma	
• Corticosteroids	
• Tetracyclines	

- Freely filtered at the glomerulus but reabsorbed in the tubules
  - Ur movement is linked to water (under vasopressin influence) in the distal nephron
  - ↓renal perfusion → ↑Ur reabsorption → disproportionate ↑Ur compared to Cr
  - Can be used to differentiate 'pre-renal' renal dysfunction (p.88).

Diagnostic imaging

To select the most appropriate investigation (and maintain healthy relations with the radiology department) the requesting clinician should understand the indications and limitations of imaging in renal disease.

Plain X-ray
- 'KUB' (kidneys–ureter–bladder). Essentially a supine AXR centred on the umbilicus.
- Main role is identification and surveillance of calcification (Table 1.2). Lateral and oblique films may differentiate calcification *in line with* as opposed to *in* the renal tract.
- The medial edges of both psoas muscles are usually visible—disappearance suggests a perinephric mass or retroperitoneal collection.
- Tomography keeps one particular image plane in focus, blurring out images in front and behind. Moving the plane can produce serial 'cuts' that detect small calculi and to establish the exact location of calcification. Superseded by CT.

Where are the kidneys on a plain AXR?

- Differences in attenuation between renal tissue and perinephric fat mean that the kidneys are (just) visible.
- Usually adjacent to the upper border of the T11 through to the lower border of L3.
- Normal renal size is 11–15cm (in adults). Kidneys appear bigger on an AXR than on ultrasound.
- Right kidney usually shorter than the left (upper limit of variation in length between right and left 1.5cm).

Table 1.2 Causes of renal tract calcification

Urinary calculi (most are radio opaque to some degree; exceptions are pure uric acid and xanthine stones)

Localized calcification:
- Tuberculosis
- Tumours

Nephrocalcinosis:
- Medullary:
  - Disturbed calcium metabolism:
    — Hyperparathyroidism
    — Sarcoidosis
    — Vitamin D excess
    — Idiopathic hypercalciuria
    — Oxalosis*
  - Tubular diseases:
    — Distal renal tubular acidosis
    — Bartter's syndrome
  - Other:
    — Medullary sponge kidney
    — Papillary necrosis
  - Cortical:
    — Trauma
    — Cortical necrosis
    — Oxalosis*

* causes both medullary and cortical calcification

Ultrasound

The front-line investigation in most forms of renal disease. Pros: non-invasive, relatively quick, and requires little patient preparation. Cons: operator dependent, poor pelvi-ureteric detail, no functional information, may miss small stones and masses.

Main uses
- Document 1 or 2 kidneys
- Diagnosis of obstruction (PC dilatation)
- Measurement of renal size in CKD
- Evaluation of renal masses (cystic vs. solid)
- Screening for polycystic disease
- Identify nephrocalcinosis and calculi
- Evaluate bladder emptying
- Estimate prostate size (may require a rectal probe)
- Guide percutaneous procedures (e.g. renal biopsy, nephrostomy)
- Doppler USS can be used to evaluate arterial and venous blood flow. Widely used for transplant assessment, but role as a screening tool in renovascular diseases uncertain (□ p.412).

Normal appearances
- Renal length 9–12cm
- Smooth outline
- Cortex >1.5cm
- Echotexture: medulla darker than cortex. ↓ corticomedullary differentiation in ↑age and parenchymal disease (e.g. acute GN)
- Pelvicalyceal (PC) system poorly visualized
- Bladder examined when full. Normal bladder wall thin and hard to delineate

Table 1.3 Causes of abnormal renal size on imaging

Large kidneys
- Unilateral:
  - Tumour
  - Cyst
  - Unilateral hydronephrosis
  - Compensatory hypertrophy
- Bilateral:
  - Polycystic kidney disease (and other cystic diseases)
  - Infiltration (e.g. lymphoma)

Small kidneys
- Unilateral:
  - Congenital hypoplasia
  - Renal artery stenosis
- Bilateral:
  - Small smooth kidneys
    — chronic glomerulonephritis
    — chronic interstitial nephritis
    — virtually any chronic renal disorder, except diabetic nephropathy
  - Small irregular kidneys
    — reflux nephropathy
    — congenital dysplastic syndromes
    — TB
    — renal infarction

Intravenous urography

Provides a good overview of the urinary tract, particularly the PC system and ureters. Good for detecting calculi.

The procedure

- Ensure good bowel prep, NBM for 4h pre-procedure. If GFR normal, a fluid restriction of ~500mL/prior 24h assists contrast concentration (⚠ dangerous if ↓GFR ∴ often avoided).
- Includes (film sequence altered according to clinical situation):
  - Plain control film (?opacities pre-contrast)
  - Post-contrast: bilateral nephrograms (delayed: poor perfusion, obstruction, ATN, venous thrombosis) renal outline (?ischaemic scars, reflux, TB)
  - Further exposures at 5 and 10min (PC filling defects: clot, tumour, sloughed papilla, stone; PC deformity: reflux)
- Mild abdominal compression delays contrast excretion and may improve PC system views.
- Post-voiding film to assess bladder outflow.
- Delayed films (2, 6, 12, and 24h) may establish a level of obstruction.

Modifications

- *IVU with frusemide:* frusemide exaggerates and distinguishes PUJ obstruction from normal anatomical variants ('baggy' pelvis).
- *High dose IVU:* used if ↓GFR limits contrast excretion. Superseded by USS and CT.

Contrast media

- Organic radio-opaque iodides excreted by glomerular filtration.
- Non-ionic, iso-osmolar agents are better tolerated than their ionic, hyperosmolar (~1500mosm/kg) predecessors.
- Minor contrast reactions (urticaria, itching, nausea, vomiting, sneezing, metallic taste) common (5–10%) esp if history of allergy. Usually self-limiting, but antihistamines may help. Not necessarily associated with reaction on re-challenge.
- Severe reactions: ↓BP, shock, pulmonary oedema, bronchospasm and anaphylaxis. ▶ Access to resus equipment mandatory. Mortality estimated between 1 in 30,000 to 1 in 75,000; lower with non-ionic media.
- Corticosteroids (e.g. prednisolone 30mg bd for 24h pre + post-procedure) are often used if history of atopy or asthma (⚠ do not guarantee non-reaction).
- Nephrotoxicity is dose dependent and ↑ if dehydration, DM, pre-existing ↓GFR, ↑age, poor CV function (🕮 p.132).

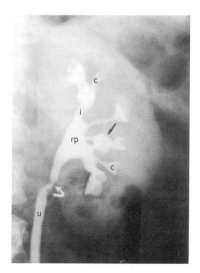

Fig. 1.5 IVU: magnified view of the left kidney. Calyx (c), infundibulum (i), renal pelvis (rp), proximal ureter (u). Calyx which projects posteriorly is seen en face (arrow). Normal fold of the ureter at the ureteropelvic junction (curved arrow). Reproduced with permission from Davison AMA, Cameron JS, Grunfeld J-P *et al.* (eds) (2005). *Oxford Textbook of Clinical Nephrology,* 3rd edn. Oxford: Oxford University Press

⚠ **Metformin**

Ingestion in the 48h prior to an IVU → ↑ risk of lactic acidosis post-procedure. ▶ Stop ≥24h beforehand in all elective cases and recheck Cr at 48h before restarting.

CT

More widespread availability, better image resolution and progressively shorter scanning times have increased the routine use of CT in the investigation of the urinary tract.

Indications

- Characterization of a renal or peri-renal mass
  - Differentiation of simple cysts from tumours (📖 p.508)
- Tumour staging
- Delineate renal or peri-renal collections and abscesses
- Renal and ureteric calculi (CT–KUB) (📖 p.432)
- Trauma
  - Defines extent of renal and associated intra-abdominal injuries
- Retroperitoneal disease
  - Abdominal aorta, adrenal glands, retroperitoneal masses, fluid collections, lymphadenopathy
  - Investigation of choice in retroperitoneal fibrosis (📖 p.506)
- Obstruction
  - Presence, level and aetiology (📖 p.498)
- Parenchymal infection
  - Pyelonephritis may not show on USS or IVU
  - Exclude associated pyonephrosis
- ☞ Renovascular disease (📖 p.412).

CT angiography (CTA)
Software reconstructs 3D images of the intra-abdominal vasculature.

Electron beam CT (EBCT)
A tool for monitoring vascular, particularly coronary, calcification (📖 p.179). Not widely available.

MRI

Indications

- Evaluation of a renal mass and tumour staging
  - Selected cases; e.g. venous invasion
- MR urography (the MR equivalent of an IVU—growing in popularity)
- Renal insufficiency
  - Gadolinium is not nephrotoxic and safe when there has been a previous adverse allergic reaction to iodinated contrast.[1]
- ☞ Renovascular disease (📖 p.412)
  - MR angiography.

---

1 Very recently, MRI contrast agents have been implicated in the development of nephrogenic systemic fibrosis, a rare, painful, and often disabling, skin lesion that can progress to involve internal organs.

Nuclear medicine

Introduction

Nuclear techniques provide functional as well as structural information and can complement other imaging modalities. Three types:

- GFR estimation (e.g. ^{51}Cr- EDTA) (🕮 p.32)
- Dynamic (e.g. ^{99m}Tc-DTPA ,^{99m}Tc-MAG 3): serial scans track renal uptake, transit and excretion of isotope. A time-activity curve is generated.
- Static (e.g. ^{99m}Tc-DMSA): isotope is taken up and retained within functioning tissue. Demonstrates non-functioning ('scarred') renal tissue.

Radiopharmaceuticals

- **^{99m}Tc-DTPA.** Filtered at the glomerulus and neither reabsorbed or secreted by the tubules. A good marker of GFR, but limited utility in renal failure (Cr>200).
- **^{99m}Tc-MAG 3.** Principally excreted by tubular secretion, so useful if ↓GFR. Less background uptake than DTPA, but more expensive.
- **^{99m}Tc-DMSA.** Filtered at the glomerulus then reabsorbed and retained in the proximal tubules. Subsequent excretion is slow. Used for parenchymal imaging.

Applications

- Split function (DTPA, MAG3, DMSA)
- Congenital abnormalities (DMSA)
  - e.g. horseshoe kidney, ectopic pelvic kidneys
- Chronic pyelonephritis and vesicoureteric reflux (DMSA) (🕮 p.430)
  - Focal scarring (more than one cause)
  - DTPA-cystogram: reflux follow up and sibling screening
- Renal transplantation
  - Perfusion and obstruction (🕮 p.252)
- Acute renal failure (🕮 p.86)
- Dilated vs. obstructed renal pelvis
  - A dilated pelvis may not indicate true obstruction
  - Diuretic renography (DTPA or MAG3) may differentiate the two
- Arterial occlusion (DTPA, MAG3)
  - Failure of perfusion
- Captopril renography in renovascular disease (🕮 p.412)
  - In renal artery stenosis, perfusion and GFR are maintained by AII mediated efferent arteriolar constriction. ACEI block this and alter uptake and excretion of DTPA or MAG3
  - +ve scan
    - Asymmetry of size and function
    - Delayed time to peak activity
    - Cortical isotope retention
  - Sensitivity ↓if bilateral disease, ↓GFR or pre-existing ACEI therapy (stop 4–5d prior).

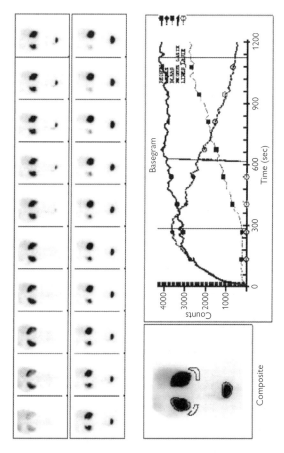

Fig. 1.6 Diuretic renogram showing 'true' obstruction of the right kidney. The collecting system does not empty and the curve remains flat (note: ↓GFR causes slow filling of the renal pelvis and ↓ response to frusemide).

Reproduced with permission from Davison AMA, Cameron JS, Grunfeld J-P et al. (eds) (2005). *Oxford Textbook of Clinical Nephrology*, 3rd edn. Oxford: Oxford University Press

Angiography and uroradiology

Angiography

Remains the gold standard investigation in renovascular disease, despite increasing promise within the chasing pack.

Technique

A retrograde catheter is passed under fluoroscopic guidance via a femoral puncture. A flush aortogram reveals number and location of renal arteries, before selective catheterization. Intravenous digital subtraction angiography (IVDSA) is generally inadequate. Contrast nephrotoxicity (📖 p.132) is a concern, but CO_2 is an alternative to iodinated media.

Indications

- Renovascular disease
  - Invasive ∴ not an ideal screening test (📖 p.412)
- Acute renal ischaemia
  - Acute emboli or thrombosis, traumatic occlusion, dissection
  - Therapeutic intervention (e.g. thrombolysis) may be possible
- Unexplained haematuria
  - Vascular lesions (e.g. AVM, angioma). May allow embolization
- Classical polyarteritis nodosa (PAN) (📖 p.464)
  - Intrarenal microaneurysms
- Renal transplantation
  - Evaluation of donor anatomy prior to live kidney donation (📖 p.246)
- Bleeding post renal biopsy
  - Identify bleeding source (±embolization).

Uroradiology

Urethrography and cystography

Contrast → urethra ± bladder. Indications: trauma, urethral stricture, bladder diverticulae or fistulae. CT cystography increasingly used.

Micturating cysturethrography (MCUG)

A contrast-filled bladder and urethra are visualized during voiding. Gold standard for diagnosis of VUR (📖 p.430). Demonstrates reflux and dilatation/distortion of the ureters and PC system. Pressure-flow video-cystometrography involves measurement of bladder pressures and urine flow rate in addition to imaging.

Retrograde ureteropyelography

The ureteric orifices are cystoscopically cannulated and contrast injected under fluoroscopic screening. The ureter, PUJ, and PC system can be visualized. May precede insertion of a retrograde ureteric stent.

Antegrade ureteropyelography (percutaneous nephrostomy)

A needle is placed percutaneously into the renal pelvis under fluoroscopic or USS guidance. Contrast media is injected to evaluate PC, ureteric, and bladder anatomy. Urine → culture and cytology. Pressure studies can be undertaken in suspected PUJ obstruction (Whitaker test). (📖 p.504)

Indications: Relief of urinary obstruction (📖 p.500), dilation of ureteric strictures, antegrade stent placement, removal of calculi.

Ileal loopography

The loop is filled with contrast following the introduction of a Foley catheter. Upper tract dilatation is common after ileal diversion and free reflux of contrast into the ureters is almost universal—if not, obstruction at the ureteric insertion (most common site) should be suspected.

Cysturethroscopy, ureteroscopy, and ureterorenoscopy

Cysturethroscopy or cystoscopy involves a visual inspection of the inside of the urethra and bladder using either a flexible (out-patient, no need for anaesthetic, little capacity to biopsy) or rigid (in-patient, anaesthetic, can biopsy if necessary) cystoscope. Undertaken by urologists rather than radiologists. Indications include:
- Micro- and macroscopic haematuria
- Recurrent UTIs
- Unexplained lower tract symptoms
- Surveillance of bladder tumours

Flexible ureterorenoscopy is a relatively new technique that involves passing a small flexible fibreoptic transurethral endoscope through the bladder and as far up as the renal pelvis. Rigid ureteroscopy does not generally reach this distance and requires a general anaesthetic, though it does allow biopsies to be taken.

Clinical syndromes

Proteinuria (📖 pp.18–19)

Protein excretion <150mg/day is normal. ~30mg of this is albumin, the rest is LMW protein, including β2 microglobulin, enzymes, and peptide hormones. A small proportion is secreted by the renal tubules, including Tamm–Horsfall mucoprotein (uromodulin).

Why is abnormal proteinuria important?

1. It is a marker of intrinsic renal disease, particularly glomerular injury.
2. It is a risk factor for the progression of renal insufficiency.
3. It is an independent risk factor for CV morbidity and mortality.

What is the relevance of a positive dipstick for protein?

- Dipsticks predominantly detect albumin (📖 p.18). +ve if protein excretion >300mg/d.
- Dipstick proteinuria has a prevalence of around 5% in healthy individuals (usually *trace* to 1+ range).
- Further evaluation is mandatory to distinguish 'benign' from 'pathological' proteinuria.

What is pathological proteinuria?

Persistent protein excretion >150mg/d implies renal or systemic disease. The amount and composition depends on the nature of renal injury. Urinary electrophoresis can distinguish the source:

- *Glomerular.* Failure of the glomerular barrier allows passage of intermediate and high MW protein. The most important cause of proteinuria in clinical practice. The predominant protein is albumin.
- *Tubular.* LMW proteins, such as Ig light chains and β_2-microglobulin, normally pass through the glomerulus and are reabsorbed by proximal tubular cells. Damage to the proximal tubule disrupts this cycle and results in tubular proteinuria. Not detectable on dipstick examination.
- *Overflow.* Overproduction of LMW plasma proteins exceeds the capacity of the normal proximal tubule to reabsorb them. Causes (i) Ig light chains in myeloma; (ii) lysozyme in monomyelocytic leukaemia. Dipstick examination will be negative—specific assays are required.
- *Secretory proteinuria.* Protein added to the urine lower in the urinary tract (e.g. bladder tumour, prostatitis). Blood (>50mL/24h) will also cause proteinuria (not albuminuria).

What is microalbuminuria?

- Albuminuria above the normal range (>30mg), but below the threshold of traditional dipsticks (<300mg).
- A misleading term, implying the albumin is of lower molecular weight–the 'micro-' prefix simply signifies the low amount.
- A sensitive indicator of (i) early renal disease and (ii) CV risk in DM, ↑BP and several other conditions.
- Detected by radioimmunoassay on a 24h urine collection, ultrasensitive dipstick, or spot microalbumin/creatinine ratio 📖 p.19.

When is proteinuria 'benign'?

Transient

- Fever
- Exercise
- Extreme cold
- Seizures
- CCF
- Severe acute illnesses

Persistent

Postural (orthostatic) proteinuria.

- Normal subjects demonstrate a small ↑ in protein excretion on standing. Postural proteinuria is an exaggeration of this.
- Relatively common in young adults (~3–5%). Rare >age 30.
- Usually <1g/24h.
- Diagnose with a 'split' urine collection: 16h daytime and 8h overnight collection (simpler: -ve dipstick on waking, +ve at night).
- Renal function remains normal, even after prolonged follow up.
- Remits with time (remains in ~50% cases at 10 years and <25% at 20 years).

Possible mechanisms: (i) trivial glomerular lesion; (ii) ↑ circulating AII and noradrenaline when upright → ↑ glomerular permeability; (iii) renal vein entrapment between aorta and superior mesenteric artery → local haemodynamic disturbance ('nutcracker' syndrome; ?also a cause of microscopic haematuria).

Table 1.4

Daily protein excretion	Cause
0.15–2.0g/24h	Mild glomerulopathies
	Orthostatic proteinuria
	Tubular proteinuria
	Overflow proteinuria
2.0–4.0g/24h	Probably glomerular
> 4.0g/24h	Virtually always glomerular

NB Proteinuria >3g does not necessarily result in the nephrotic *syndrome* but is often referred to as nephrotic *range*. Proteinuria with accompanying microscopic haematuria strongly suggests glomerular disease.

Clinical consequences

Mild proteinuria does not produce clinical sequelae. When more severe (>3–5g/day) a distinct clinical entity—the nephrotic syndrome—may result. Heavy proteinuria may cause a frothy urine ($\downarrow$ surface tension).

The nephrotic syndrome (📖 p.386)

Urine albumin loss → $\downarrow$serum albumin → oedema (through a variety of mechanisms). The concomitant loss of other serum proteins → hyperlipidaemia, thrombotic tendency, $\uparrow$ susceptibility to infection.

Selectivity

Selectivity refers to size discrimination at the glomerulus.

- Highly selective proteinuria
  - Only albumin and proteins of similar MW
- Non-selective proteinuria
  - Larger proteins, including Igs.

Calculated by comparison of IgG and albumin (or transferrin) clearance. Requires a sample of plasma and 'spot' urine specimen.

$$\text{Selectivity index} \quad \frac{\text{urine IgG} \times \text{serum Alb}}{\text{serum IgG} \times \text{urine Alb}} \times 100$$

$\leq 10\%$ highly selective
11–20% moderately selective (limited discriminatory value)
$\geq 21\%$ poorly selective

- May have a limited prognostic value—non-selective proteinuria denoting more severe injury to the glomerular apparatus.
- In children: identifies the highly selective proteinuria of minimal change disease, circumventing the need for biopsy.

Microalbuminuria and cardiovascular risk

- Microalbuminuria is a marker of CV risk.
- Applies to the general population, not just DM or $\uparrow$BP.
- The mechanisms underpinning this association are poorly understood, but microalbuminuria, endothelial dysfunction, and chronic inflammation are interrelated processes that develop and progress together.
- Microalbuminuria can be correlated to the risk of stroke, MI, LV dysfunction, PVD, and death.
- BP reduction is the key to microalbuminuria reduction—RAS blockade with ACE inhibitors or ARBs (or both) appears to be the treatment of choice.
- There is no present consensus on microalbuminuria screening in non-diabetics, though screening of hypertensive patients (and other high risk groups) is increasingly advocated.

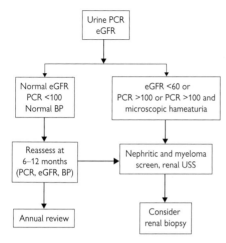

Fig. 1.7 Suggested management of asymptomatic proteinuria. NB Nephritic and myeloma screen: ANA, ANCA, anti-GBM antibodies, complement components, hepatitis B and C serology, protein electrophoresis, immunoglobins, urinary Bence–Jones proteins (📖 p.84)

Haematuria

Can result from bleeding at any site in the urinary tract. Causes range from benign to serious (Table 1.5).

Classification

Macroscopic vs. microscopic

- *Macroscopic*: blood is visible to the naked eye. Gross haematuria startles the patient and ∴ presents early—the patient may not recognize blood and report discolouration (pink, smoky, cola, or tea-like).
  ▶ Macroscopic haematuria always requires investigation (presenting complaint in 85% of bladder and 40% of renal tumours). Heavy bleeding with clot formation almost never occurs in glomerular disease.
- *Microscopic*: blood only visible under high-powered microscopy. Often found on dipstick examination in an asymptomatic patient.

Glomerular vs. non-glomerular

Provides a framework for considering pathology. Both can present with macro- or microscopic bleeding (particularly non-glomerular haematuria). Locally agreed nephrological and urological referral and investigation pathways are desirable.

Transient' haematuria
- Exercise ('joggers' nephritis')
- Menstruation
- Sexual activity
- Viral illnesses
- Trauma

Table 1.5 Important causes of haematuria by age and source

Origin	< age 40	≥ age 40
Glomerular	IgA nephropathy	IgA nephropathy
	Thin basement membrane disease	Alport's syndrome
	Alport's syndrome	Mild focal GN of other causes
	Mild focal GN of other causes (e.g. lupus nephritis)	
	Other GN (variably present in membranous and diabetic nephropathies)	
Non-glomerular		
Upper urinary tract	Renal stones	Renal stones
	Pyelonephritis	Renal-cell carcinoma
	Polycystic kidney disease	Polycystic kidney disease
	Medullary sponge kidney	Pyelonephritis
	Hypercalciuria/ hyperurico-suria ± stones	Transitional-cell tumour
	Renal trauma	Papillary necrosis
	Papillary necrosis	Renal infarction
	Ureteral stricture and hy-dronephrosis	Ureteral stricture and hy-dronephrosis
	Sickle cell trait or disease in black patients	Renal TB
	Renal infarction or arterio-venous malformation	Renal vein thrombosis
	Renal TB (?HIV)	
	Renal vein thrombosis	
Lower urinary tract	Cystitis, prostatitis, and urethritis	Cystitis, prostatitis, and urethritis
	Benign bladder, ureteral polyps, and tumours	Bladder cancer
	Bladder cancer	Prostate cancer
	Prostate cancer	Benign ureteral/bladder tumours
	Urethral stricture	
	Schistosoma haematobium	
Uncertain	Exercise haematuria	Exercise haematuria
	Unexplained haematuria Over-anticoagulation (usually warfarin)	Over-anticoagulation (usually warfarin)
	Factitious haematuria	

History
- How much bleeding? Is the urine discoloured or frankly bloody?
- Recent trauma? May be relatively trivial, e.g. contact sports.
- Previous episodes?
- History of stone disease?
- Relevant medications? Anticoagulants should not cause haematuria if the INR is in the required range.
- Recent instrumentation of the urinary tract?
- Any associated urinary symptoms? Urinary infection?
- Pain? Sudden onset of colicky flank pain suggests a stone. Suprapubic pain may indicate infection or clot colic. ▶ Painless macroscopic haematuria indicates a tumour until proven otherwise.
- What part of the stream?
  - Initial haematuria suggests an anterior urethral lesion.
  - Terminal haematuria usually arises from the posterior urethra, bladder, bladder neck, or trigone.
  - Continuous haematuria usually originates at or above the level of the bladder.
  - Cyclical haematuria in ♀ suggests endometriosis of the urinary tract.
- Risk factors for urothelial malignancy (📖 p.512)?
- Recent skin or throat infection—post-streptococcal GN.
- Episodic macroscopic haematuria with throat infections is a classical presentation of IgA nephropathy 📖 p.374.
- Recent travel? Schistosomiasis is the most common cause of haematuria worldwide (don't swim in lake Malawi!).
- Systemic symptoms (e.g. arthralgia, rashes) to suggest an underlying inflammatory disorder?
- Family history of deafness (Alport's).

Physical examination (signs usually scarce)
- Haemodynamically stable?
- Anaemia
- Bruising/bleeding (bleeding diathesis)
- Skin or throat infections
- Rashes, swollen joints
- Cardiorespiratory
  - Endocarditis
  - ↑BP and oedema (glomerular disease)
- Abdomen
  - Flank tenderness (stone disease, pyelonephritis)
  - Masses
  - Bruit (AVM)
  - Testicles and prostate
  - ±VE (?misinterpreted vaginal bleeding).

Investigation of macroscopic haematuria

- Urinanalysis.
  - A −ve dipstick in a patient with documented macroscopic haematuria should not stop further investigation.
  - In heavy bleeding the dipstick often tests +ve for protein: interpret with caution.
- Urine M, C+S. Verify dipstick. Evidence of infection? Ova of *Schistosoma haematobium* (if relevant)?
- Urine cytology. Malignant cells? Casts & dysmorphic cells?
- FBC, U&E, clotting, G&S (± cross-match when severe), PSA, Hb electrophoresis in black patients.
- Imaging. CT is the investigation of choice. If unavailable, USS + IVU.
- Cystoscopy (in all patients) ± ureterography 📕 p.44
- ± Angiography. May demonstrate a vascular lesion.

Microscopic haematuria

Definition

Arbitrary. >2 red cells/hpf (📖 p.20) (~10^7 red cells/24h). It is usually a +ve dipstick, not a cell count, that triggers investigation (dipsticks detect 2–5 cells/hpf).

Epidemiology

Reported prevalence varies widely (0.19%–16.1%), reflecting differences in the definition used and population screened (particularly age). Common in both adults and children.

Predictive value

The proportion who have (or develop) significant disease depends on group studied and thoroughness of investigation. Overall risk of malignancy (2–10%) is less than macroscopic haematuria (5–22%), but ↑ with age.

Table 1.6

↑ chance of malignant lesion	↑ chance of glomerular lesion
• Age>40	• Proteinuria
• History of gross haematuria	• Dysmorphic red cells and red cell casts (📖 p.20)
• Analgesic abuse	• Renal impairment
• Smoking	• ↑BP
• Alcohol abuse	
• Occupational exposures (📖 p.512)	
• Pelvic irradiation	
• Previous cyclophosphamide treatment	

Evaluation

- See Fig. 1.8, opposite.
- Casts and dysmorphic cells (📖 p.20).
- Imaging: CT is the investigation of choice. If unavailable, a combination of USS (alone: may miss small stones and renal tumours <3cm diameter) and IVU (alone: may miss tumours not involving the PC system) is used.
- Nephrology work up: measure BP, FBC, U&E, eGFR, quantify proteinuria, consider nephritic screen (📖 p.84) ± renal biopsy (📖 p.642).
- 'High risk': left hand column in Table 1.6, above.

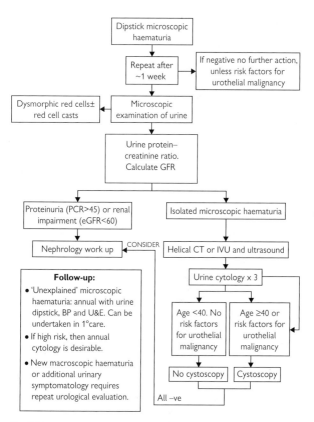

Fig. 1.8 Suggested management of microscopic haematuria. See notes opposite.

Chronic kidney disease (see Chapter 3)

The end result of any process causing renal parenchymal damage. Implies irreversible reduction in the number of functioning nephrons and characterized by progressive inability of the kidneys to fulfill their homeostatic responsibility. ⚠ Make sure reversible factors have been excluded.

Definition

Previously termed chronic renal failure, with an arbitrary definition. Recently clarified by K/DOQI (📖 p.142).

Table 1.7 Introduction to CKD

Stage	Description	GFR mL/min 1.73m^2
1	Asymptomatic urinary abnormalities	>90
2	Mild CRF	60–89
3	Moderate CRF	30–59
4	Severe CRF	15–29
5	Approaching ESRD	<15 or on dialysis

Nomenclature

Uraemia (or uraemic syndrome): the constellation of symptoms and signs produced as GFR declines (originally chosen to imply retention of urine in the blood). A multisystem disorder with a complex pathophysiological basis (📖 p.158). Correlation of Ur and Cr with symptomatology is poor, so the diagnosis is part clinical, part biochemical.

Azotaemia, a popular term in the USA, used to imply retention of nitrogenous compounds. Usually refers to early CKD, sparing uraemia for symptomatic patients. Also attempts to play down the role of Ur itself.

End-stage renal disease (ESRD): generally defined as a GFR ≤5mL/min. The initiation of renal replacement therapy (RRT) is required for the patients continued well-being (note: RRT does not have to wait until the patient is symptomatically uraemic 📖 p.159).

The uraemic syndrome

Water, electrolyte, and acid–base balance

- Breathlessness 2° to volume overload and Kussmaul breathing 2° to acidosis
- Postural hypotension caused by volume depletion
- Effects of ↑ or ↓ potassium

Haematological system

- Symptomatic anaemia and bleeding tendency

Cardiorespiratory

- Cardiac failure associated with fluid overload, ↑BP, anaemia, and impaired LV function
- Accelerated atherosclerosis (angina, stroke, PVD) and vascular calcification
- Pleuropericarditis
- Cardiac arrhythmias 2° electrolyte disturbances

Musculoskeletal

- Weakness, bone pain, and deformity 2° osteodystrophy
- Gout

Nervous system

- Hypertensive stroke and encephalopathy
- Anxiety, depression, and other psychological disturbances
- Impaired cognitive function
- Peripheral and autonomic neuropathy
- Involuntary movements (including restless legs)
- Decreased conscious level and seizures (late)

Gastrointestinal

- Nausea, anorexia, and malnutrition
- GI bleeding (↑ peptic ulceration and angiodysplasia)
- Fetor, constipation, and diarrhoea

Skin

- Dry skin, nail changes, and pruritis
- Bullous eruptions
- Pallor, pigmentation, and uraemic frost (late)

Eyes

- Conjunctival calcium deposits and retinal vascular disease

Immunity

- Impaired cellular and humoral immunity (↑ infection and malignancy)

Endocrine

- Aberrant vitamin D and PTH metabolism
- Impaired IGF-1 production (growth retardation in children)
- Hyperprolactinaemia (gynaecomastia in ♂)
- Multiple other subclinical abnormalities

Sexual function

- Sexual dysfunction
- Decreased fertility

Other clinical syndromes

The nephritic syndrome (📖 p.364)

Acute post-infectious GN, particularly following pharyngitis or cellulitis with group A β-haemolytic streptococci, provides a historical prototype but is now uncommon in developed countries. May be associated with a variety of other conditions (📖 p.378).

Clinical features
- Haematuria (usually microscopic)
- Proteinuria
- ↑BP
- Oliguria
- Circulatory overload and oedema
- ↓GFR.

Rapidly progressive glomerulonephritis (RPGN)
The dramatic end of the nephritic spectrum with a rapid ↓GFR and (usually) oligo-anuria. Caused by an aggressive glomerular lesion with extensive crescent formation (📖 p.362). Other renal diseases can produce an identical clinical picture (e.g. thrombotic microangiopathy).

▶ Seek expert help. Recovery of renal function is rare without early treatment.

Hypertension (📖 Chapter 5)
Hypertension in renal disease
- Underlying renal disease is found in a minority of patients with ↑BP, although the possibility should always be considered.
- ↑BP may be a feature of any renal disease, though particularly common in glomerular and vascular diseases.
- Hypertension has an important bearing on the progression of renal disease (📖 p.150).

Renal disease in hypertension
- The normal kidney plays an important role in the pathogenesis of essential hypertension (📖 p.283).
- The kidney is an important site of end-organ damage caused by ↑BP.
- The kidney has been described as both 'villain and victim' in ↑BP.

Acute renal failure (ARF) (📖 Chapter 2)

Pulmonary renal syndromes

The combined presentation of acute GN and pulmonary haemorrhage is one of the most dramatic in clinical medicine.

Causes

ANCA +ve vasculitis (📖 p.458) ~60% cases. Anti-GBM disease also known as Goodpasture's disease (📖 pp.466–7) ~20%. Also SLE (📖 p.468), Henoch–Schönlein purpura (📖 p.378), and rheumatoid vasculitis (📖 p.476).

History

The first report of a condition simultaneously affecting lungs and kidney was presented in 1919 by Ernest Goodpasture following post-mortem studies during the 1918–19 influenza pandemic. Four decades later the eponymous term Goodpastures Syndrome was adopted to describe comparable clinicopathological presentations. Subsequent realization that pulmonary renal syndromes are not a single clinical entity brought about further refinements to nomenclature—Goodpastures *disease* is now reserved for lung haemorrhage and crescentic GN in the context of anti-GBM disease (📖 p.466). With hindsight it is likely that Goodpastures original patient had a systemic vasculitis and not the disease that now bears his name.

Clinical features

- Acute nephritic syndrome (rapidly progressive renal failure with an active urinary sediment).
- Features of an underlying systemic condition may be present; (e.g. cutaneous vasculitis, sinusitis, arthritis).
- Pulmonary haemorrhage:
  - Cough
  - Dyspnoea
  - Haemoptysis (extensive bleeding)
  - Anaemia (and iron deficiency)
  - Hypoxaemia and respiratory failure
  - CXR: diffuse or patchy alveolar shadowing (indistinguishable from pulmonary oedema/ARDS)
  - CT: confirms air space filling
  - Lung function: ↑ diffusion capacity for carbon monoxide (KCO)
  - Bronchoscopy: bloody bronchoalveolar lavage.

Other 'pulmonary renal' syndromes

Pulmonary haemorrhage is rare, but respiratory dysfunction and/or CXR abnormalities are common in ARF.

- Pulmonary oedema
- Infection
  - ARF may accompany pneumonia and vice versa
  - A vasculitis patient receiving immunosuppressive therapy will be at risk of opportunistic infections including fungi, viruses and TB
  - Hantavirus
- Pulmonary emboli
- Acid–base disturbances
- Acute respiratory distress syndrome (ARDS)

Changes in urine volume
- Polyuria: >3L/24h
- Oliguria: <400mL/24h
- Anuria: <100mL /24h.

Polyuria

Excretion of a urine volume in excess of normal; >3L/day is an arbitrary cut-off. H_2O excretion is tightly controlled, so daily volumes vary widely in an individual.

It is usually frequency of micturition (especially overnight) 2° to the larger volume, rather than the volume itself, that causes the patient to present (though most patients with frequency do not have polyuria). Obtain a 24h urine collection for volume before undertaking further investigation.

Polyuria is seen in three clinically important situations:
1. Excessive fluid intake.
2. Increased tubular solute load; e.g. hyperglycaemia.
3. Failure of the renal tubules to concentrate the urine (diabetes insipidus 📖 p.527).

Oliguria

Passage of a urine volume inadequate for excretion of the end products of metabolism. <400mL/24h (~20mL/h). The causes of oliguria (and anuria) are analogous to those of ARF.

Anuria

Passage of <100mL/24h, or the absence of urine flow.
▶ Address the following questions urgently if anuria:
1. Is the urinary tract obstructed?
2. Are the kidneys perfused?

Pain

Loin pain

Renal pain is usually experienced in the loin near the costovertebral angle. Anterior radiation may cause confusion with intraperitoneal pain. It may also radiate to the genitalia. Usually associated with distension of the renal capsule and described as a constant dull ache.

Differential: nerve root irritation (commonly T10–T12).

△ An aggressive and destructive renal disease may be painless.

Ureteric colic

Sudden onset, extremely severe (pale, distressed, unable to settle) colic. Caused by a combination of ureteral stretching, local inflammation and hyper-peristalsis (spasm of ureteral smooth muscle). Pain may not completely fade between exacerbations.

Causes

Passage of a stone (common), blood clot, or sloughed papillae. Ureteral pathology that develops slowly or produces only partial obstruction may be painless (small stone → excruciating colic; large, non-obstructing, staghorn calculus → no pain)

Pattern of referred pain can sometimes help determine the level of ureteric obstruction.

- Upper ureter → loin
- Midureter → ipsilateral iliac fossa. May → testicle in ♂, labium in ♀, and upper thigh in both.
- Lower ureter → bladder irritability (frequency, dysuria, urgency), and suprapubic discomfort. May → urethra and tip of penis.

The bladder

Suprapubic pain

- Usually over-distension of the bladder (acute retention) or local inflammation (cystitis).
- Cystitis: signs of bladder irritability (below) and sharp, stabbing pain towards the end of voiding (strangury).
- Slowly progressive distension (e.g. neurogenic bladder) may cause no pain.
- Constant suprapubic pain, unrelated to retention, may not originate in the bladder. In ♀ consider gynaecological causes.

Bladder irritability

- Dysuria, frequency, and urgency among the commonest symptoms encountered in clinical practice.
- Urinary infection, causing inflammation of the urethra, trigone and bladder, is (by far) the most frequent cause (📖 p.424).
- △ About one-third of patients with bladder cancer present with bladder irritability.

Tubular syndromes

A degree of tubular dysfunction may occur with any renal injury (though the clinical picture is usually dominated by ↓GFR). Several distinct clinical syndromes result from tubular defects in the context of a normal GFR.

Generalized tubular dysfunction (Fanconi syndrome)

Multiple tubular defects produce a distinct clinical phenotype referred to as the Fanconi syndrome. Components may be present to a variable degree.

- *Phosphaturia and bone disease.* Impaired PO_4 reabsorption → phosphaturia → hypophosphataemia. This, and impaired 1α hydroxylation (activation) of 25-hydroxyvitamin D_3 in proximal tubular cells, produces skeletal abnormalities including rickets (children), osteomalacia (adults) and osteoporosis.
- *Aminoaciduria.* Amino acids are usually filtered at the glomerulus before reabsorption by multiple transport carriers in the proximal tubule. Fanconi syndrome → all amino acids appear in the urine in excess. No clinically significant sequelae and supplementation unnecessary.
- *Glycosuria.* Amount varies but serum glucose usually normal. Clinical sequelae are rare, though hypoglycaemia occurs in some forms (e.g. Fanconi–Bickel syndrome/glycogenosis).
- *Renal tubular acidosis (RTA).* Defective bicarbonate reabsorption in the proximal tubule results in systemic acidosis (a form of type II RTA 🕮 p.556).
- *Na^+ loss.* If severe → postural ↓BP, ↓Na^+, and metabolic alkalosis result. Salt supplementation occasionally necessary.
- *Hypokalaemia.* ↑ delivery of Na^+ to the distal tubule → Na^+ reabsorption at the expense of K^+. Acidosis and RAS activation by volume depletion also → K^+ loss. Clinical sequelae common (muscle weakness, constipation, polyuria, cardiac arrhythmias) and supplementation often required.
- *Proteinuria.* LMW proteinuria is common ($β_2$-microglobulin, lysozyme, and other tubular proteins), though excretion rates are usually low–moderate.
- *Polyuria.* Polyuria, polydipsia, and dehydration can be prominent. Caused by ↓K^+ and impaired concentrating ability in the distal tubule.
- *Hypercalciuria.* Rarely → nephrolithiasis/calcinosis (?protective effect of polyuria), although these may be precipitated by treatment with vitamin D metabolites (further ↑ urinary Ca^{2+}). Serum Ca^{2+} usually normal.

Isolated tubular defects

Renal glycosuria

- ↓ proximal tubular glucose reabsorption → glycosuria (despite normal blood glucose).
- Clearance studies allow differentiation into different patterns implicating several defective tubular transport mechanisms.
- The amount can be quite significant (normally 1–30g/24h), but generally a benign condition with no clinical sequelae.
- ⚠ Always needs to be distinguished from DM.
- Genetic mechanisms involved, but inheritance unpredictable.

Aminoaciduria

- Causes
  - Inborn error of metabolism → ↑ plasma levels and 'overflow'.
  - Renal aminoaciduria → defective tubular transport mechanisms. Amino acid transport is complex, involving transporters specific to single or chemically related groups of amino acids.
- The most important isolated aminoaciduria is cystinuria, a cause of recurrent cystine stone formation. Autosomal recessive (📖 p.432).

Phosphaturia

- Defective phosphate transport → phosphaturia, hypophosphataemia, and disorders of the skeleton.
- Several described, including X-linked hypophosphataemic rickets (vitamin D resistant rickets).

Bladder outflow obstruction

Main causes shown opposite. The likelihood of each is influenced by age and sex. Presentation is with:
- Acute retention of urine
- Lower urinary tract symptoms (LUTS)

LUTS are divided into two groups. Symptoms correlate poorly with underlying urinary pathology, so it is best to remain as descriptive as possible.

Table 1.8

Obstructive (voiding) symptoms	Storage (filling) symptoms*
• Impaired size or force of stream	• Nocturia
• Hesitancy or straining	• Daytime frequency
• Intermittent or interrupted flow	• Urgency
• Sensation of incomplete emptying	• Urge incontinence
	• Dysuria

*also called irritative

'Prostatism' is no longer favoured to describe outflow symptoms (age matched ♀ report similar symptoms).

Examination

Palpate for bladder enlargement, rectal examination, pelvic examination in ♀, examine the legs neurologically, and test anal tone/sensation.

Investigations

Urine M,C&S, U&E and PSA (in males >40 years).
- *Imaging.* Bladder USS to measure residual volume post micturition (correlation to outflow obstruction is poor).
- *Uroflowmetry.* Full bladder emptied into a flowmeter to generate a flow curve (rate vs. time). Normal max flow >20mL/s. Further urodynamic assessment will distinguish non-obstructive causes of low flow (e.g. detrusor failure).
- *Pressure-flow studies (cystometrography).* More sensitive and specific but invasive. Bladder and rectal catheters record filling and voiding bladder pressures (normograms relate pressure to flow).
- *Videocystometrography.* Fluoroscopic screening of the ureters, bladder, and urethra. Useful in the investigation of neurological bladder dysfunction.
- *Retrograde urethrography.* ?urethral stricture.

Causes of bladder outflow obstruction
- Congenital
  - Urethral valves and strictures
- Structural
  - Benign prostatic hyperplasia
  - Carcinoma of the prostate
  - Bladder neck stenosis
  - Urethral stricture
- Functional
  - Bladder neck dyssynergia
  - Neurological disease—spinal cord lesions, MS, diabetes
  - Drugs—anticholinergics, antidepressants

Prostatic enlargement (📖 p.514)
- Prostate size correlates poorly with degree of obstruction on urodynamic assessment.
- Impaired flow is a function of two separate components.
  - Dynamic: ↑ sympathetic tone of prostatic smooth muscle.
  - Static: mass effect of enlargement.

Acute renal failure

Definition and epidemiology

Acute renal failure (ARF) is the syndrome arising from a rapid fall in GFR (over hours to days). It is characterized by retention of both nitrogenous (including Ur and Cr) and non-nitrogenous waste products of metabolism, as well as disordered electrolyte, acid–base, and fluid homeostasis.

Definition

- Despite its relative insensitivity to acute changes in GFR, most definitions have been based on serum Cr, either as an absolute value or as a change from baseline. Other definitions incorporate urine output (UO) or need for dialysis support.
- Until recently, there has been no consensus on a clinical definition of ARF, making it difficult to compare and interpret studies of prevention, incidence and treatment. A survey of 598 participants at a critical care nephrology conference in 2004 revealed 199 different criteria to define ARF, and 90 for initiating RRT[1].

The RIFLE classification

- In 2004, a multilayered definition of ARF was proposed by the Acute Dialysis Quality Initiative (ADQI). In this model, ARF is stratified into 5 stages based on severity and duration of injury: **R**isk, **I**njury, **F**ailure, **L**oss and **E**nd-stage disease (RIFLE), as shown opposite.
- More recently, as a modification of the RIFLE criteria, the concept of Acute Kidney Injury (AKI) has emerged and is likely to be widely adopted as the standard over the next few years.

Acute Kidney Injury (AKI) classification

- AKI is defined as functional or structural abnormalities, or markers of kidney damage (including abnormalities in blood, urine, tissue tests or imaging studies), present for <3 months.
- Diagnostic criteria: an abrupt (within 48 hours) reduction in kidney function as classified below. Assumes adequate fluid resuscitation and that obstruction has been excluded.

Acute Kidney Injury (AKI) classification

Stage	Cr criteria	UO criteria
1	↑Cr of ≥25µmol/L (≥0.3mg/dL) or ↑ to ≥150-200% baseline	<0.5mL/kg/h for >6h
2	↑Cr to >200-300% baseline	<0.5mL/kg/h for >12h
3	↑Cr to >300% baseline or Cr≥350µmol/L (≥4.0mg/dL) with an acute rise of at least 45µmol/L (0.5mg/dL). Or on RRT.	<0.3mL/kg/h for 12h or anuria for 12h

Only 1 criteria (i.e. Cr or UO) needs to be met. If both are present then select the one that places the individual in the higher stage.

---

1 Ricci et al. (2006). NDT, **23**, 690–6.

	GFR criteria	Urine output criteria
Risk	Cr increased 1.5x	<0.5mL/kg/h for 6h
Injury	Cr increased 2.0x	<0.5mL/kg/h for 12h
Failure	Cr increased 3.0x or Cr>355µmol/L when there was an acute rise of >44µmol/L	<0.3mL/kg/h for 24h or anuria for 12h
Loss	Persistent ARF; complete loss of kidney function for >4 weeks	
End-stage renal disease	ESRD for 3 months	

The RIFLE (**R**isk of renal dysfunction, **I**njury to the kidney, **F**ailure of kidney function, **L**oss of kidney function and **E**nd-stage kidney disease) classification of ARF[1]. Acute renal failure is divided into three severity categories: risk, injury and failure, and two clinical outcome categories: loss and end-stage renal disease. Criteria can be fulfilled through changes in Cr, urine output (UO) or both (the measure leading to the more severe ranking is used). Note: the F component of RIFLE is present even if the ↑ in Cr is <3x, as long as the new Cr is >355µmol/L (4.0mg/dL) with an acute ↑ of at least 44µmol/L (0.5 mg/dL). The designation RIFLE$_{FC}$ is used to denote acute on chronic disease. Similarly, when RIFLE$_F$ is achieved by UO criteria, a designation of RIFLE$_{FO}$ is used to denote oliguria.

1 2nd International Consensus Conference of the Acute Dialysis Quality Initiative (ADQI) Group; Bellomo R, Ronco C, Kellum J A, *et al.* (2004). *Critical Care* **8**(4), R204–12.

Incidence

Depends on the population studied and definition used.

Hospital
• 7% of general admissions.
• 20–25% of patients with sepsis and ~50% with septic shock.
• By AKI criteria, ~65% of ITU admissions (▶ mortality 43–88%).

Community
• Community based studies in the UK (Cr>300µmol/L) estimate 486–620 per million population (pmp). Incidence is age- and comorbidity-related (17 pmp in age <50 and 949 pmp age 80–89).
• Dialysis dependent ARF: ~200 pmp annually.

Prognosis

Mortality: overall mortality in dialysis-requiring ARF remains >50% (reflecting a high incidence in the elderly and those with multi-organ failure). This is despite improvements in many aspects of clinical care (particularly nutrition and dialysis support). Using the new AKI classification[2]:

Rise in Cr	Odds ratio for hospital mortality
≥27µmol/L (0.3mg/dL)	4.1
≥45µmol/L (0.5mg/dL)	6.5
≥90µmol/L (1.0mg/dL)	9.7
≥180µmol/L (2.0mg/dL)	16.4

2 Chertow G M, Burdick E, Honour M, *et al.* (2005). *J AM SOC Nephrol*, **16**, 3365–70.

Recovery of renal function: depends on underlying diagnosis. Irreversible in ~5% (~16% in the elderly).

Causes and classification

ARF is caused by, or complicates, a wide range of disorders and may be the result of multiple precipitants. Three clinical syndromes can be used to direct diagnosis and therapy.

1. Prerenal ARF

- ↓ renal blood flow (RBF) → ↓GFR.
- ↓ RBF may be 2° hypovolaemia per se, ↓ effective RBF (↓ cardiac output, vasodilatation in sepsis), or intrarenal vasomotor changes (e.g. NSAIDs and ACEI).
- Easily reversed by restoration of RBF.
- Kidneys remain structurally normal.

2. Intrinsic renal ARF

- The renal parenchyma itself is damaged through injury to the renal vasculature, glomerular filter, or tubulo-interstitium.
- The commonest cause (by far) is acute tubular necrosis (ATN), itself the end product of an ischaemic or nephrotoxic injury (▢ p.96).
- The diagnosis of ATN implies:
  - Glomerular, vascular, and other interstitial diseases are not responsible for ARF. Be cautious; these disorders often require specific treatment and a delay in their diagnosis can have severe consequences for long term kidney function. They may co-exist with ATN. ▶ Seek expert help if you are uncertain.
  - Recovery of renal function should occur if supportive measures are adequate (so make sure that they *are* adequate).
  - A potentially reversible phase has passed during which ATN could possibly have been avoided.

3. Postrenal ARF (▢ p.500)

- The kidneys produce urine, but there is obstruction to its flow.
- ↑ back pressure → ↓ tubular function
- Obstruction may occur at any level in the urinary tract.
- ARF results when both kidneys are obstructed or when there is obstruction of a solitary kidney.
- Obstruction eventually causes structural (and ∴ permanent) damage.

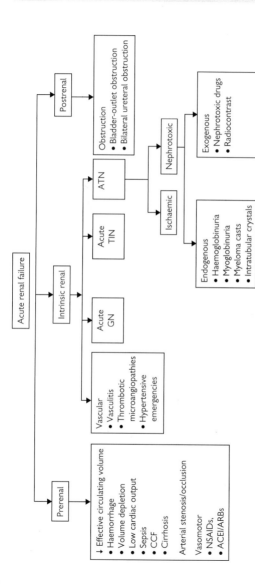

Fig. 2.1 Classification and major causes of acute renal failure.

Prevention

▶ Many cases of ARF should never occur in the first place.

Who is at risk?

- ↑ age.
- Pre-existing renal disease.
  - ↑Cr, ↓eGFR or proteinuria (dipstick positive).
- Surgery (esp if with another risk factor).
  - Trauma and burns surgery (hypovolaemia, sepsis, myoglobinuria).
  - Cardiac surgery (poor LV function, intra-operative haemodynamic instability, cardiopulmonary bypass, aprotinin use).
  - Vascular surgery (suprarenal aortic cross-clamping disturbs renal perfusion ± atheromatous emboli to kidneys). Risk of emergency AAA repairs > elective (25% vs. <5% ARF).
  - Hepatic and biliary surgery (over 70% of hepatic transplants complicated by ARF) Biliary surgery ± jaundice also high risk.
- Diabetes mellitus (esp. if established diabetic nephropathy with ↑Cr).
- Volume depletion (NBM, bowel obstruction, vomiting, burns).
- LV dysfunction and other CV disease.
- Other causes of ↓ effective arterial volume (cirrhosis).
- Drugs that cause renal vasomotor changes (NSAIDs, ACEI, ARB).
- Jaundice (hyperbilirubinaemia).
- Multiple myeloma (● may just be that these patients are often dehydrated with a degree of renal insufficiency to start with).

Common nephrotoxins

- NSAIDs, COX-2 inhibitors.
- Diuretics, ACEI, ARB esp. in volume depleted patients.
- Antibiotics: aminoglycosides, vancomycin.
- Amphotericin B (lipid preparation is ONLY ~50% less nephrotoxic than non-lipid, and may still cause ARF).
- Immunosuppressants (e.g. ciclosporin, tacrolimus) and chemotherapeutic agents (e.g. cisplatin).
- IV contrast (▢ p.132).

Using nephrotoxic drugs

⚠ Use with caution:

- Definite indication.
- No therapeutic alternative.
- Precautions to minimize toxicity undertaken.
- Renal function closely monitored.
- Regular drug levels where possible (e.g. gentamicin)

Reducing risk perioperatively

Three principles

1. Avoid dehydration (▶ Use 0.9% NaCl as replacement).
2. Avoid nephrotoxins (⚠ Contrast, NSAIDs, aminoglycosides).
3. Review clinical status and renal function in those at risk.

- Optimize volume status pre-operatively
  - No patient should ever go to theatre dehydrated.
  - Review daily weights, chart input/output, check postural BP ± CVP
  - Calculate losses, esp. in patients NBM.
  - ▶ Use correct IV fluid replacement (0.9% NaCl, not 5% dextrose).
- Optimize blood sugar control in diabetics (▶ sliding scale).
- Optimize nutrition (with par/enteral nutrition if indicated).
- Catheterize those with prostatic disease.
- Avoid surgery if possible immediately after a contrast procedure .
- Stop antihypertensive agents (esp. diuretics, ACEI/ARB) for 24–48 hr.
- Find out how the procedure and patient progressed in theatre. Check intraoperative records for blood loss and fluid and drugs administered.
- Review the patient early post-op.

Clinical approach to ARF

Introduction

There is a lot to get to grips with in a patient with ARF. It occurs in the context of a wide range of underlying conditions and the patient is often extremely unwell.

Recognize the problem

Patients may be asymptomatic during the early stages of ARF, despite nearly non-functional kidneys. They may be very unwell by the time the diagnosis is apparent. This is why it is so important to be familiar with at risk patients in high risk situations (📖 p.74).

Presenting features of ARF

Usually
- ↑Ur and ↑Cr
- ↓UO (UO <400mL/d is frequent [~50%] but not invariable).

Frequently
- Volume depletion OR
- Volume overload → pulmonary oedema
- Hyperkalaemia (→ arrhythmias or cardiac arrest)
- Non-specifically sick patient.

Rarely
Uraemic symptoms (📖 p.57).

▶ Check renal function and K^+ in all acutely unwell patients, esp. if:
- Falling or low UO, or anuria.
- Persistent nausea and vomiting, or prolonged NBM.
- Drowsiness or impaired conscious level.
- Signs of systemic sepsis.
- Hypertension or hypotension, particularly if severe.
- Pulmonary + peripheral oedema.
- Puzzling ECG abnormalities (▶ T wave changes and conduction delays).
- Metabolic acidosis.

▶▶ Make the patient safe

Evaluate if critically unwell as per protocol: airway, breathing, circulation. The standard priorities of resuscitation override thoughts as to the underlying cause. Two specific questions must be addressed urgently:

▶ How high is the K^+?

▶ What is the volume status?

Hyperkalaemia (📖 p.102) and pulmonary oedema (📖 p.108) will kill your patient quickly.

Look for a reversible cause of ARF

Consider the following questions first; relatively straightforward interventions can have a big impact in such situations.

- Is the patient septic?
- Is the patient passing urine—if so, how much? What does it look like?
- Is it pre-renal (📖 p.91)?
  - Are there pre-disposing factors in the history?
  - Carefully assess the patient's volume and haemodynamic status
    (▶ lying and standing BP).
  - Is invasive monitoring going to be needed? (It rarely is...)
- Is it post-renal (📖 p.500)?
  - Are there pre-disposing factors in the history?
  - Is there a *palpable bladder* or symptoms of prostatism?
  - Arrange an urgent USS.
- What's on the drug-chart (📖 p.74)?
  - Stop all nephrotoxins. Check random levels of suspected culprits
    (gentamicin).
- Has any contrast been administered, and if so, what volume?
- Have you dipsticked the urine (📖 p.80)?
  - Do it now—you may forget later.

If ↑Cr or↓eGFR, is it ARF or acute on chronic renal failure?

See overleaf, 📖 p.78.

Acute or chronic renal failure?

Patients are often found to have ↑Cr or ↓eGFR ± oliguria on presentation with unrelated medical or surgical conditions. Differentiating true ARF from stable (longstanding) CKD, or even an acute deterioration on pre-existing renal impairment is often very important.

Much is made of the ability to distinguish the two after an initial clinical assessment and blood tests. Many of these features, even when present, are at best suggestive and, at worst, misleading. The only two consistently useful discriminators are:

1. Previous measurements of renal function.
   • Where might this be documented? Admitted before?
   • Search your pathology system and pull hospital notes.
   • Ask the patient's GP to check their records.

2. Ultrasound.
   • Long-standing renal disease leads to loss of renal parenchyma and ↓ renal size.
   • Small (< 9–10cm length), echobright and often cystic kidneys are characteristic of CRF.

⚠ Normal sized kidneys should arouse suspicion of ARF. An exception is diabetic nephropathy (📖 p.438).

Laboratory findings suggesting ARF rather than CKD

These are *rarely* as helpful as textbooks imply. Err on the side of caution (assume ARF until proven otherwise).

• Anaemia might suggest chronic under-synthesis of erythropoietin by scarred kidneys: a *normal* Hb argues against CKD, but anaemia occurs in both ARF and CRF

• ↓Ca^{2+} and ↑PO_4 suggest impaired vitamin D synthesis (as found with CKD). Not so: disturbances of mineral metabolism occur *rapidly* in ARF.

▶ In many situations, particularly when renal size is normal, a biopsy may be necessary to determine the nature of the renal lesion and the extent of reversibility. (📖 p.87)

Assessing ARF

Urinalysis

▶ The only excuse for not doing a urine dipstick is if a patient is not making any. Always exclude bladder outflow obstruction. Different urinary findings lead to a diagnosis, particularly when suspecting glomerulonephritis. See. Fig. 2.2 opposite.

After collecting a urine sample for dipstick:

- ▶ Send an MSU for microscopy (or do it yourself) and culture.
- Consider, protein: creatinine ratio, urine electrolytes.

Urine biochemistry

In pre-renal ARF, tubular function is intact with avid salt retention, whereas in ATN the resorptive and concentrating capacity of the kidney is lost. Urinary biochemical indices can ∴ differentiate the two.

- 'Typical' pre-renal ARF
  - ↓u-Na+, ↑Ur, ↑Cr in the urine. u-osmolality high.
- 'Typical' ATN
  - ↑u-Na+, ↓Ur and ↓Cr in the urine. u-osmolality relatively low.

⚠ In everyday practice, these indices are of limited value.

- They are not sufficiently sensitive or specific.
- Diuretics confound the analysis (→ dilute urine with a ↑Na⁺ content).
- There are exceptions that biochemically appear prerenal, but are not:
  - Hepatorenal syndrome
  - Contrast nephropathy
  - Early obstruction
  - Acute GN and vasculitis.
- They will often not influence management.

Urine biochemistry in ARF

	Prerenal ARF	ATN
Urine specific gravity	>1.020	<1.010
Urine osmolality (mOsm/kg H₂O)	>500	<350
Urine:plasma osmolality	>1.5	<1.1
Urinary Na⁺ (mmol/L)	<20	>40
Fractional Na⁺ excretion % (FE_{Na⁺})[1] best index!	<1	>2
Fractional urea excretion % (FE_{urea})	<35	>35
Plasma urea:creatinine ratio	>10	<15
Urine:plasma urea ratio	>8	<3
Urine:plasma creatinine ratio	>40	<20
Renal failure index[2]	<1	>1

1 (urine Na⁺/plasma Na⁺)/(urine Cr/plasma Cr) × 100.
2 urine Na⁺/(urine creatinine/plasma creatinine) × 100.

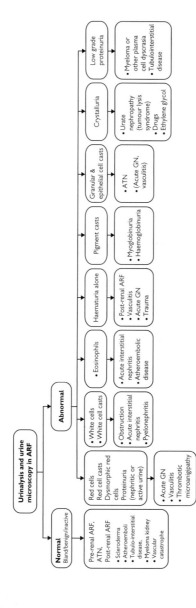

Fig. 2.2 The findings on urinanalysis and urine microscopy in ARF

Blood work

Managing and diagnosing renal impairment requires regular and informed testing. Order investigations sensibly and cumulatively, rather than simply requesting everything below.

Haematology

- FBC and ESR.
  - ↓Hb develops early, typically 8–11g/dl. ⚠ Haemolysis, GI bleeding.
  - ↑WCC: infection (rarely tissue infarction or vasculitis). Eosinophilia is a rare feature of TIN. ↓WCC: severe sepsis (rarely SLE).
  - ↓Plt: DIC or thrombotic microangiopathy (→ check clotting and ask for a blood film). ↑Plt: vasculitis.
  - Pancytopenia: ?marrow infiltration (?myeloma or other malignancy).
  - ↑ESR with any inflammatory condition, but esp myeloma and SLE.
- Clotting.
  - ?Liver disease (↑INR) or DIC (↑PT, ↑APTT, ↑D-dimers).
- Group and save if anaemic.
- Blood film if ↓plts, or ?microangiopathy .
  - Fragmented red cells. If found, send LDH, haptoglobins, retic count.

Biochemistry

- U&E (including venous bicarbonate, Cl^- and Cr).
  - ↑plasma Ur:Cr ratio may indicate prerenal ARF (but see 📖 p.33).
  - ↑K^+ ▶▶ Needed urgently.
  - Na^+ usually normal; ↓Na^+ occurs if volume overload or diuretics.
  - ↓Venous HCO_3^- from metabolic acidosis (may not need ABG).
- LFTs.
  - ↓albumin may imply GN.
  - ?↑bilirubin, ?hepatorenal syndrome (📖 p.126), ?paracetamol OD.
  - ⚠ ↑transaminases may be of muscle origin → check the CK.
- Ca^{2+} and PO_4.
  - ↑Ca^{2+} is a cause of ARF (?myeloma, sarcoidosis, malignancy).
  - ↓Ca^{2+} and ↑PO_4 present in most cases.
- CRP as a marker of any infection or inflammation. Procalcitonin?
- Creatine kinase (CK) if rhabdomyolysis likely.
- Urate if tumour lysis or pre-eclampsia possible.
- Lactate to assess tissue ischaemia or under-perfusion.
- PSA.

Microbiology

- Urine and blood culture if any clinical suspicion of sepsis.
- Hepatitis serology.

Arterial blood gas

A venous HCO_3^- is usually enough to assess the acidosis of ARF, particularly if O_2 sats are normal. However, have a low threshold for ABG, esp. in deteriorating or critically ill patients.

A minimum ARF panel
- Dipstick of the urine.
- FBC, U+E, Ca^{2+}, phosphate, albumin, LFT, CK, and CRP.
- Venous HCO_3, or ABG

The nephritic and myeloma screen

▶ Request urgently if an intrinsic cause of ARF (but not ATN) suspected, but use common sense. These are costly (and often unnecessary) assays that careful clinical assessment can put in perspective.

Anti nuclear antibodies (ANA)

ANAs are the serological hallmark of many autoimmune diseases. Further defined by specific assays against target antigens.

Antigen	Association
Double stranded DNA	SLE
Sm (Smith)	SLE
Ro/SSA and La/SSB	SLE, Sjogren's syndrome
Scl-70	Diffuse systemic sclerosis (SS)
Centromere	CREST syndrome (limited SS)
RNA polymerase	Renal involvement in systemic sclerosis
RNP	Mixed connective tissue disease (overlap)

If a clinical suspicion is strong, the specific assay may be necessary despite a negative ANA. ⚠ False +ve ANAs are common

Anti neutrophil cytoplasmic antibodies (ANCA)

A set of autoantibodies directed against components of neutrophil cytoplasm, characteristic of small vessel vasculitis (📖 p.458). Two patterns:
- Cytoplasmic ANCA (cANCA). Diffuse cytoplasmic staining on immunofluorescence. Antigen usually proteinase 3 (PR3).
- Perinuclear ANCA (pANCA). Several antigens—myeloperoxidase (MPO) the most important.

Anti glomerular basement membrane antibody (anti-GBM)

Highly sensitive and specific for anti-GBM disease (📖 p.466).

Anti-streptolysin O titres (ASOT)

Post-streptococcal GN is the historical prototype for the acute nephritic syndrome, though incidence is falling (📖 p.378). Sensitive for the diagnosis of streptococcal pharyngitis, but less so for skin infections.

Protein electrophoresis (serum and urine)

- Serum: M band in multiple myeloma.
- Urine: monoclonal light chains (Bence–Jones proteinuria).
- Free serum light chains may be indicated (📖 p.446)

Immunoglobulins

Serum IgG, IgA and IgM.
- Immune paresis in myeloma.
- Diffuse increase in vasculitis, SLE (and other connective tissue disorders). IgA raised in ~50% IgA nephropathy (📖 p.374).
- Polyclonal ↑Ig in HIV infection.

Rheumatoid factor

May be positive in vasculitis associated with RA (📖 p.476), or cryoglobulinaemia (📖 p.484)

Viral serology

Hepatitis B surface antigen (if positive, full HBV profile ± viral DNA), anti-hepatitis C antibody and anti-HIV antibody.
- Hepatitis B is associated with PAN (📖 p.464).
- Hepatitis C with mixed essential cryoglobulinaemia (📖 p.484).
- HIV may present in many ways, not least in the kidney.

It is also advantageous to know hepatitis status prior to haemodialysis.

Cryoglobulins (📖 p.484)

Not routine. Send if unexplained rash, peripheral neuropathy, hypocomplementaemia (see box below), known Hep C, known lymphoproliferative disorder or +ve RhF (a useful screening test). The sample needs to be transported at 37°C, so bleed the patient and take the sample to the lab yourself (in a water bath—armpit 2nd best) within minutes. Warn them it is coming.

Antiphospholipid antibodies

Not routine. Associated with the primary anti-phospholipid syndrome (📖 p.472). Request IgG and IgM anticardiolipin antibodies, anti-β_2 glycoprotein I and the lupus anticoagulant

Complement

Common investigations are immunoassays for C3 and C4 and a functional assay for the total haemolytic component (CH50). C3 and C4 can be used to screen for abnormalities in the classical and alternative pathways, with diseases associated with high levels of circulating immune complexes associated with hypocomplementaemia. CH50 measures red cell lysis and is a good screen for overall complement activity (e.g. a patient with recurrent infections).

Disorder	C3 & C4
SLE	↓C3, ↓C4, ↓CH50
Infective endocarditis	↓C3, ↓C4, ↓CH50
Shunt nephritis	↓C3, ↓C4, ↓CH50
Post-strep GN	↓C3, ↓/↔ C4, ↓CH50
Essential mixed cryoglobulinaemia	↔C3, ↓C4, ↓CH50
MCGN type II	↓C3, ↔C4, ↓CH50
	?C3 nephritic factor (📖 p.380)

Assessing ARF: imaging and histology

►► Get a CXR (pulmonary oedema, infection, pulmonary haemorrhage) Any clinical indication in its own right (tachypnoea, ↓O_2 sats, haemoptysis, occult infection or suspected associated primary lung disease) obviously merits CXR, but much important information about ARF may be gathered:
- Cardiac contour—?LVH consistent with longstanding ↑BP.
  ? Pericardial effusion.
- ?upper lobe venous diversion or frank pulmonary oedema.
- Hilar lymphadenopathy, lytic lesions.

►► Get an USS of the renal tract as soon as possible.

Imaging rarely makes a specific diagnosis. It has two principal aims:
- To exclude reversible obstruction (post-renal failure).
- To confirm the presence of two kidneys and quantify renal length. Renal length is used as a surrogate for the time course of renal impairment. Longstanding CKD → parenchymal scarring and loss of volume.
  - >10–11cm = normal (∴ probable ARF).
  - <8–9cm (► acquired cysts strongly suggest CKD) suggests CRF .

► 📖 p.498 for imaging in suspected acute obstruction.

Isotope studies in ARF

Not first line, but can occasionally be useful.
- Acute loss of renal perfusion associated with renal artery occlusion or embolism can be diagnosed with nuclear scans.
- Cortical necrosis (after severe haemorrhagic shock, particularly post-partum) is readily demonstrated.
- Early vascular complications in the immediate post-renal transplantation setting can be evaluated.
- In experienced hands, recovery from ATN can be assessed, though is rarely clinically useful.
- In partial obstruction, delayed transit in the ureteric phase can be helpful, 📖 p.42.

Renal biopsy in ARF

Only consider once pre- and post- renal factors addressed. Required in a minority of cases. Most intrinsic ARF is caused by ATN—histological confirmation will not alter management and prognosis for renal recovery is generally good. The aims of biopsy should be to:

- Establish a tissue diagnosis
- Assess prognosis (?is renal function salvageable)
- Guide therapy.

Potential indications

- Unexplained ARF (initial assessment unhelpful/equivocal)
- Suspected glomerular disease (haematuria ± casts, marked proteinuria)
- Serological or other evidence of systemic disease
  - ANCA, ANA, anti-GBM, paraprotein, HIV
- Suspected thrombotic microangiopathy (HSP/TTP)
- Marked ↑BP (⚠ control BP first)
- Presumed ATN persists >2 weeks (esp. if anuric)
- Pre-existing glomerular disease
- Suspected TIN/drug allergy
- Suspected athero-embolic disease.

Intrinsic renal disease presenting as ARF

- Acute primary GN (📖 p.364)
- Systemic vasculitis affecting the kidney (📖 p.456)
- Infection-associated GN (📖 p.378)
- Thrombotic microangiopathies (📖 p.400)
- ATN
- Acute TIN (📖 p.406)
- Myeloma cast nephropathy (📖 p.446)
- Athero-embolic disease (📖 p.416).

Pre-renal ARF

Any cause of *apparent* volume depletion may compromise renal perfusion, as ↓RBF → ↓GFR. The kidneys are structurally intact, but functionally compromised. As a general rule, the metabolically susceptible proximal tubule can withstand relative under-perfusion (and hypoxia) for a period of days (and often as much as 5 days) before true cellular injury supervenes (ATN).

Causes of hypo-perfusion

Hypoperfusion is *not* the same as volume depletion. Renal perfusion is a product of effective circulating volume, cardiac output and peripheral vascular resistance.

⚠ Any cause of a fall in effective arterial blood volume (📖 p.90) will cause pre-renal failure, despite the hydration status of the patient:

- Hypovolaemia
- Cardiogenic shock (or cardiac failure)
- Systemic vasodilatation (as in sepsis).

Physiological response to hypo-perfusion

Systemic response

Systemic hypo-perfusion is sensed as a ↓ in arterial BP by carotid and arteriolar baroreceptors. Activation of the sympathetic nervous system (SNS) and renin–angiotensin–aldosterone axis (RAS), as well as ↑vasopressin release then acts in concert to maintain BP and preserve blood flow to vital organs. This is accomplished by:

- Vasoconstriction in 'dispensable' vascular beds (e.g. cutaneous)
- ↑cardiac output and heart rate
- ↑ thirst and ↓ sweating
- ↑ renal conservation of salt and water.

Renal response (renal autoregulation)

GFR is initially maintained because intra-glomerular pressure is preserved despite the fall in systemic BP through renal auto-regulation and is dependent on the balance between dilatation of the pre-glomerular afferent arteriole (prostaglandins and NO) and constriction of the efferent post-glomerular arteriole (mainly angiotensin II).

If perfusion continues to fall pre-renal ARF results. As RBF drops, so glomerular filtration and urine output fall as well. Below a mean arterial pressure (MAP) of ~80mmHg, GFR ↓ rapidly. Lesser degrees of hypotension may provoke pre-renal ARF in susceptible individuals:

- The elderly.
- Those with pre-existing afferent arteriolar pathology (e.g. hypertensive nephrosclerosis or diabetic nephropathy).
- Those taking ACEI or ARBs, where constriction of the efferent arteriole is blocked.

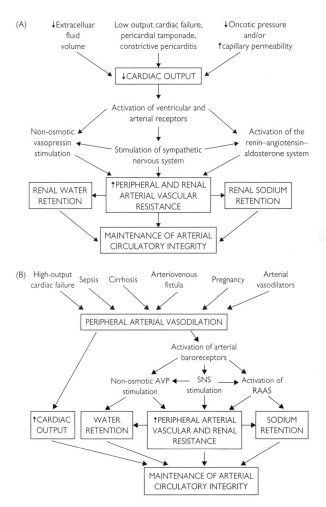

Fig. 2.3 (A) Sequence of events in which reduced cardiac output intiates renal sodium and water retention. (B) Sequence of events in which peripheral arterial vasodilatation intiates renal sodium and water retention.

Reproduced with permission from Schrier RW *et al.* (2004). *Neuroscience*, **129**, 897–904.

Causes of pre-renal ARF

Hypovolaemia

Any cause of ↓ intravascular volume.
- ECF depletion (usually both Na^+ and H_2O depletion—when losses are predominantly H_2O, ECF volume is usually preserved until late).
  - Inadequate fluid intake: limited access to fluid (children, elderly patients with poor mobility, endurance sports), NBM, inadequate IV fluids (everyone on a drip is at risk).
  - GI losses: D&V, NG drainage, GI bleeding.
  - Renal losses: diuretic therapy, uncontrolled DM (osmotic diuresis), salt losing nephropathy (rare—📖 p.522), post relief of urinary obstruction, diabetes insipidus .
  - Skin losses: excessive sweating, febrile patients, burns.
- Haemorrhage.
  - Trauma, surgery (and surgical drains), GI bleeding.
- 'Third-space' compartmental losses*.
  - Intestinal obstruction, peritonitis, pancreatitis, major fractures.

*'Third space' was originally coined to refer to a fluid compartment that is not in equilibrium with the ECF.

Impaired cardiac output

- Cardiac pump failure → ↓BP → ↓RBF.
  - Ischaemic heart disease → angina or MI.
  - Dysrhythmias (incl. rapid AF).
  - New or established LV dysfunction (incl. myocarditis and cardiomyopathy of any cause).
  - Pericardial disease: ⚠ Tamponade.
- In CCF the ECF volume may be normal or ↑ (with oedema and ascites) but the kidneys respond as though it were inadequate (↓ 'effective circulating volume'). See 📖 p.88 and 📖 p.520.

Peripheral vasodilatation

- Septic shock causes failure of peripheral circulatory control (📖 p.136). Systemic vasodilatation → ↓MAP → ↓RBF → ARF.
- Interactions between intraglomerular vaso-dilating and -constricting mediators resulting from sepsis also contribute to ↓GFR.

Intrarenal vasomotor changes

- NSAIDs impede prostaglandin-mediated afferent arteriolar dilatation. ▶ Post-op patient prescribed NSAIDs.
- ACEI and ARB oppose angiotensin II-induced efferent arteriolar constriction. ▶ Dehydrated elderly patient still taking an ACEI.
- Radiocontrast administration (📖 p.132).
- Renovascular disease (📖 p.412).

Is it pre-renal ARF?
- Is the patient volume deplete?
- Is cardiac function good?
- Is the patient septic ± vasodilated?

Physical examination

Many signs have been described as representing volume depletion. Some are absolutely key to diagnosis.
- Blood pressure: check lying and standing if possible.
- Heart rate.
- Peripheral perfusion.
  - Warm with bounding pulse → vasodilatation(? sepsis).
  - Cold and shut down with ↓capillary refill → volume depletion or low cardiac output.
- JVP: may be elevated with pump failure. *Not* ↑ with hypovolaemia or vasodilatation
- Urine output.

Poor signs
- Dry mucous membranes (most sick patients mouth breathe).
- ↓Skin turgor (better sign in children).
▶▶ Proceed to try and elicit a cause for the signs.

Classically

1. Volume depletion (hypovolaemic or haemorrhagic shock):
- (Postural) hypotension
- May be peripherally shut down
- JVP ↓.

2. Poor cardiac output (cardiogenic shock)
- Hypotension with narrow pulse pressure
- Peripherally shut down (often very)
- JVP ↑.

3. Systemic vasodilatation (septic shock)
- Hypotension with ↑pulse pressure
- Peripherally warm
- JVP ↓.

Volume replacement in pre-renal ARF

Prompt fluid resuscitation reverses pre-renal ARF. The key to fluid management is repeated clinical assessment of a patient's volume status.

Which fluid?

Crystalloids

0.9% NaCl (normal saline) is the initial treatment of choice in virtually all patients. Even in critically unwell patients with capillary leak, early resuscitation with 0.9% NaCl is indicated.

⚠ Hartmann's and Ringer's solutions contain K^+ ∴ avoid in ARF.

Sodium bicarbonate

'Weak' $NaHCO_3$ solutions (e.g. 1.26% or 1.4%) can be useful in volume depleted, acidotic (pH < 7.15), hyperkalaemic patients (📖 p.102). Use with 0.9% NaCl, usually in a ratio of 1 litre $NaHCO_3$ to 2–3 litres of saline.

⚠ Avoid stronger (4.2% or 8.4%) solutions, and monitor for ↓Ca^{2+}.

Hypotonic crystalloids

0.45% ('half-normal') saline and 5% dextrose distribute rapidly throughout total body water and are of limited use for the restoration of intravascular volume. Avoid unless true water depletion (hypernatraemia).

Synthetic colloids

Contain oncotically active ingredients (e.g. hydroxyethyl starch or gelatin) that remain in the intravascular compartment and pull in extravascular water. Effective volume expanders, but no evidence of specific benefit in ARF (☜ some studies suggest they may ↓GFR). Often used when significant ↓BP mandates rapid resuscitation. The most familiar are Gelofusine® and Haemaccel®—both gelatin based. The use of ≥1000–1500mL may deplete clotting factors and ↑bleeding risk.

Human albumin solutions

'Physiological colloid'. Expensive. Although a Cochrane meta-analysis concluded that its use was associated with ↑mortality in the critically ill, the more recent (and well designed) SAFE study suggested equivalence with saline. Many favour it when volume depletion occurs in the context of hypoalbuminaemia. Proven benefit in one situation alone—ARF in the context of cirrhosis with spontaneous bacterial peritonitis (📖 p.126).

- Isotonic (4–5%). Usually 100–500mL bottles. Used to restore circulatory volume.
- Concentrated (20–25%). Usually 50–100mL bottles. Used to expand circulatory volume when general salt and water restriction is desirable; i.e. an oedematous, hypoalbuminaemic patient who is intravascularly depleted (e.g. nephrotic syndrome, cirrhosis).

How much fluid?

The volume required to restore euvolaemia is the amount that improves clinical signs of volume depletion. These might include:

- Improving tachycardia.
- Better peripheral perfusion.
- Improving BP (▶ postural drop). If ↓BP despite apparently adequate filling, consider cardiogenic or septic shock.
- Visible JVP.
- Improving UO.

⚠ Beware volume overload: ↑BP, ↑RR, basal lung crackles, ↓O_2 sats.

How quickly?

Resuscitation

Infusion of fluids (± blood products) to restore BP and tissue perfusion. If in doubt, trial of 200–300 mL 0.9% NaCl fast IVI, and re-assess clinical parameters. Repeat as required.

Replacement

If (once) a patient is not shocked, the optimal infusion rate depends on:

- Degree of hypovolaemia
- Ongoing losses
- Whether oligo-anuric
- Cardiovascular status.

The following is a *rough* guide to getting things underway:

- First litre over 2 hours, *then reassess.*
- Second litre over 4 hours, *then reassess.*
- Third litre over 6 hours, *then reassess.*

⚠ Slower in the elderly and in those with poor LV function.

In the face of ongoing losses (e.g. diarrhoea), input should aim to exceed measured and unmeasured (insensible, ~30mL/h) losses by 100mL/h. If you think you have overdone it, stop all fluids and reassess the patient.

Maintenance

Once euvolaemic, and assuming no other losses, match UO + 30mL on an hourly basis. Insensible losses will be higher if febrile.

⚠ Reassess the patient at least twice a day.

When do you need a central line?

- Not often.
- Managing pre-renal failure rarely requires a CVP. Accurate bedside assessment is not difficult. If you are not experienced enough to assess volume status clinically, then you are probably not experienced enough to use invasive monitoring correctly.

▶ Putting central lines into hypovolaemic patients is not easy, and offers a real risk of complication.

However, a CVP may be useful in ARF in conjunction with:

- Septic shock and capillary leak.
- Cardiogenic shock, or where the CV status is precarious and you feel it would be dangerous or unwise to give significant fluids without a more accurate baseline and continuous monitoring.
- Target for euvolaemia is a CVP of 8–12cm H_2O.

Intrinsic renal ARF

Encompasses all causes of ARF in which the renal parenchyma has been damaged. ▶ ATN accounts for 80–90% of all intrinsic ARF.
⚠ Exclude or correct prerenal ± postrenal factors prior to diagnosis.

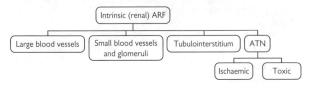

Fig. 2.4 Classification of intrinsic ARF

Differential diagnosis of acute intrinsic renal failure

- Larger renal vessels:
  - ACEI + bilateral renovascular disease (📖 p.412)
  - Renal artery occlusion due to thrombosis or dissection
  - Cholesterol emboli (📖 p.416)
  - Renal vein thrombosis (📖 p.416)
- Diseases involving the small renal vessels and glomeruli:
  - Glomerulonephritis (📖 p.366)
  - Vasculitis (📖 p.456)
  - Thrombotic microangiopathies (📖 p.400)
  - Malignant hypertension (📖 p.350) or scleroderma renal crisis (📖 p.474)
- Diseases of the tubulointerstitium:
  - Acute interstitial nephritis (📖 p.406)
  - Cast nephropathy (complicating multiple myeloma) (📖 p.416)
  - Contrast nephrotoxicity (📖 p.132)
  - Tumour lysis or acute urate nephropathy (📖 p.134)
- Acute tubular necrosis (📖 p.96)

Is it intrinsic renal ARF?

▶ Have pre- and post-renal causes been excluded?

Large renal vessels

History
- Cardiovascular:
  - Risk: smoking, diabetes, lipids, ↑BP, age.
  - Disease: claudication, stroke, IHD.
  - Intervention: invasive radiological procedures or vascular surgery.
- Source of embolus: AF, prosthetic valve, cardiomyopathy.
- Nephrotic syndrome: renal vein thrombosis (📖 p.416).

Examination
AF, missing pulses, dilated heart, bruits, aortic aneurysm, ischaemic toes,
↑BP (though very non-specific), oedema (?nephrotic).

Small renal vessels and glomeruli

History

- No other cause evident.
- Recent infection: particularly skin or throat (post streptococcal GN).
- Symptoms suggesting a deep seated infection: fevers, night sweats.
- Known systemic disorder: e.g. SLE, scleroderma, vasculitis.
- Symptoms suggesting an underlying connective tissue disorder or vasculitis (📖 p.3).

Examination

Rash, ↑BP, oedema, synovitis, arthropathy, uveitis, mouth ulcers, epistaxis or hearing loss, stigmata of endocarditis, evidence of scleroderma or other connective tissue disorder, abnormal respiratory findings (pulmonary-renal syndrome)

Investigations

- Urinalysis (📖 p.80).
- Abnormality in nephritic/myeloma screen (📖 p.84).
- Renal biopsy often necessary.

Tubulointerstitium

History

- Drugs (📖 p.5).
- Systemic infection: many are associated, including TB (📖 p.488).
- Systemic diseases: myeloma, sarcoidosis, Sjogren's syndrome, SLE.
- Uveitis: tubulointerstitial nephritis and uveitis (TINU) syndrome (📖 p.406).

Examination

Fever or rash, easy bruising multiple myeloma (MM), eosinophiluria.

Acute tubular necrosis (ATN)

ATN is is by far the most commonly encountered cause of intrinsic ARF. It is widely seen in hospitalized patients, and is predictable in high-risk clinical scenarios (so it is often preventable).

The diagnosis implies that pre-renal and post-renal factors have been excluded (or corrected) and that other causes of intrinsic ARF, such as vasculitis or TIN, are deemed unlikely. It suggests that recovery of renal function is likely—but only if the causative insult is removed and adequate supportive measures are put in place. The kidneys are particularly susceptible to nephrotoxic injury because of their rich blood supply and a propensity to concentrate toxic substances within their cortex.

ATN subdivided by cause

Ischaemic (incl. septic)	ANY cause ↓renal perfusion:
	 • Hypotension
	 • Shock
	   • Haemorrhagic
	   • Cardiogenic
	   • Septic
	 • Devascularization (incl. aortic cross-clamping)

Nephrotoxic	• Myoglobin • Haemoglobin • Aminoglycosides • Contrast • Amphotericin B • Cisplatin

Presentation

ATN presents as ARF: ↓GFR → uraemia and disordered salt, water, and electrolyte homeostasis.
► ATN may be oliguric or non-oliguric.
It is a continuum from pre-renal failure, though now with:
• Actual structural injury to the renal parenchyma.
• Limited (or no) resolution upon restoration of renal perfusion.
• Differentiation between pre-renal ARF and ATN can be difficult.
Helpful features include (*not* uniformly present):
• Clear evidence of sepsis, hypotension or nephrotoxin exposure
• Bland urine on dipstick (or minor proteinuria)
• Urine biochemistry (*often* not helpful, 📖 p.80)
  • ↑u-Osm <350mOsm/kg
  • FE_{Na} >2
  • u-Na^+ >40mmol/L.

Histology

▶ A kidney biopsy is rarely required for diagnosis

ATN is a misnomer—frankly necrotic tubular cells are uncommon. There may be few histological changes even with marked functional renal impairment. Typical features: tubular cell flattening, wide spacing of tubules 2° to interstitial oedema, tubular cell vacuolation, loss of proximal tubular cell brush border, tubular cell sloughing into the lumen (→ obstruction), mitotic figures in regenerating epithelial cells ± and leucocyte infiltration. Glomeruli are normal.

Prognosis

ARF 2° ATN imparts a significant in-hospital mortality of ~19–37%. The renal prognosis is that:

- 60% can expect a full recovery.
- 30% can expect a recovery short of baseline.
- 5–10% will eventually require long-term renal replacement therapy.

Pathophysiology of ATN

Vessels and endothelium

- Blood flow is not uniform within the kidney—pO_2 falls progressively from cortex (6.65–13.3 kPa) to medulla (1.3–2.9 kPa), despite higher metabolic activity in the latter. ▶ The proximal tubular S3 segment and the medullary thick ascending loop of Henle are found in the medulla.
- Any cause of ↓RBF or endothelial injury may ↓delivered O_2, rendering vulnerable segments of the nephron relatively hypoxic.
- As a result of endothelial cell injury:
  - ↑afferent arteriolar cytosolic Ca^{2+} → ↑sensitivity to vasoconstrictor and sympathetic stimulation → impaired glomerular autoregulation .
  - Endothelial cell swelling compounds ↓flow → ↓O_2 delivery.
  - Injured endothelium (or endothelium under the influence of pro-inflammatory mediators (TNF-α, IL-18) → ↑endothelial adhesion molecules (ICAM-1, VCAM, P-selectin) → ↑leucocyte-endothelial interaction → medullary vascular congestion → medullary hypoxia.
  - Activated leucocytes → local inflammation and local injury.
  - ↓endothelial nitric oxide production + ↑endothelin and prostaglandin synthesis → enhanced vasoconstriction, further ↓RBF.
- The net result is impeded flow and ↓O_2 delivery to metabolically active and relatively hypoxic tubular segments: demand exceeds supply.

Tubular cells

- Hypoxic proximal tubular cells (PTC) now become ↑energy deplete.
- Injured PTC generate pro-inflammatory mediators → recruitment of leucocytes into the interstitium with subsequent inflammation.
- ↓O_2 delivery leads to ↑Ca^{2+} entry into energy-depleted cells.
- ↑Ca^{2+}-dependent cysteine protease activity → actin breakdown → cytoskeletal disruption → loss of cell polarity.
- Loss of polarity → ↓basolateral Na^+/K^+-ATPase pumps and ∴ ↓proximal Na^+ absorption.
- More Na^+ is delivered to the distal nephron, and sensed at the macula densa. This triggers *tubuloglomerular feedback* (🕮 p.616) → ↓GFR.
- Apical relocation of integrins → loss of cell–cell adhesion → tubular cell desquamation and cast formation → tubular obstruction → ↓GFR.
- Desquamation of PTC exposes the basement membrane and provides a route for mis-directed filtrate, further ↑interstitial congestion.
- Necrosis ± apoptosis (*both* are present—ATN is a misnomer)
  - ATP depletion + ↑reactive O_2 species + intracellular acidosis + ↑cytosolic Ca^{2+} + ↑phospholipase activity → cell necrosis.
  - Apoptotic stimuli → caspase activation → cell apoptosis.
- Nitric oxide
  - Hypoxia → ↑ PTC iNOS expression → NO release → cell death.
  - NO scavenged by O_2 radicals → toxic peroxynitrite generation.
  - (eNOS in the afferent arteriole *protects* against ischemic injury).

Repair

Post reperfusion, sub-lethally injured cells undergo repair and proliferation.

- Non-viable cells die (necrosis and apoptosis) and exfoliate.
- Poorly differentiated epithelial cells appear (?a population of renal stem cells).
- Viable cells enter the cell cycle under regulation of cyclin-dependent kinase inhibitors (especially p.21).
- Growth factors (IGF-1, EGF, HGF, TGF-β) → proliferation and differentiation of tubular cells, restoring the epithelium to health.

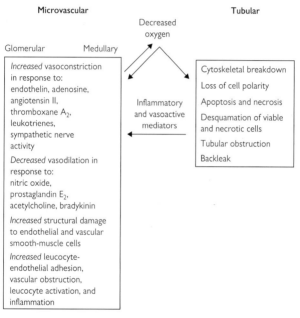

Fig. 2.5 Pathophysiology of ATN

Reproduced with permission from Bonventre JV, and Weinberg JM (2003). *Journal of the American Society of Nephrology* **14**: 2199–210.

Management of ARF 1: a checklist

The management of ARF depends on the cause—nevertheless as all failing kidneys fail to maintain salt, water, electrolyte, acid–base homeostasis, general principles of management can be described.

Where is information on...

- Resuscitating volume deplete pre-renal failure? (📖 p.92)
- Managing hyperkalaemia? (📖 p.102)
- Managing volume overload and pulmonary oedema? (📖 p.108)
- Managing acidosis? (📖 p.110)
- Maintaining nutrition? (📖 p.114)
- Instituting dialysis? (📖 p.118)
- Specific causes of ARF?:
  - ATN? (📖 p.96)
  - Hepatorenal syndrome? (📖 p.126)
  - Contrast nephrotoxicity? (📖 p.132)
  - Tumour lysis? (📖 p.134)
  - Septic shock and ARF? (📖 p.138)
- Post-renal failure and acute obstruction? (📖 p.500)

Have you...

- Seen the result of the serum K^+ and acted appropriately?
- Assessed the patient's volume status and
  - satisfied yourself that, clinically and radiologically, the patient is not in pulmonary oedema?
  - adequately corrected volume depletion?
- Taken a full history and examined the patient from head to toe?
- Excluded a palpable bladder?
- Seen a list of *all* the patient's drugs? If they are an in-patient, have you checked their drug chart, including the 'prn' side?
- Stopped nephrotoxins?
- Performed a urinalysis and sent an MSU for M,C+S?
- Arranged an urgent ultrasound?
- Checked the Hb ± sent a group and save?
- Tried to find any historical tests of renal function?
- Checked serum Ca^{2+} and PO_4 ± written up a phosphate binder?
- Checked acid–base status and intervened appropriately?
- Arranged for the patient to be nursed in a sufficiently high dependency environment, with strict monitoring of fluid intake and output?
- Spoken to your dietitian?
- Discussed the patient with your local renal unit if needs be?
- If intrinsic ARF is suspected, sent off a nephritic and myeloma screen?

What you will be asked when you speak to a renal unit

- What's the story?
- What's the potassium?
- What is the patient's volume and haemodynamic status?
- Is there anything else of note on clinical examination?
- What is the patient's acid–base status?
- What drugs has the patient been on?
- What did the urine dipstick show?
- Has the patient had a renal ultrasound?
- Is the patient passing urine? If so, how much?
- Do you have any record of a previous serum creatinine?
- What co-morbidity does the patient have?
- Is the patient fit for transfer? Are you sure?

Management of ARF 2: dangerous hyperkalaemia

In excitable tissues, $\uparrow K^+ \rightarrow$ depolarization of the membrane resting potential $\rightarrow$ Na^+ channel inactivation $\rightarrow$ $\downarrow$membrane excitability $\rightarrow$ neuromuscular depression and cardiac dysrhythmias.

What is dangerous $\uparrow K^+$?

Chronically hyperkalaemic patients may tolerate $\uparrow K^+$ of 6.0–7.0mmol/L (but should certainly be treated if >6.5mmol/L). Acute $\uparrow K^+$ is much less well–tolerated, particularly if at risk:

- Elderly
- Associated cardiac disease (esp. arrythmias)
- Oliguric patients (cannot excrete $\uparrow K^+$).

Monitor all patients with $\uparrow K^+$ acutely >6.0 and enhance K^+ wasting (🕮 p.106). Treat to urgently lower if $\uparrow K^+ \geq 6.5$mmol/L.

⚠ Always repeat U+E to exclude haemolysis or artefact. In the interim, put the patient on a cardiac monitor and start treatment.

The hyperkalaemic ECG

ECG manifestations of $\uparrow K^+$ are manifold. ⚠ Mild ECG changes can progress to life-threatening disturbances very quickly. All may be exacerbated by co-existing $\downarrow Ca^{2+}$ and acidosis.

⚠ A normal ECG does *not* rule out cardiac instability.

- Peaking of T waves ('tenting')
- Flattening and disappearance of P waves
- Prolonged PR interval (1° heart block)
- Progressive widening of the QRS complex
- Deepened S waves and merging of S and T waves
- Idioventricular rhythm
- Sine wave pattern
- VF and asystolic cardiac arrest.

Rising K^+

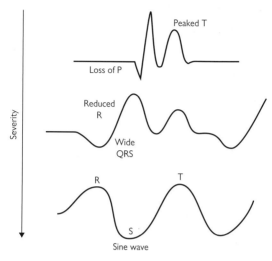

Fig. 2.6 The ECG changes of hyperkalaemia

Treatment of dangerous hyperkalaemia
The following will reduce serum K^+ acutely, but NOT affect the elevated total body K. Longer term measures described overleaf are needed in conjunction with emergency treatment.

Calcium
- If $K^+ \geq 6.5$mmol/L or ECG changes.
- Antagonizes membrane effects of $\uparrow K^+$ by a poorly understood mechanism.
- 10ml 10% calcium gluconate (usually 1 ampoule—calcium gluconate contains 220µmol Ca^{2+}/mL), *or*
- 5ml 10% calcium chloride (usually ½ an ampoule—$CaCl_2$ contains 680µmol Ca^{2+}/mL).
- Give over 2–5min. Repeat if no ECG improvement after 5min (up to 40mL calcium gluconate).
- Acts within minutes but *protective effect lasts <1 hour*.
- ⚠ Can induce digitalis toxicity ($\rightarrow$ a pragmatic approach: half the initial dose and give more slowly if taking digoxin).
- ►Ca^{2+} is cardioprotective—it does not $\downarrow K^+$.

Insulin and glucose
- If $K^+ \geq 6.5$ mmol/L or ECG changes.
- Insulin in binding its cellular receptor $\rightarrow \uparrow$Na-K-ATPase activity, moving K^+ into cells. Glucose alone will $\downarrow K^+$ through endogenous insulin release, but insulin/glucose more effective.
- 15 IU of actrapid in 50mL of 50% glucose/dextrose IVI over 10min.
- Expect effect within 15–30min (peak ~60min), lasts for 2–4hr. Expect a $\downarrow$ of 0.5–1.5mmol/L.
- Check BMs regularly for 6hr and infuse 10% dextrose IVI if $\downarrow$glucose.
- Can be repeated after 4hr.
- 50% glucose is extremely viscous and irritant. Find a large vein and flush with saline afterwards.

Sodium bicarbonate
- If $\uparrow K^+$ in the presence of acidosis ($HCO_3^- <16$) and volume depletion.
- $\uparrow Na^+/H^+$ exchange $\rightarrow \uparrow$intracellular $[Na^+] \rightarrow \uparrow$Na-K-ATPase activity (i.e. K^+ in for Na^+ out). Additional pH independent mechanisms.
- 1.26% or 1.4% solutions as 200–500ml over 15–60min IVI
- In cardiac arrest: 50–100ml of 4.2% or 50ml of 8.4% (1 ampoule) IVI.
- Action within hours, not minutes.
- Presents an appreciable Na^+ load (150mmol Na^+⚠Volume overload).
- Rapid correction of acidosis in a patient with $\downarrow Ca^{2+}$ may induce tetany and seizures as ionized calcium drops rapidly as pH$\uparrow$.

Why not to use β₂-agonists (salbutamol, etc.)
10–20 mg (i.e. big dose) of nebulised salbutamol will $\downarrow$ serum K^+ by up to 1 mmol/L, but has *no* additive benefit beyond insulin/dextrose (it acts via the same Na–K–ATPase, and has a slower onset of action.
⚠ It may precipitate arrhythmias in those with underlying cardiac disease.

Management of ARF 3: reducing total body K⁺

Once (if) the immediate arrhythmic danger is past, the aim should be to reduce total body potassium to prevent further hyperkalaemic episodes.

1. Urinary K⁺ wasting: diuretics

- Only useful in patients expected to pass urine, and urine into which K⁺ can be excreted. Particularly useful if also volume overloaded.
- Act on the renal tubule—K⁺ loss one of several effects.
- Furosemide 40–120mg IVI as a slow bolus, or 10–40mg/hr to a maximum of 1000mg/day. Bumetanide offers a better absorbed oral alternative.
- Effect depends on onset of diuresis. Can lose substantial amounts of K⁺ over 24 hours with a UO>2L/day.
- *Much* less effective as GFR deteriorates.

2. Gut K⁺ wasting: cation exchange resins

Over-used, particularly orally.

- Exchange Na⁺/Ca²⁺ for K⁺ in the gut, so does remove K⁺ rather than just redistribute it.
- Calcium polystyrene sulphate (CPS) (Calcium Resonium®) or sodium polystyrene sulphonate (SPS) (Resonium A® or Kayexalate®). Can give 15g orally (supplied as a powder to be suspended in water) up to qds or 15–30g suspended in 2% methylcellulose and 100mL water rectally up to qds, retained for at least 2 (preferably >4) hours. May require saline irrigation through a catheter to remove the resin from the colon.
- Rectal route is more effective, as there is more K⁺ available for exchange : colonic [K⁺] = 60–90mmol/L, whereas upper GI tract = 5–10mmol/L.
- The constipating effect of these agents given orally may paradoxically prevent K⁺ losses in the stool—equally, the laxatives (lactulose 10–20mL tds) given with these agents may be more efficacious than the agent itself!
- Modest effect seen within 24–48hr.
- May cause colonic ulceration and necrosis (recognized with SPS when given with sorbitol as a hyperosmotic laxative—a common practice in the USA. Post-op patients with an ileus at highest risk).

3. Extracorporeal K⁺ wasting: dialysis

- If K⁺>6.0 and renal function cannot rapidly be restored.
- Lowers K⁺ within minutes.
- Haemodialysis (HD) can process 20–60L of blood against a dialysate K⁺ of 1–2mmol/L, and as such is potent means of removing K⁺.
- Haemofiltration (□ p.118) with returned infusate free of K⁺ can do much the same thing, though much slower.
- Peritoneal dialysis is effective, but rarely indicated acutely (□ p.122).
- Does require dialysis access and transfer to a dialyzing facility.

- ⚠ Never transfer a dangerously hyperkalaemic patient—if they have not responded to the emergency measures, speak to your ITU.

4. Further management

The aim is to prevent further dangerous rises.
- Restrict oral K$^+$ intake to <2g per day. ► speak to your dietitian (📖 p.190). K$^+$ content of enteral and parenteral feeds may need modification.
- No K$^+$ in IV fluids.
- Avoid K$^+$ sparing diuretics, ACEI, ARB, spironolactone and NSAIDs.
- Refractory ↑K$^+$ is an indication for dialysis.
- If ↑K$^+$ persists despite dialysis then:
  - Review dietary intake and compliance.
  - Triple check the drug chart.
  - Check for GI or occult bleeding (reabsorbed red cells are rich in K$^+$).
  - Exclude concealed tissue or muscle damage (eg, compartment syndrome).
  - Review dialysis access and adequacy (📖 p.210) and check the dialysate K$^+$ concentration (📖 p.206).

Transfusion

⚠ Caution is needed when transfusing a patient with ARF, particularly if oligo-anuric. The volume and K$^+$ content of red cell transfusions can precipitate pulmonary oedema and hyperkalaemia respectively. If the patient requires renal support, then transfusions are safest given on dialysis.

Management of ARF 4: pulmonary oedema

Oliguric or anuric patients rapidly accumulate salt and water unless (and even if) tightly fluid restricted. Volume overload, often exacerbated iatrogenically, remains a relatively common presentation of ARF.

In ARF the heart is often structurally normal, but salt and water overload push the heart inexorably along the Starling curve. Many patients with ARF may also have poor underlying cardiac reserve, so mortality is high.

Findings

Cool, clammy, agitated patient. Tachycardia, tachypnoea, ↑JVP, ↑BP (↓BP in this context is worrying), gallop rhythm, respiratory crackles and wheezes. Possibly: ascites, pleural effusions and oedema.
Investigations:
- Poor O_2 saturation
- Hypoxaemia on ABGs (PaO_2 < 8 kPa)
- Widespread alveolar shadowing on CXR.

Management

- Sit the patient up and stop all IV infusions.
- *Oxygen*: maintain S_aO_2 > 95%. It should be possible to achieve an FiO_2 > 60% using a well-positioned high flow (e.g. Venturi) mask with an O_2 flow rate of 6L/min. Combine with nasal prongs if necessary. Masks with reservoir bags may allow FiO_2 > 80%. Consider ward CPAP if available (e.g. Boussignac system).
- *Opiates*: give IV diamorphine (1.25–2.5mg) or morphine (2.5–5mg) as an anxiolytic and venodilator (+ 5mg metoclopramide as anti-emetic). Can be repeated after 15min, but opiates accumulate in ARF so resist giving further doses.
- *Nitrates*: if the systolic BP ≥90mmHg start intravenous GTN 2–10mg/hr. Start low and titrate every 10min as tolerated. Give 2 puffs of sublingual GTN while the pump is being set up. If systolic BP is <90mmHg (i.e ?cardiogenic shock) warn ITU and consider inotropes.
- *Diuretics* (☐ p.116)): give 250mg furosemide over 1hr (or partial dose) at a rate not exceeding 4mg/min to avoid ototoxicity. If this initiates a diuresis then follow with a further 250mg or start a continuous infusion (10–40 mg/hr). If no response, refer for dialysis.
- *Dialysis*: oligo-anuric patients are likely to need renal support (☐ p.118)
⚠ If renal facilities are not on site then ensure the patient is fit for transfer—discuss with ITU.

How to give loop diuretics in ARF

Give 250mg (25mL ampoule) furosemide IV made up to 50 mL (syringe driver) or 100mL (infusion pump) over 1hr (rate not exceeding 4mg/min to avoid ototoxicity). Bumetanide 5mg an alternative.
- If this initiates a diuresis, give a further 250mg.
- If no response, further doses are likely to be futile. (▶ Dialysis?)

If there is a reasonable, but transient, response, then a continuous infusion 10–40mg/hr over 24hr may promote ongoing diuresis

Consider respiratory support if
- Continuing severe breathlessness.
- Falling respiratory rate (tiring patient).
- PaO_2 <8KPa, rising $PaCO_2$
- Worsening acidosis (pH < 7.2)

Continuous positive airways pressure (CPAP)
Provides a constant positive pressure support throughout the respiratory cycle (typically 5–10cm H_2O) allowing delivery of a higher FiO_2 (80–100%) and ↓ the work of breathing.
⚠ Patients must be conscious, able to protect their airway, and possess sufficient respiratory muscle strength.

Endotracheal intubation and mechanical ventilation
On ITU. Probably with PEEP. A preset pressure is added to the end of expiration to prevent airway/alveolar collapse and open up atelectatic and fluid-filled lung. The trade off is a potential ↓ in cardiac output (through ↓ venous return).

Venesection
- Exceptional circumstances + Hb≥10g/dL + SBP≥120mmHg.
- 250mL blood removed from a large vein with venesection kit.
- Ideally the blood should be saved to transfuse back when the patient is more stable (or on HD).

Management of ARF 5: electrolytes and acidosis

Hyperphosphataemia

↓urinary PO_4 excretion → ↑serum PO_4 Particularly marked elevations occur in rhabdomyolysis (📖 p.128), tumour lysis syndrome (📖 p.134), and haemolysis (tissue injury and cell death → release of intracellular PO_4).

Acute ↑PO_4 is important because it:
- Contributes to ↓Ca^{2+} (by a poorly understood mechanism).
- Encourages 2° hyperparathyroidism.
- Promotes soft tissue/vascular calcification (esp. Ca x PO_4 product >4.4).
- Makes the patient feel itchy, uncomfortable and anorexic.
- May cause arrhythmias.

Treatment (see also 📖 p.176)
- Dietary restriction of phosphate (< 800mg/day, 📖 p.190).
- Removal on dialysis.
- Oral phosphate binders (reduce intestinal absorption of phosphate)
  - If both ↓Ca^{2+} and ↑PO_4^{2-}, start calcium carbonate or calcium acetate (500mg).
  - If PO_4<2.0, 1 tablet with each meal.
  - If PO_4 2.0–3.0, 2 tablets with each meal.
  - If PO_4 > 3.0, 3 tablets with each meal.
- If Ca^{2+}≥ 2.4 use sevelamer HCl (0.8–2.4g with meals) or alucaps (1–3 capsules with meals).
- Severe ↑PO_4 is unlikely to correct until the patient dialyses or recovers renal function.
- If the patient is being NG or parenterally fed, speak to your dietitian.

Hypocalcaemia

Common in prolonged or severe ARF. Caused mainly by ↓1, 25-dihydroxyvitaminD$_3$ synthesis, but also by ↑PO_4 Usually in the corrected range of 1.6–2.0mmol/L. Clinical sequelae (e.g. paraesthesia, tetany and seizures) are rare, partly because concomitant acidosis protects by increasing the ratio of ionized to protein bound Ca^{2+}.

⚠ Rapid correction of acidosis with oral or IV HCO_3^- can precipitate symptomatic ↓Ca^{2+}.

Calcium is supplemented orally (as above)—the dual phosphate binding role of calcium salts makes life simple. IV Ca^{2+} (e.g. calcium gluconate) is virtually never required. If Ca^{2+}<2.0mmol/L (and PO_4 <1.5mmol/L) start α-calcidol 0.25–0.5μg po daily.

⚠ In rhabdomyolysis (📖 p.128), Ca^{2+} can precipitate in injured muscle causing necrosis and ischaemic contractures—resist administration of Ca^{2+} unless symptomatic.

Other electrolyte abnormalities found with ARF

Hypokalaemia: rare in ARF, but can accompany non-oliguric ATN caused by tubular toxins (e.g. aminoglycosides, amphotericin, cisplatin). May also develop as GFR recovers, especially if polyuria.

Hypomagnesaemia: $\downarrow Mg^{2+}$ occasionally complicates non-oliguric ATN. Usually asymptomatic, but can → neuromuscular instability, cramps, arrhythmias, resistant $\downarrow K^+$ and resistant $\downarrow Ca^{2+}$.

Metabolic acidosis

ARF is usually associated with a raised anion gap metabolic acidosis:
- As GFR falls, unmeasured anions (such as HSO_4^- and HPO_4^-) from dietary and metabolic sources accumulate.
- As H^+ is buffered, HCO_3^- is consumed. The struggling kidney is unable to reclaim filtered HCO_3^- from the urine (proximal tubule) or generate new HCO_3^- (through production and excretion of NH_4^+).

The degree of acidosis is usually modest in uncomplicated ARF (serum HCO_3^- >10, pH >7.2) but more problematic in the critically ill, where it may contribute to circulatory compromise. ⚠ If unexpectedly severe, consider 2° cause—especially lactic acidosis (sepsis, cardiogenic shock), ketoacidosis (diabetes and alcohol) and poisoning (salicylates, methanol, ethylene glycol).

Acidosis per se may be an indication for dialysis, particularly if pH < 7.0–7.1, with evidence of cardiovascular compromise.

Management of ARF 6: other strategies

Anaemia

▶ Don't always assume anaemia is part of the uraemic syndrome. Beware bleeding—especially from the GI tract, or haemolysis.

An Hb of ~8–11g/dL is a frequent finding in ARF—it does not help distinguish between ARF and CRF. Major contributing factors are impaired erythropoiesis (↓renal EPO production), ↓red cell life span, haemolysis (↑red cell fragility), haemodilution (from fluid overload) and blood loss.

Erythropoietin is rarely effective in ARF, so transfusion may be necessary, particularly if ↓CV reserve means the ↓Hb is poorly tolerated. See 🕮 p.107 for transfusion in oligo-anuric patients.

Bleeding

ARF is associated with a bleeding tendency 2° to platelet dysfunction. Uraemic toxins disrupt the interaction between platelet GPIIb/IIIa, and adhesion molecules such as von Willebrand factor (vWF) and fibrinogen. ↑Plt nitric oxide synthesis may also inhibit aggregation.

Clinical manifestations are typically mild: spontaneous bruising, bleeding at venepuncture sites, though occasionally more troublesome. Usually found if urea >25 mmol/L for several days.

INR, APTT and platelet count are usually normal (if abnormal → look for other causes). The bleeding time is prolonged.

Correcting the bleeding tendency of ARF

The two situations that require specific intervention are:
● Active bleeding or poorly controlled persistent oozing.
● Prior to an invasive procedure (including renal biopsy).

Management
● Stop aspirin, clopidogrel, anticoagulants.
● Correct anaemia (transfusion of packed cells). A haematocrit (Hct) ≥25–30% ↓bleeding time.
● DDAVP (desmopressin): a synthetic analogue of ADH that probably works by ↑amount of available vWF. Easy to administer and works. Give 0.3µg/kg (roughly 20µg or 5 ampoules in an adult) IV in 100mL of 0.9% NaCl over 30min. Effective within 1hr, lasts 4–24 hr. Less effective on repetitive dosing. Can also be given subcutaneously (same dose) and intranasally (3µg/kg). ⚠ Rarely causes coronary vasospasm—avoid if unstable angina.
● Cryoprecipitate: 10 units every 12–24hr. **Not** usually required, unless catastrophic bleeding
Dialysis: improves bleeding time, presumably through removal of uraemic toxins. ▶ Dialysis usually requires anticoagulation to prevent clotting of the extracorporeal circuit (🕮 p.212).

Infection

▶ Sepsis is an important cause of morbidity and mortality in ARF (76% mortality if ARF + sepsis). It occurs in 3 contexts:

- ARF is the consequence of a specific infection (e.g. post-infectious GN, endocarditis, malaria, leptospirosis).
- Septicaemia → circulatory compromise → prerenal ARF → ATN.
- Localized or systemic infection arises in those with pre-existing ATN.

Approach

- Take signs of infection such as fever, ↑WCC, ↑CRP seriously—as a minimum re-examine the patient thoroughly.
- Culture (and re-culture) blood, urine, sputum, and other secretions.
- Make use of imaging. Repeat CXRs frequently. If the source of sepsis remains obscure, consider abdo USS ± abdo/chest CT.
- Attention to microbiological detail; chase up samples, review sensitivities, carefully consider antibiotic options and speak to your microbiologist regularly about resistance patterns.
- ⚠ Many antibiotics require dose adjustment in renal impairment.
- Strict aseptic technique for central line, dialysis catheter and bladder catheter insertion. Consider prophylactic antibiotics when inserting a line or catheter into a febrile patient. Don't leave bladder catheters in place longer than necessary. In the majority of cases, accurate monitoring of UO does not require a catheter. Antibiotic cover for removal if the urine is a likely source of sepsis.
- Inspect IV cannula sites regularly and look under dressings.
- Consider removing lines as soon as feasible.

▶▶ Treat proven infection aggressively.

Management of ARF 7: nutrition

Both pre-existing and hospital-acquired malnutrition → ↑morbidity and mortality in the critically ill. Preventing malnutrition preserves (respiratory) muscle function, ↑wound healing and ↑resistance to infection.

General rules

- If pre-existing nutritional status is normal and a normal diet is likely to be resumed in ≤5 days, support is not initially indicated.
- If the patient is malnourished, ignore this 5 day rule and start feeding.
- If hypercatabolic (sepsis, trauma, burns), initiate support early.
- Avoid feeding within the first 24hr: there is evidence of harm (feeding during the 'insult phase' ↑O$_2$ requirements and worsens tissue injury).
- Modify nutritional support with changes in GFR and with dialysis.
- Don't over-prescribe—you *can* have too much of a good thing.
- Enteral nutrition is always preferable to parenteral (not mutually exclusive).

Step 1: determine the nutritional status of the patient

- Body weight: recent unintentional loss >10% body weight is a bad sign.
- Determine body mass index (BMI, as mass in kg/height in m^2). Normal range 20–25 kg/m^2. ⚠ Beware fluid retention falsely ↑weight
- Serum albumin (< 30g/L worrying), though inflammation may be a confounder. Pre-albumin, transferrin and cholesterol also used.
- Subjective global assessment (SGA): combines clinical parameters with albumin, anthropometry, clinical judgement and others.

Step 2: estimate energy requirements

- Standard formulae (>200 published), e.g. Schofield[1] revolve around gender-based weight-adjusted formulae. Ask your dietitian.
- Energy expenditure in 'uncomplicated' ARF is actually within the normal range. Energy requirements for those with 'complicated' ARF is determined by associated disorders (e.g. sepsis): nevertheless, it is rare for energy requirements to exceed 130% basal.

▶ Broadly speaking: ♂ should receive 25–30 non-protein kcal/kg/day and ♀ 20–25kcal/kg/day.

Step 3: estimation of protein (and amino acid) requirements

Depends on associated catabolic stress. Hypercatabolism → ↑Ur, which can be used to estimate nitrogen balance. Rules of thumb:

- For 'uncomplicated' ARF daily protein or amino acid requirement is near the recommended allowance of 0.8g/kg/day for normal adults.
- In complicated ARF, the requirement is ~1.0–1.2g/kg/day.
- If dialysis necessary, add 0.2g/kg/day.
- Critically ill patients may need more (up to 1.5g/kg/day).
- ≥1.5g/kg/day will aggravate the situation by stimulating formation of urea and other nitrogenous waste products.

Step 4: decide on route of administration: see table opposite

Step 5: ensure volume and electrolyte content appropriate for ARF

Low volume ± low electrolyte feeds are required if on intermittent haemodialysis. Standard feed can be used for those on CRRT (⬛ p.118).

1 Schofield WN (1985). *Hum Nutr Clin Nutr*, **39**(1), 5–41.

Route	What's in it?	Notes	Concerns in ARF	Complications
Oral • Nutrition dense oral diet • Supplementary sip feeding	Modest protein and energy content.	• Many patients can tolerate an oral diet. • Supplementation with nutrition drinks useful if appetite poor.	Observe restrictions: • K^+ • PO_4 • Volume	
Enteral	Enteral feeding formulas specifically for ARF are available; e.g. Nepro® (Ross), Nova source renal® (Novartis). • Ensure correct position of NG tube (aspirate pH or CXR). • Start at 30mL/h. Allow 4hr bowel rest in every 24hr.	Enteral feeding maintains the structural integrity of the gut and protects against translocation of GI bacteria.	• A tailored regimen (i.e. non-standard feed) may be necessary if the above restrictions apply. • To prevent refeeding syndrome in a malnourished patient, PO_4, K^+, and Mg^{2+} must be checked and corrected prior to commencement.	*Mechanical:* dislodged tube. *Gastrointestinal:* abdominal distension, nausea, cramps and diarrhoea. *Infectious:* aspiration pneumonia *Metabolic:* hyper/hypo-glycaemia, electrolyte abnormalities.
Parenteral	*Amino acids:* combined essential and non-essential (the latter often become 'conditionally' essential in the context of ARF) *Energy:* principally given as glucose, although >5g/kg/day causes ↑CO_2 production (increasing respiratory demands), ↑lipogenesis (fatty liver) and hyperglycaemia. Lipids are used to provide the remainder (usually ≤1g/kg/day to avoid hyperlipidaemia). *Vitamins,* trace elements, electrolytes (and sometimes insulin) are added as necessary.	• IV lipids have a low osmolality and can be given into peripheral veins. • They do not meet all energy requirements so are mainly a short term measure. • Full TPN must usually be given centrally (via a dedicated line). • If possible a small amount of enteral feed is run concurrently.	• Start feed slowly. • Continuous renal replacement techniques (e.g. CVVHF) assist the delivery of feeding.	*Catheter insertion:* pneumothorax etc. *Catheter infection* *Metabolic:* requires close laboratory monitoring

Management myths

Loop diuretics

Theory: (i) ↑urinary flow 'washes out' cellular debris, casts and nephrotoxins from tubules; (ii) blockade of active transport processes → ↓tubular O_2 consumption and protects against ATN; (iii) vasodilator action → ↑RBF.

Evidence: none to suggest improved renal or patient outcome in any ARF setting. In particular, the natural history and prognosis of ATN remains unchanged. Some studies have suggested **harm**. May increase diuresis.

▶▶ Give as part of the treatment of pulmonary oedema (🕮 p.108).

- Never give diuretics until you have corrected volume depletion.
- If oliguria persists despite correction of pre-renal factors, diuretics may ↑UO, simplifying fluid balance and easing fears of pulmonary oedema.

Mannitol

An osmotic diuretic previously used for the prevention of ATN in high risk CV surgery. A lack of evidence means the practice is in decline. Can paradoxically cause pulmonary oedema through volume expansion. Avoid.

✿ Dopamine

Despite a lack of evidence for efficacy, dopamine has proved a difficult habit to kick. **Do not use it** for treatment or prophylaxis of ARF.

Theory: dopamine (DA) is synthesized in the proximal tubule from circulating L-dopa and helps regulate Na^+ excretion and renal vasodilataion through specific DA1 and DA2 receptors. Exogenously administered 'low dose' dopamine should → renal vasodilatation → ↑RBF → ↑natriuresis and mild ↑GFR. All potentially beneficial in ATN.

µg/kg/min	Effect
0.5–3	Selective DA (mainly DA1) receptor activation → ↑renal (and mesenteric) blood flow
3–10	Both DA and β_1 receptors are activated, the latter → ↑cardiac output (mainly by ↑SV).
10–20	β_1 effect predominates. Start to activate α adrenoceptors.
>20	α adrenergic (vasoconstrictive) effect takes over with ↑ SVR.

Evidence: largely anecdotal or from inadequate studies. Larger trials (e.g. ANZICS) failed to show benefit.

⚠ It may cause **harm:**
- Tachycardia, arrhythmias, myocardial ischaemia
- Blunted hypoxaemic drive
- Splanchnic vasoconstriction (→ bacterial translocation)
- Digital ischaemia
- Impaired pituitary function
- Electrolyte disturbances (even at 'renal' dose)
- Dopamine accumulates in renal failure.

Hope for the future? Putative reno-protective agents

- N-acetylcysteine (see 📖 p.132 for full discussion)
- Fenoldopam
- Erythropoietin
- NGAL (neutrophil gelatinase-associated lipocalin).

▶ Some of the above may yet become useful agents in managing or preventing ARF—many, many more have been tried, shown to work in animal models, and been found to have no effect in humans (see table below).

Pathogenetic mechanism	Interventions of unproven benefit in humans
Renal vasoconstriction	Low-dose dopamine
	Calcium channel blockers
	Atrial natriuretic peptide
	Endothelin receptor antagonists
	Leukotriene receptor antagonists
	PAF antagonists
	iNOS antisense oligonucleotides
Inflammation	Anti-ICAM-1 monoclonal Ab
	Anti-IL-18 monoclonal Ab
	N-acetylcysteine and or other free radical scavengers
	α-MSH
Tubular obstruction	Diuretics
	RGD peptides
Tubular regeneration	Insulin-like growth factor
	Thyroxine
	Epidermal growth factor
	Hepatocyte growth factor
	Osteopontin
	Protease (e.g. caspase) inhibitors

PAF: platelet activating factor; RGD peptides: peptides containing the arginine–glycine–aspartic acid motif (involved in adhesion); ICAM-1: intercellular adhesion molecule-1; α-MSH: α-melanocyte-stimulating hormone.

Novel bio-markers and techniques are being tested that may **predict** ARF before established, and discriminate between pre-renal impairment and ATN. Some of these include:
- Blood oxygen level-dependent MRI (a non-invasive method of measuring actual tissue pO_2, useful to describe medullary ischaemia in ATN).
- KIM-1 (kidney injury molecule-1) or IL-18, as urinary markers of injured proximal tubular cells.
- NGAL (neutrophil gelatinase-associated lipocalin).

Renal replacement therapy in ARF

Opinion differs on the indications, when to start, when to stop, what method to use and what 'dose' to give. Some generalizations can be made:

Absolute indications

▶ Hyperkalaemia
- K^+ ≥6.5mmol/L or rapidly rising, regardless of ECG changes

▶ Volume overload
- Pulmonary oedema with inadequate response to diuretics particularly if occurring in an oligo-anuric patient

The remaining indications for dialysis are *urgent*, rather than *emergent*. An important distinction—it is always better to perform dialysis as a planned procedure during the day. Dialysing a patient is not without potential problems, including:
- Complications of dialysis access insertion (□ p.630).
- Placing a haemodynamic strain on an already sick patient.
- Dialysis disequilibrium (□ p.121).
- ❧ Prolonging ARF duration.

Relative indications
- Intractable acidosis (pH < 7.1), especially if haemodynamically unstable.
- Uraemia.
  - Uraemic pericarditis or encephalopathy
  - Uraemic symptoms, especially if Ur >40mmol/L (⚠ There is no absolute figure that equates with 'uraemia' and much inter-patient variability is seen).
- Critically unwell patients (usually on ITU)
  - Start before accumulation of toxins → circulatory compromise.
  - Allows safer administration of volume: feeding, transfusion, other blood products, antimicrobials, other drugs.
  - Diuretic-resistant cardiac failure.
- Poison or toxin removal (lithium, ethylene glycol etc.).
- Hyperthermia.

Modalities (□ p.204)
- Generally, intermittent haemodialysis (HD) is performed on renal units and continuous haemofiltration (CVVHF) and variants of continuous therapies on ITUs.
- None is demonstrably superior in ARF, and selection tends to depend on availability.
- However, shocked patients with SBP ≤90, and those with raised intracranial pressure are better managed using continuous therapies.

□ p.204 for explanation of the techniques of renal replacement therapy.

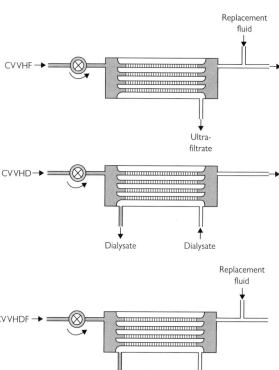

Fig. 2.7 Principles of different CRRT modalities. Replacement fluids can be given before or after the haemofilter (pre-or post-dilution)

Reproduced with permission from Levy J, Morgan J, and Brown E (2004). *Oxford Handbook of Dialysis*, 2nd edn. Oxford: Oxford University Press

Prescribing acute haemodialysis (HD)

▶ The dialysis nursing staff may know a great deal more than you.

⚠ Rapid overcorrection of uraemia may → dialysis disequilibrium. The first dialysis should aim to take the edge off uraemia ($\downarrow$Ur ≤30%) only.

- Time: 1st session 2hr, 2nd 3hr, and subsequent 3–4hr.
- Blood flow: slow, ~150–200mL/min ($\uparrow$ by 50mL/min/session).
- Frequency: Ur rebound is common, so dialyse daily against symptoms and chemistry for the first 2–4days. Catabolic patients (e.g. sepsis) may need to remain on a daily regimen.
- Dialyser (📖 p.208): small dialyser (≤1.4 m^2) preferable.
- Fluid removal (ultrafiltration, UF, rate).
  - ▶ Assessment of the patient's volume status is crucial.
  - Hypovolaemia: administer saline (1–2L)—no UF.
  - Euvolaemia: no UF
  - Overload: up to 2–3L can be removed over 2hr. If further UF necessary (patient still in pulmonary oedema), it can be removed by isolated UF (→ dialysate flow turned off leaving fluid removal, not biochemical control, as 1° goal).
- Anticoagulation-free: minimize (avoid) heparin, acutely unwell ARF patients are at risk of bleeding: arterial puncture during line insertions, GI bleeding, $\uparrow$BP, pericarditis (which may → haemorrhagic tamponade).
- Dialysate
  - Dialysate Na$^+$ of 145mmol/L is typical. If serum Na$^+$<125mmol/L use a dialysate Na$^+$ ≤ 20mmol/L higher to avoid rapid correction.
  - Serum K$^+$ decides dialysate K$^+$. ⚠ Overcorrection → arrhythmias.

Serum (mmol/L)	Dialysate (mmol/L)
>5.5	2.0
3.5-4.5	4.0
<3.0	4.5

K$^+$ free dialysate can be used if $\uparrow\uparrow$K$^+$.

- ◆ Adequacy. Some evidence that daily dialysis → better outcomes. Kt/V (📖 p.210) is unreliable in ARF, but $\uparrow$Kt/V may → $\uparrow$survival. Aim to keep Ur <25mmol/L. The urea clearance using intermittent HD is about 160mL/min.

Modifications of HD

Modifications of IHD using standard HD equipment may improve tolerability, though overall benefits appear marginal.

- Extended duration dialysis (EDD): 6–8hr treatments with blood and dialysate flows of 200–300mL/min and 300mL/min respectively. Well-tolerated and can achieve good UF volumes (~3L).
- Sustained low efficiency dialysis (SLED): 12hr treatment with blood and dialysate flows of 200mL/min and 100mL/min respectively. Well-tolerated, but circuits are prone to clotting.

Dialysis disequilibrium

A syndrome thought to be 2° to cerebral oedema: blood urea drops rapidly on dialysis, but not as readily across the blood–brain barrier and within cells → water influx into the brain and cerebral oedema ± cerebral acidosis.

- Rare if first dialysis precautions opposite observed.
- Those with Ur >60mmol/L at particular risk.
- Symptoms (during or shortly after dialysis): nausea, dizziness, headache, visual disturbance, agitation, confusion, ↓GCS, seizures.
- Exclude hypoglycaemia, ↓Na⁺, drug toxicity, and intracerebral bleeding.
- ♦ Prophylaxis: phenytoin 15mg/kg loading dose, then 200–300mg/d. Treatment: stop dialysis & supportive (improvement should occur within 24hr). Mannitol 10–15g IV and diazepam IV if fitting.

Prescribing CVVHF

See 📖 p.204 for explanation of technique.
- *Time*: continuous.
- *Blood flow*: usually 150–200 mL/min.
- *Filter*: high flux (synthetic) membrane.
- *Fluid removal*: UF rates of 10–45 mL/kg/hr are typical. Fluid removal is achieved by the UF rate exceeding replacement fluid (*not* dialysate) per hr (e.g. net 100 or 200mL UF/hr). Replacement fluid (usually supplied in 5L bags) contains:
  - Buffer: usually lactate (liver metabolism to HCO_3^-), but HCO_3^- based solutions preferable if lactate intolerant (liver disease, shock).
  - K⁺ generally 0–2mmol/L and adjusted to serum K.
  - Also contain Na⁺ (132–140mmol/L), Ca^{2+}, Mg^{2+}, and Cl⁻.
- *Anticoagulation*: heparin or prostacyclin (📖 p.212) usually preferred.
- *Adequacy*: the urea clearance using CVVHF is about 10mL/min, increasing to 25–30mL/min with continuous haemodiafiltration.
- ♦ ↑ volume of filtration (35–45mL/kg/h) may → better outcomes.

Peritoneal dialysis (PD) in ARF

Rarely used for ARF in Europe and North America, but an important treatment worldwide. Until recently, it was also the most popular technique for the treatment of ARF in children.

Potential advantages
- No need for a specialist renal set-up.
- Technically (relatively) straightforward.
- Minimizes haemodynamic instability (making fluid removal easier).
- Gentle correction of biochemical abnormalities. No need for vascular access or systemic anticoagulation.
- Dextrose in PD fluid boosts caloric intake

Potential disadvantages
- Bowel perforation during catheter insertion (esp. if previous surgery → adhesions).
- ⚠ Infection: peritonitis and catheter exit site.
- Relatively slow correction of uraemia and $\uparrow K^+$.
- Unpredictable UF rate (inter-patient variability).
- Protein and amino acids lost in dialysate.
- Catheter problems: migration, poor inflow/outflow, leakage.
- Abdominal distension → diaphragmatic splinting → respiratory compromise.
- Hyperglycaemia (PD fluid uses glucose to generate hypertonicity).
- Contraindicated by recent abdominal surgery.

Catheter placement
Semi-rigid ('stab PD')
Pros: inserted at the beside under LA (usually via a Seldinger technique).
Cons: non-cuffed, therefore high infection rates. Uncomfortable and easy to dislodge. Higher incidence of bowel perforation. Usually requires removal after 48–72hr (→ repeated insertions often necessary).

Cuffed catheter (similar to those used in chronic PD)
Pros: cuff prevents bacterial migration ∴ ↓ infection rates. Softer catheter, so more comfortable with less risk of bowel perforation. More compatible with automated cyclers.
Cons: Insertion requires more expertise (though LA still possible).

Haemodialysis, haemofiltration, or PD for ARF?
Studies are limited. A recent comparison suggested a worse outcome than for CVVHF—though second-rate PD equipment (rigid catheters, home made fluids, acetate buffer, no automated cyclers) was judged against first-rate CVVHF technology in highly catabolic patients. Cannot be considered a front line treatment for ARF, but may be life saving if HD/CRRT unavailable.

Prescribing acute PD

- Commercially available dialysate solutions preferable. Warm to body temperature prior to infusion.
- A correctly positioned catheter should allow inflow and outflow times of <10–15min. Both proceed under gravity. Ensure complete drainage (remember: more drains out than in if UF has occurred).
- Dwell times of 1hr are typical (<30 min a waste of time and effort).
- With non-cuffed rigid catheters peritonitis risk ↑ dramatically after 72hr. Cuffed catheters offer uninterrupted treatment.
- Aim for 20–24 exchanges/day (logistically often difficult).
- Record the number of exchanges and bag input:output.
- Continuous equilibrium PD (CEPD), which is similar to standard CAPD, is an alternative. Dwell times are 4–6hr, allowing more time for solute equilibration between blood and dialysate. Less time 'hands on' the catheter → ↓ risk of infection.
- Dialysate volume: most patients tolerate 2L exchanges. Larger volumes (up to 3L) can → catheter leaks, hernias, and diaphragmatic splinting.
- Dialysis dose is increased by ↑dialysate volume ± exchange frequency
- Fluid balance. If the patient is euvolaemic, mildly fluid overloaded, or haemodynamically unstable, a 1.5% dextrose concentration ('light bag') is appropriate. Check the subsequent drainage volume to assess UF. Use this figure in combination with repeated clinical assessment to direct the need for higher dextrose concentrations (2.5% or 4.25%).
- Heparin (200–500U/L) can be added to the dialysate to prevent plugging of the catheter with fibrin clots. It is not absorbed systemically.
- Commercial PD solutions don't contain K^+, so if the patient is hypokalaemic, or the serum K^+ is rapidly falling, potassium chloride can be added (usually 2–4mmol/L).

The hepato-renal syndrome (HRS)

HRS occurs in advanced liver dysfunction, usually cirrhosis, in conjunction with ascites and portal hypertension. HRS has been split into 2 types based on (i) rapidity of onset, (ii) severity of ARF, and (iii) prognosis (see box below).

▶ Not all concomitant renal and hepatic impairment is due to the HRS—it isn't even top of the list.

Common causes of combined hepatic and renal dysfunction

● Hypovolaemia (GI haemorrhage, diuretics) → ATN
● Sepsis → ATN
● Nephrotoxins (drugs and ↑bilirubin → ATN)
● Glomerulonephritis (e.g. MCGN with Hep C).

Pathophysiology

Liver disease is associated with marked splanchnic (and systemic) vasodilatation (→ arterial underfilling and ↓SVR) in part due to excess local NO production (↑shear stress in portal hypertension), ↑bacterial translocation and ↑vasoactive gut peptides (glucagons, prostacyclin). As a result, the effective arterial blood volume is sensed to have fallen, leading to intense α-agonism, 2° hyperaldosteronism, and non-osmotic ADH release (hence salt and water overload). Catecholamine, angiotensin, and endothelin excess result in profound and intense renal vasoconstriction (→ ↓RBF). The kidneys are structurally *normal* and the renal impairment is entirely pre-renal in nature—tubular integrity and function is preserved:

● Kidney biopsies are normal (in practice unnecessary and hazardous).
● Kidneys from HRS patients have been successfully transplanted.

Classification of HRS	
Type I	ARF the dominant clinical feature
	Rapid ↓GFR (Cr >221μmol/L or CrCl falling to <20mL/min in less than 2 weeks)
	Progressive oligo-anuria (often profound)
	Median survival 2 weeks
Type II	Ascites (often refractory) the dominant clinical feature
	Protracted clinical course
	Renal impairment less acute and severe
	Can convert to type I
	Median survival 6 months

HRS: diagnostic criteria

Major criteria

- Acute or chronic liver disease with advanced hepatic failure and portal hypertension.
- Renal impairment: serum Cr ≥133µmol/L or CrCl <40mL/min.
- Absence of shock, GI fluid losses, excessive diuresis*, or ongoing bacterial infection (▶ spontaneous bacterial peritonitis).
- No recent nephrotoxic drugs (e.g. NSAIDs, aminoglycosides).
- No sustained improvement in renal function (serum Cr ↓ to <133µmol/L or ↑ in CrCl >40mL/min).
- Proteinuria <500mg/dL and no evidence of obstruction or renal parenchymal disease on US.

Additional criteria

- Urine volume <500mL/day
- Urine Na$^+$ <10 mmol/L
- Urine osmolality >plasma osmolality
- Urine red blood cells <50/HPF
- Serum Na$^+$ <130 mmol/L.

* Weight loss >500g/day for several days in ascitic patients without (or 1kg/day in those with) peripheral oedema.
From Arroyo V et al. (1996) Hepatology; **23**:164–76.

Recognizing deteriorating renal function may not be easy, as cirrhotics often have a ↓muscle mass (serum Cr may overestimate GFR). Urea is influenced by GI bleeding, low hepatic production ± variable dietary protein intake and ∴ unhelpful. The diagnosis depends on the exclusion of other causes of ARF.

Clinical features

- Advanced liver disease: ascites, stigmata of chronic liver disease, portal hypertension (beware GI bleeding), encephalopathy, jaundice (degree variable), coagulopathy.
- Cardiovascular: oedema (Na$^+$ and water retention) and ↓BP (both SVR and effective circulating volume are ↓).
- Infection: ↑ susceptibility to sepsis (⚠ pneumonia, line infections and spontaneous bacterial peritonitis).
- Electrolyte disorders: dilutional ↓Na$^+$ is almost universal (disproportionate retention of Na$^+$ compared to water).
- Nutritional state: usually poor and deteriorating.
- Urine output: oligo-anuria the norm in type I HRS, with urine volumes decreasing as the condition progresses. Anuria is a bad sign.
- Urinalysis bland, with no proteinuria/haematuria.
- Tubular function preserved so the kidneys excrete concentrated urine that is low in Na$^+$ (<10mmol/L) (indistinguishable from prerenal ARF). Heavily emphasized in the past, but now considered minor criteria.
- Normal renal ultrasound.

Management of HRS

Identify those at risk on admission to hospital. Risk factors include:
- Cirrhosis + ascites = 40% 5 year probability of HRS.
- Large volume (>5L) paracentesis without concurrent plasma expansion. (☞ Give 100mL 20% human albumin per 1.5L ascites removed.)
- Over-diuresis (possibly—see diagnostic criteria).
- GI bleeding (variceal bleeding is a well-known precipitant).
- Sepsis: especially spontaneous bacterial peritonitis (SBP) (~ 20% develop HRS). Any cirrhotic with ascites should be assumed to have SBP until tapped and proven otherwise.
- Surgery

> **Preventative measures**
> May be effective in specific situations:
> - Spontaneous bacterial peritonitis. Administration of IV albumin 1.5g/kg at diagnosis and 1g/kg 48hr later in addition to antibiotics (as below) appears to decrease risk.
> - Alcoholic hepatitis: pentoxifylline (a TNF inhibitor) 400mg tds orally.

Managing established HRS

▶ Seek expert help early.
- Volume assessment:
  - IV 20% albumin (salt-poor) for a CVP of 5–10cmH$_2$O
  - Na$^+$ (80mmol/24hr) and fluid restriction (<1L/24hr) if overloaded
- Culture blood, urine, and ascites. Empirical IVI cefotaxime 1g bd or piperacillin/tazobactam 4.5g 8hr.
- Consider therapeutic paracentesis if tense ascites with ascitic pressure >30cm H$_2$O (↑intrabdominal pressure transmitted to kidneys (↑renin release, ↓GFR) and ureters (relative obstruction).

Specific rescue therapies

- Vasoconstrictors → constrict the splanchnic bed → improve circulatory (and ∴ renal) function. Given in combination with albumin 20–40g daily for 15 days. Aim for MAP >75mmHg.
  - Vasopressin analogues (acting via splanchnic V$_1$ receptors). Terlipressin (0.5–1mg/4–6hr IVI) is the most used. Renal response slow but real, and improvements generally persist. Repeat courses are effective and responders have a better prognosis. Nonadrenalin (1–10µg/min) is an alternative.
  - α-agonists: midrodine (7.5–12.5mg po tds) is a selective α$_1$ agonist that may be beneficial in combination with octreotide (100–200µg SC tds). Aim to ↑MAP by 15mmHg.
- Trans-jugular intrahepatic portosystemic shunts (TIPS) may have a role in combination with vasoconstrictors and in selected patients when pharmacotherapy has failed.
- N-acetylcysteine 100mg/kg bd IVI may be beneficial.

Renal replacement therapy

⚠ RRT does not improve outcome and should be viewed as a bridge to liver transplantation: only consider if liver transplantation intended. Continuous RRT (haemofiltration) is better tolerated than intermittent HD. Standard indications apply (📖 p.118).

Molecular adsorbent recirculating system (MARS) is an extracorporeal albumin dialysis technique still in relative infancy. Dialysate recirculates through charcoal and anion-exchanger columns (removing potential HRS mediators; e.g. TNF, IL-6, and NO).

Liver transplantation.

The most (only?) effective therapy, but many patients die before transplantation possible. Organ allocation differs between countries, but in many systems (e.g. MELD) HRS patients accorded high priority. Most patients have ↑GFR after transplantation, although the majority do not regain normal renal function (10% incidence of ESRD at 11 years). Patients with pre-transplant renal impairment have a ↓long-term survival compared with those with normal GFR.

Rhabdomyolysis

First described as 'crush syndrome' during the London blitz of WWII. Rhabdomyolysis is a clinical syndrome caused by release of cellular contents after significant striated muscle injury.

Injury is caused by either energy-depletion and cell death, or more commonly, at reperfusion in ischaemic skeletal muscle. Infiltrating leucocytes release oxidant species which cause myonecrosis. If cell death is widespread, intracellular elements and membrane products are released into the circulation: creatine kinase (mainly MM isoenzyme, but also MB), LDH, myoglobin, purines ($\rightarrow$ hyperuricaemia), electrolytes (esp. K^+ and PO_4) and aminotransferase enzymes.

Myoglobin (Mb)

The main nephrotoxin. A 19kD weak O_2 carrier (similar to Hb but with a single haem moiety), Mb is usually bound to plasma proteins. When in excess the ferric form (Fe^{3+}) is freely filtered and concentrated $\rightarrow$ intraluminal cast formation. Tubular degradation generates highly toxic ferryl-Mb (Fe^{4+}) $\rightarrow$ direct oxidant tubular cell injury. A key feature of rhabdomyolysis is the large quantities of fluid retained in inflamed muscle, $\rightarrow$ profound hypovolaemia in addition to toxic renal injury.

▶ Not all rhabdomyolysis $\rightarrow$ ARF (particularly if you act quickly).

Clinical presentation

Variable, but myalgia, weakness and dark urine are rare (~50% have no muscle pain at presentation). Maintain high index of suspicion, esp. if ↑ALT/AST, ± ↑Cr and ↓UO with dipstick positive haematuria.

⚠ Examine the limbs carefully—don't miss a compartment syndrome. Recurrent rhabdomyolysis after mild exertion $\rightarrow$ an underlying myopathy.

Investigations

Dipstick cannot distinguish between myoglobin and haemoglobin. Classically urine is dipstick +ve for blood, but with no red cells on microscopy. ~20% of patients will have a −ve urinalysis. ▶ Urinary myoglobin +ve (not present in normal urine). ↓ u-Mb can be used to monitor treatment.

- U+E (Cr:urea ratio often very high), ↑Alb if volume deplete, or hypoalbuminaemia if capillary leak.
- ↑CK (better indicator of amount of muscle damage than likelihood of ARF). ↑ALT, AST, LDH.
- ↑K^+ (⚠ often ↑↑), ↑↑PO_4, ↑urate, ↑lactate and ↑AG acidosis (organic acids).
- ↓↓Ca^{2+}, often with avid calcium sequestration in injured muscle.
- Mild DIC frequent (↓Plt, ↑D-Dimers).
- Consider toxicology screen for drugs, viral screen, TSH if cause not apparent.

Causes of rhabdomyolysis

Physical causes	Drugs and toxins
Trauma and disasters (crush injury)	Alcohol, heroin, amphetamines, cocaine and ecstasy
Prolonged immobility	
Compartment syndrome	Statins & fibrates
Muscle vessel occlusion	Antimalarials
Sickle cell disease	Zidovudine
Shock and sepsis	Snake and insect venoms
Excessive exertion	Infections
Delirium tremens	Pyomyositis and gas gangrene
Electric shock	Tetanus, legionella, salmonella
Status epilepticus or asthmaticus	Malaria
Neuroleptic malignant syndrome	HIV, influenza and coxsackie
Malignant hyperthermia	**Electrolyte abnormalities**
Myopathies	$\downarrow K^+$, $\downarrow Ca^{2+}$, $\downarrow PO_4$, $\downarrow Na^+$, $\uparrow Na^+$
Polymyositis/dermatomyositis	**Endocrine disorders**
McArdles' disease and other inherited myopathies	Hypothyroidism
	Hyperglycaemic emergencies

Management of rhabdomyolysis

Prevention of ARF

In the early phase of the disorder, vigorous resuscitation may protect patients from many of the subsequent complications.
- Aim to resuscitate to euvolaemia
  - As much as 12L may be required/day (and more if severe injury).
  - If clinical doubt of volume status, aim for CVP 8–12 cm H_2O.
  - Alternate 1L 0.9% NaCl with 1L 1.26–1.4% $NaHCO_3$.
  - If the Na^+ load → ↑Na^+, use 1L 5% dextrose or 1L 0.45% NaCl containing 50mL 8.4% $NaHCO_3$ to ↓ total Na^+ load.
- Maintain a UO ≥150mL/hr, or ≥300mL/hr with traumatic injuries.
- Continue therapy until disappearance of urinary myoglobin.

Urinary alkalinization and mannitol

✍ The role of urinary alkalinization (stabilizes oxidizing form of myoglobin) and forced diuresis (↑urine flow → ↓tubular precipitation) remains controversial. ▶ The priority is to volume resuscitate the patient.
- ⚠ Alkalinization → systemic alkalosis and thus symptomatic ↓Ca^{2+}. Aim for a target u-pH > 6.5 by using alternating NaCl and $NaHCO_3$ as above, but increasing the frequency of $NaHCO_3$ if need be. Evidence is weak that it has a meaningful clinical impact, and volume overload a real risk unless UO good.
- Diuretics may ↑flow, thus limiting tubular precipitation. Loop diuretics acidify the urine, and should be avoided. Mannitol an osmotic diuretic, is preferred: give as a bolus (e.g. 12.5–25g as a bolus [= 62.5–125mL of 20% (200mg/mL) mannitol solution]) or as an infusion (10mL/hr of 15–20% mannitol). ⚠ mannitol ↑osmolar gap and may worsen ARF.

⚠ Once overt renal failure has developed, the only reliable treatment is dialysis. The prognosis is good, if causative insult removed. Physiotherapy to debilitated muscles will be required. Renal function returns to normal in the majority, even if dialysis dependent.

Compartment syndrome in rhabdomyolysis

May occur in two circumstances:
- If the blood supply to particular limb has been compromised (immobility after fits, drug overdose etc.).
- Generalized muscle injury and inflammation (toxic, viral).

Inflammation and oedema within a closed muscle compartment →↑intra-compartment pressure → ↓O_2 delivery → myonecrosis.

▶ Always examine the major muscle groups for the characteristic 'woody hard' feeling of an evolving/established compartment. Prophylactic fasciotomy in these circumstances may save limb function.

If in doubt, stick a needle in: using an attached tonometer, an intra-compartment pressure >50mmHg with a normal BP, or 30–50mmHg in hypotensive patients is worrying. If in doubt, re-check every 6hr.

Hypocalcaemia

Don't attempt to correct $\downarrow Ca^{2+}$ unless it is symptomatic (tetany, arrhythmias)—there is a risk the administered calcium will precipitate in injured muscle. Rebound hypercalcaemia is common during the recovery phase.

⚠ Symptomatic $\downarrow Ca^{2+}$ may complicate $NaHCO_3$ administration

Haemoglobinuric ARF

Occurs in the context of massive intravascular haemolysis.
- Transfusion reactions (ABO incompatibility)
- Falciparum malaria (blackwater fever, 📖 p.492)
- Haemolytic anaemias (drug induced, autoimmune)
- Mycoplasma infection
- Snake, insect, and spider venoms.

Free Hb does not enter the urine as freely as myoglobin, so ARF is relatively rare.

Investigations

$\downarrow$Hb, $\downarrow$haptoglobins, $\uparrow$bilirubin, $\uparrow$LDH, $\uparrow K^+$, urine is dipstick +ve for blood, plasma appears dark.

Management

Treat underlying disorder, volume resuscitation to establish a diuresis.

Radio-contrast nephropathy (RCN)

Accounts for ~10% of in-hospital ARF and is associated with significant mortality (x 5.5 odds adjusted risk of death), and may irreversibly ↓GFR (esp. in those with pre-existing CKD). Associated with ↑length of stay. Overall incidence is ~3.5%, but rises to >30% if starting Cr >265μmol/L.

Why is contrast toxic?
- Direct toxicity: oxidant injury to proximal tubular cells
- Vasomotor effects: contrast (perhaps through its osmolality) alters afferent/efferent tone and thus perfusion
- ▶ ATN is the result.

Precautions
- Specific measures are listed in the box opposite
- Identify those at risk (📖 p.74). Don't do high-risk patients as a 'day case'.
- Is the procedure really necessary? Is there an alternative 'non-contrast' technique? Speak to your radiologist.
- Use iso-osmolar, non-ionic contrast
- Minimize contrast volume (< 140mL if possible).
- Optimize volume status pre-study.
- Stop all other nephrotoxins prior to procedure.
- Where possible, stop diuretics, ACEI and ARB (●⃰ Some data suggests ACEI may be protective for 2 days). If they can't be stopped for any reason (e.g. uncontrolled BP or CCF), consider postponement.
- Space out multiple procedures whenever possible.
- Inform the renal team of high-risk cases (beforehand!)

Clinical features
- ↓GFR begins immediately (though Cr may be unchanged initially).
- The earliest (and often only) sign may be oliguria (so ensure UO is being measured).
- ARF may not be apparent until renal function is rechecked the following day (so make sure it is checked and that you see the result).
- Unlike other causes of ATN, fractional excretion of Na^+ is <1%

Treatment
Once established treat for ATN as for any other cause Ensure the patient remains well-hydrated and avoid additional nephrotoxins. Dialysis support may be necessary.

Prognosis
- In the majority, renal dysfunction is mild and transient (though still associated with ↑ mortality).
- Recovery within a week is usual. Those with pre-existing advanced CKD are most susceptible to a permanent ↓GFR.

Strategies to prevent RCN

Hydration

IV fluids correct volume depletion and ↑RBF. They also minimize the pre-renal effects of a post-contrast diuresis. Evidence supporting their use is strong.

- 0.9% NaCl 1mL/kg/hr for 12hr pre- and 12hr post-procedure (recommended).
- 0.45% NaCl 1mL/kg/hr for 12hr pre- and 12hr post-procedure.
- 1.26% $NaHCO_3$ 3mL/kg/hr for 1hr pre- and 1mL/kg/hr for 6hr during and post-procedure (may be as good as 0.9% NaCl).

Examine the patient first—if overtly dehydrated then larger volumes are required and the procedure may require postponement. If already volume overloaded then further fluids are ill-advised.

◆ N-acetylcysteine (NAC)

Used for its anti-oxidant properties, *always in conjunction with IV hydration*. Evidence base is not yet robust: as many randomized trials and meta-analyses have suggested benefit as no effect. NAC may even ↓Cr independently of GFR, through interference with tubular handling.

▶ Inexpensive with few side effects.

- 600–1200mg po bd for 24hr on either side of the procedure

Others

- Theophylline: antagonizes adenosine-mediated ↓RBF. Evidence of benefit, but only in low-risk groups. Further study required.
- Haemofiltration/haemodialysis: prophylactic removal of circulating contrast. No large-scale evidence of benefit.
- Fenoldopam: specific dopamine₁ receptor agonist that ↑RBF. No clear current evidence of benefit.

▶ Any unit undertaking large numbers of contrast studies should have a locally agreed protocol, usually based on fluid ± NAC administration.

Differential diagnosis

Many patients undergoing invasive vascular studies have diffuse atherosclerotic disease and are at risk of renal atheroemboli. These can occur as a distinctive clinical syndrome (📖 p.416), but often go unrecognized until the expected recovery of renal function doesn't occur.

Tumour lysis syndrome

Tumour lysis usually occurs at initiation of treatment (chemo- or radio-therapy, or even corticosteroids) of lymphoproliferative (and less commonly solid) malignancies, but may occur spontaneously with a large tumour burden or at later stages of treatment. Classically, it is a complication after chemotherapy for high-blast count acute lymphocytic leukaemias, lymphoma, myeloma or germ cell tumours.

It is a result of treatment-induced necrosis of large numbers of purine-rich (actively proliferating) malignant cells, with intracellular and membrane products released abruptly into the circulation. Uric acid in particular causes renal failure:

Acute uric acid nephropathy

Uric acid is freely filtered, and in excess precipitates in the tubular lumen to form obstructing crystalline casts. This is more likely in volume deplete patients with low urinary flow rates ($\uparrow$urate concentration) or if u-pH$\downarrow$.

Clinical findings

In the context of recent therapy, symptoms and signs are due to electro-lyte abnormalities ($\triangle$ $\uparrow K^+$ and dysrhythmias) and ARF.

Investigations

Within 6–72hr of therapy:
- $\uparrow K^+$: often rapid $\uparrow$ of >2 to >7mmol/L.
- $\uparrow PO_4$: avidly binds calcium, precipitating hypocalcaemia and calcium phosphate deposition in the vasculature and kidney. $\downarrow Mg^{2+}$ for same reason.
- $\uparrow$uric acid: purine nucleotides are metabolized to hypoxanthine, xanthine, and then uric acid, often rising to >1mmol/L.
- U+E, $\uparrow$LDH, Ca^{2+}, PO_4 twice daily, lactate, urate. Urinary urate. Microscopy for urate crystals.

Prevention

1. Identify at-risk patients (typical or large bulk tumours, first treatment)
2. Pre-hydration:
    - 0.9% NaCl 3–5L/day for 48hr pre- and post-therapy for UO >2.5 L/day
3. Prevent uric acid formation:
    - If risk low–moderate: allopurinol 300mg 12–24 hourly 2 days prior to therapy inhibits xanthine oxidase, preventing the metabolism of hypoxanthine to xanthine (and then uric acid and its salt, urate)
    - If risk of TLS high, pre-emptive rasburicase (see opposite).

Treatment of established tumour lysis
- Continue volume expansion with 0.9% NaCl and maintain high urine flow.
- Continue allopurinol.
- ☛ Alkalinize the urine: 50mL 8.4% $NaHCO_3$ in 1L 0.45% NaCl or 5% dextrose (depending on sodium load and serum Na^+), aiming for u-pH >7.0. Simply maintaining UO at 3–4 L/day may be as good as ↑pH.
- Rasburicase: a recombinant form of the enzyme urase oxidase that occurs in most species, but not higher primates. It oxidizes uric acid to soluble allantoin. It rapidly ↓uric acid levels (within 4 hr often to undetectable), and has been shown to prevent dialysis-requiring tumour lysis syndrome. Give as 200 µg/kg IVI over 30 min daily for 5 days. ⚠ Avoid if G6PDH deficient.
- Institute daily intermittent haemodialysis early if oliguric (or uncontrolled electrolyte abnormalities), and aim for high clearances.

ARF in sepsis

What is the sepsis syndrome?

Sepsis accounts for 2% of all hospital admissions, but 10% of admissions to ITU. ARF is a frequent complication of the sepsis syndrome, increasing in incidence as the severity of sepsis increases. Patients whose renal failure is sepsis-related have a mortality of 75%. With sepsis, there is evidence of (usually local) infection with systemic signs of inflammation (↑temp, ↑HR). This progresses to the sepsis syndrome if organ dysfunction ensues: typically confusion, oliguria, hypoxia, and acidosis. Full-blown septic shock implies hypotension refractory to volume resuscitation.

Causes of significant sepsis

- Gram +ve organisms
  - Staphylococci (incl. *S. aureus,* MRSA and *S. epidermidis*) 20–35%
  - *Streptococcus pneumoniae* 10%
  - Other Gram +ve 10–20%
- Gram −ve organisms
  - *E. coli* 10–25%
  - Other Gram −ve 5–20%
- Others
  - Fungi (candida) 3%, viruses 3%, parasites (malaria) 1–2%

How sepsis becomes shock

Engulfed pathogens are lysed, liberating membrane products (classically lipopolysaccharide, LPS, or exotoxin), proteins, and DNA. These fragments are recognized by specific host receptors on cells (toll-like receptors) which → NFκ-B-dependent cell activation. Activated cells release pro-inflammatory mediators (IL-1, TNF, interferon), stimulating local and systemic host defence networks.

Systemically activated leucocytes now orchestrate the immune response, while local leucocyte recruitment into inflamed tissue is encouraged. At the same time, anti-inflammatory and resolution pathways (negative feedback) are induced: inappropriate regulation of these pathways often leads to a deleterious prolongation of systemic inflammation.

Within inflamed tissue, and then generally, endothelium up-regulates cellular adhesion molecules and tissue factor to encourage recruitment of effector cells. Inducible nitric oxide synthase generates large quantities of NO, and the integrity of intra-cellular tight junctions is compromised.

Clinically, this translates into

- ↓Systemic vascular resistance (NO is a potent vasodilator, and renders angiotensin II and adrenalin less efficacious).
- ↑Capillary leakiness (tight junctions impaired).
- Local tissue injury (neutrophil recruitment with elastase release and oxidant burst).
- ↑Sympathetic activity.
- Activation of the renin–angiotensin–aldosterone axis (AII as a vasoconstrictor, aldosterone to promote Na^+ retention, 📖 p.286).
- Non-osmotic ADH (vasopressin) release (vasoconstrictor).

► Vascular smooth muscle becomes less sensitive to vasoconstrictors, so despite high circulating levels of adrenalin, angiotensin, and endothelin, the vascular tree remains (maximally) dilated.

The kidney in sepsis

Noradrenalin vasoconstricts the afferent arteriole dropping the trans-glomerular perfusion pressure → ↓GFR and Na^+ retention. High systemic NO levels → down-regulation of intra-renal NO production, altering RBF further, particularly in the metabolically vulnerable outer medulla. Inflammatory cells produce oxidants and proteases that injure renal endothelium (remember 20% of cardiac output is to the kidney), and a local coagulopathy → intra-glomerular thrombus formation.

This → ↓O_2 delivery, and ATN (as described 📖 p.98).

Managing septic shock and ARF

Definitions

Systemic inflammatory response syndrome (SIRS)

- Temperature >38.5° or <35.0°
- HR >90
- RR >20, pCO_2 <4.2kPa or the need for ventilation
- WCC >12 or <4 (or blasts > 10%).

Sepsis: SIRS +

- Positive cultures or local infection identified (e.g. cellulitis).

Severe sepsis: sepsis + one of

- Skin mottling
- Capillary refill ≥ 3 seconds
- UO <0.5mL/kg/hr or the need for dialysis
- Lactate >2mmol/L
- Altered mental status (or abnormal EEG)
- Plt <100 or DIC
- Acute lung injury (ARDS)
- Impaired cardiac function.

Shock: severe sepsis + one of

- MAP <60 (80 if known hypertensive) after 40–60mL/kg 0.9% NaCl or 20–30mL/kg colloid.
- Requiring adrenalin/nor-adrenalin >0.25µg/kg/min or >5µg/kg/min dopamine to maintain MAP >60.

General priorities

There is an evidence base suggesting better mortality data for:

1. Early goal-directed therapy (maintain tissue perfusion):
   - Start volume resuscitation within 6hr of diagnosis.
   - Fill for target CVP 8–12cm H_2O and MAP ≥65mmHg.
   - Transfuse for Hct ≥ 30% if central SvO_2 (or $ScvO_2$) ≤ 70%.
   - Despite these measures, if if central SvO_2 (or $ScvO_2$) remains ≤ 70% → dobutamine.
2. Culture and institute broad-spectrum antibiotics, surgical treatment of localized infection (treat sepsis).
3. Insulin infusion for target glucose 4.4–6.1mmol/L (hyperglycaemia impairs leucocyte function ± less well-understood effects?).
4. ☛ Hydrocortisone 50mg IVI 6 hrly + fludrocortisone 50µg po/NG daily if blunted adrenal response: random cortisol <415nmol/L, or with synacthen no ↑ >250nmol/L above baseline (relative insufficiency).
5. Low tidal-volume ventilation 6–7mL/kg ideal BW (limits ventilator induced lung injury—barotrauma).
6. ☛ Drotrecogin-α (activated protein C) in high-risk (APACHE II >24) patients without clinical improvement and no bleeding risk.

Renal priorities

Obviously, maintain independent renal function if possible.

- No convincing data to suggest any particular vasopressor or volume expander is better or worse for the kidneys (hydroxyethylstarch was implicated in ↑ARF).
- Avoid reno-protective strategies that lack an evidence base (📖 p.116)—low-dose dopamine!
- Continuous veno-venous haemofiltration is easier to use in critically unwell patients, but is not demonstrably superior to intermittent HD.
- 'High-dose' CVVHF, aiming for an UF rate of 45mL/kg/min, may improve outcomes—the evidence is **not** conclusive.
- A larger delivered dialysis dose (adequacy, Kt/V) may improve outcomes—the evidence is **not** conclusive.

Calculating MAP

Mean arterial pressure is expressed as DBP + [SBP–DBP]/3.

Chronic kidney disease

What is chronic kidney disease (CKD)?

Definition

The US NKF-DOQI (National Kidney Federation—Kidney Dialysis Outcomes Quality Initiative) classification of chronic kidney disease (CKD) has rapidly been adopted internationally. It is both simple and useful, dividing CKD into 5 stages, according to GFR[1].

CKD stage	GFR (ml/min/1.73 m^2 surface area)	Description
1	>90*	Normal renal function, but other evidence of kidney damage
2	60–89*	Mild reduction in renal function, with other evidence of kidney damage
3	30–59	Moderately reduced GFR
4	15–29	Severely reduced GFR
5	<15	End-stage, or approaching end-stage renal failure

* Early CKD is not diagnosed on GFR alone. There must also be evidence of chronic kidney damage (see below). Patients with a GFR of 60–89 ml/min, with no evidence of kidney disease, do not have CKD, but are classified as having a ↓GFR (± ↑BP).

- Patients with a GFR >60mL/min should not be considered to have CKD unless there is concomitant evidence of kidney damage, suggested by:
  - Abnormal urine findings (proteinuria, haematuria).
  - Structural abnormalities (e.g. abnormal renal imaging).
  - Genetic disease (e.g. APKD).
  - Histologically proven disease.
- Chronic renal failure (CRF) is now an outmoded term denoting an irreversible decline in GFR.
- The exact prevalence of CKD in the general population is currently unknown. However, early stages of CKD appear common and represent a significant disease burden.
- Many cases of early and asymptomatic CKD are unrecognized and ∴ untreated.
- CKD prevalence increases with age.
- The most common identifiable causes are diabetes and vascular disease (including ↑BP).
- CKD is more common in many ethnic minorities.
- ▶ The majority of patients with CKD stages 1–3 do not progress to ESRD. Their risk of death from CV disease is higher than their risk of progression

1 National Kidney Foundation (2002) *Am J Kidney Dis*, **1**, S1–S266

eGFR for diagnosis and management of CKD

- Cr has a non-linear relationship with GFR. In early CKD, Cr may remain within the 'normal' range and be misleading (📖 p.29)
- eGFR is calculated from formulae that adjust the Cr for age, sex and race (📖 p.30)
- The most widely used is the MDRD equation, since it appears the most reliable and reproducible in individual patients
- Normal GFR is ~100mL/min/1.73m^2, so eGFR roughly gives a percentage kidney function
- CKD stages 1–5 are based on eGFR

Cautions

- It is only an estimate (confidence intervals are wide; 90% of patients will have a GFR within 30% of their eGFR)
- eGFR is likely to be inaccurate at extremes of body habitus (malnourished, obese), as well as in pregnant ♀ and amputees
- It is not validated <age 18
- Race: only validated in Caucasians and blacks, though probably acceptable for use in South Asians (⚠ check whether your own lab corrects for race, otherwise use a correction factor of x1.21 for black patients)
- MDRD equation tends to underestimate normal renal function
- It is not validated if the GFR is rapidly changing

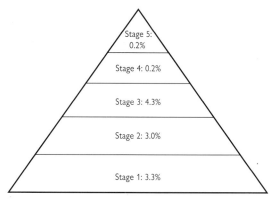

Fig. 3.1 The burden of chronic kidney disease in the population. Data taken from NHANES study in United States population[1]. ESRD represents just the tip of the iceberg -note the large numbers in stage 1–3 compared to 4 and 5. Early stages have significantly increased CV risk.

1 Coresh J, Astor BC, Greene T, *et al.* (2003) Prevalence of chronic kidney disease and decreased kidney function in the adult US population: Third National Health and Nutrition Examination Study. *Am J Kidney Dis*, **41**(1), 1–12.

Pathogenesis of CKD

Causes of kidney disease

Accurate data on the causes of early CKD are scarce. Registry data focuses on causes of ESRD. As only patients whose disease progresses (and who live long enough) reach dialysis or transplantation, it is difficult to extrapolate back to early CKD. UK causes are given below, though there is considerable variation worldwide.

Common causes of ESRD in the UK

- Diabetes (19%)
- Glomerulonephritis (13%)
- Reflux nephropathy (10%)
- Renovascular disease (7%)
- Hypertension (7%)
- Polycystic kidney disease (7%)

There is a tendency for renal dysfunction to progress. A series of interacting processes eventually results in:

- Glomerulosclerosis (glomerular scarring and obsolescence).
- Proteinuria.
- Tubulointerstitial fibrosis.

Mechanisms

Raised intra-glomerular pressure

- As nephrons scar and 'drop out', remaining nephrons undergo compensatory adaptation, with ↑blood flow per nephron attempting to 'normalize' GFR (the Brenner hypothesis).
- ↑Glomerular capillary wall permeability is a feature of glomerular diseases.
- Renal vasodilatation may be an initiating event, with the glomerulus exposed to a higher capillary pressure.

Glomerular damage

- ↑Intraglomerular pressure → ↑wall stress and endothelial injury.
- ↑Strain on mesangial cells → ↑matrix deposition mediated (in part) by angiotensin II and cytokine release (TGF-β, PDGF).

Proteinuria may be due to an underlying glomerular lesion, or result from raised intraglomerular pressure. Protein or factors bound to filtered albumin (such as fatty acids, growth factors or metabolic end-products) may lead to:

- Direct proximal tubular cell injury.
- Local cytokine synthesis (→ recruitment of interstitial inflammatory cells).
- Pro-fibrotic factors → interstitial scarring.
- Trans-differentiation of tubular cells into fibroblasts.

Tubulointerstitial scarring

The degree of tubulointerstitial damage correlates better with long-term prognosis than glomerular damage. Proteinuria may itself be harmful to the tubulointerstitium, but chronic ischaemic damage is also important: tissue oxygen tension is relatively low in the renal medulla, making tubules sensitive to hypoxic injury. Chronic ischaemia occurs with:

- Damage to glomerular capillaries (glomerulosclerosis → altered peritubular perfusion).
- RAS activation → intrarenal vasoconstriction.
- Intratubular capillary loss and increased diffusion distance between capillaries and tubular cells, leads to a vicious cycle of hypoxia.

Diagnosing CKD

▶ Always assume a ↓eGFR represents acute renal failure until proven otherwise. If uncertain, repeat within 5 days and refer as necessary.

Why is it important to identify patients with CKD?

- CKD predisposes to ↑CV risk. Modifying other CV risk factors (▶↑BP) is likely to ↓morbidity and mortality.
- Some patients will benefit from further investigation (e.g. renal biopsy).
- It may be possible to slow progression to ESRD.
- Complications of CKD (e.g. anaemia and bone disease) can be identified and treated early.
- Those (relatively few) patients who will reach ESRD and require dialysis or transplantation need to be properly prepared.

Screening for CKD?

There is currently no evidence that screening of the general population for CKD saves lives or money. Screening should be targeted at those patients at most risk (see below), and repeated annually.

Who:
- Patients with known CKD
- ↑BP
- Unexplained oedema
- CCF
- Atherosclerotic disease (coronary, cerebral, peripheral)
- Diabetes mellitus
- Multisystem disease with possible renal involvement (e.g. SLE, myeloma)
- Bladder outflow obstruction, neurogenic bladder or diversion surgery; renal stone disease
- Chronic nephrotoxin use (e.g. NSAIDs, lithium, ciclosporin, ACEI, ARBs)
- Urologically unexplained haematuria

How:
- Urinalysis for blood and protein (± PCR if positive)
- BP
- eGFR

Why is proteinuria so important?

- It is a marker of chronic kidney damage.
- It has prognostic value in the progression of CKD.
- It may itself cause progression of CKD (❖).
- It is a good surrogate treatment target.
- It is an independent CV risk factor.

The importance of BP

- Hypertension does not usually lead to significant renal disease. However the prevalence of hypertension in the population is so high that hypertensive nephropathy remains a relatively common renal diagnosis (especially in black patients)
- Renal disease is a powerful risk factor for the development of hypertension (most patients with CKD have ↑BP).
- Blood pressure control slows progression of CKD.
- Any patient with hypertension should be examined for the presence of renal disease (UA, eGFR), and the BP should be regularly monitored in all patients with renal disease.

Detection and quantification of proteinuria (📖 pp.46–7)

- There is no need to perform 24h urine collections for quantification of proteinuria.
- If dipstick ≥ 1+, send an MSU to exclude UTI, and send a sample (preferably early morning) to clinical biochemistry (ideally 2 samples, 2 weeks apart): Positive result:
  - Protein/creatinine ratio (PCR) ≥ 45mg/mmol.
  - Albumin/creatinine ratio (ACR) ≥ 30mg/mmol.
  - PCR is adequate in most instances. ACR is more sensitive for early disease screening in high risk groups (e.g. diabetes).
  - ACR ≥ 2.5mg/mmol (♂) or 3.5mg/mmol (♀) represents microalbuminuria.

Progression of CKD

Once CKD is established it tends to progress, regardless of underlying cause. Decline in GFR tends to be linear over time, unless clinical circumstances change. Progression of CKD is more often due to 2° haemodynamic and metabolic factors, than underlying disease activity.

Factors influencing progression of CRF

Non-modifiable
- Underlying cause of kidney disease (tubulointerstitial disease tends to progress more slowly than glomerular disease).
- Race (progression faster in blacks).

Modifiable
- BP.
- Level of proteinuria.
- Plus:
  - Nephrotoxic agents
  - Underlying disease activity (e.g. SLE, vasculitis)
  - Further renal insults (superimposed obstruction, UTI)
  - Hypovolaemia or intercurrent illness
  - Dyslipidaemia
  - Hyperphosphataemia
  - Uncontrolled metabolic acidosis
  - Anaemia
  - Smoking
  - Blood glucose control (if diabetic).

1. What can be done to prevent or slow progression?

- Diagnose the cause of CKD:
  - Helps determine prognosis.
  - Is specific intervention/treatment possible?
  - History: systemic disease (e.g. DM, SLE myeloma), lower urinary tract symptoms, stone disease, inherited renal disease, review all medications.
  - Examination: BP, hypovolaemia, atherosclerosis, palpable bladder, stigmata of inflammatory disease.
  - Investigation: UA (haematuria and/or proteinuria may suggest a renal or systemic disease that might benefit from specific intervention), USS renal tract (🕮 p.36), renal biopsy (🕮 p.636).

2. Influence mediators of progression

- BP (🕮 p.150).
- Other factors (🕮 p.152).

Preventing progression: blood pressure

Hypertension may be cause or effect in CKD. Either way, it should be treated aggressively as poor BP control causes (i) a more rapid decline in GFR (↑BP → ↑glomerular filtration pressure and ↑proteinuria → ↑renal injury) and (ii) ↑CV risk. BP targets are more stringent in CKD (and lower still for patients with proteinuria).

Blood pressure targets in CKD

- Without proteinuria (PCR <100mg/mmol)
  - Treat at 140/90
  - Target 130/80
- With proteinuria (PCR >100mg/mmol)
  - Treat at 130/80
  - Target 120/75
- Diabetes mellitus
  - Target 120/75.

What drug?

Several studies have shown a beneficial preservation of renal function in proteinuric renal disease using ACEI and ARB. This may be 'added value', over and above their antihypertensive effect. The evidence is not conclusive (esp. for non-proteinuric CKD), but there is general consensus for first-line use. Putative mechanisms include:

- ↓Efferent arteriolar tone → ↓intraglomerular pressure and ↓proteinuria.
- ↓AII activity → AII-induced inflammation → ↓ fibrosis and scarring.
- ACEI affect both angiotensin type 1(A1) and type 2 (A2) receptors, but may not completely inhibit AII formation (📖 p.342).
- ARBs block A1 receptors, but not A2.
- There is growing evidence that ACEI + ARB (dual blockade) is an effective therapeutic combination (📖 p.344).

Anti-hypertensives in CKD: a suggested batting order

Expect to need ≥ 3 agents (warn the patient this is likely to be the case).
- First, limit Na^+ intake and recommend other lifestyle measures (📖 p.190).
- ACE inhibitor (especially if PCR >100mg/mmol).
- Loop diuretic (e.g. frusemide) if evidence of salt and water overload. Thiazide diuretics may be effective in early CKD.
- Add ARB if PCR remains >100mg/mmol.
- Dihydropyridine calcium channel blocker (e.g. nifedipine, amlodipine).
- Beta blocker (e.g. atenolol, bisoprolol).
- Centrally acting agent (e.g. moxonidine).
- Alpha blocker (e.g. doxazosin).
- Vascular smooth muscle relaxant (e.g. minoxidil).

Black patients may benefit from a different combination of drugs (📖 p.322).

Preventing progression: other measures

Dyslipidaemia

Experimental work suggests that hyperlipidaemia accelerates ↓GFR. ⚡ It is not yet clear whether treating dyslipidaemia with statins limits progression (or ↓CV risk in CKD). However, lipid lowering is recommended for diabetics with CKD and for CKD patients with a history of myocardial events as 2° prevention.

- All the large studies of cholesterol lowering have excluded patients with CKD. The ongoing SHARP study has been designed to redress this issue.
- Current consensus is that dyslipidaemia in CKD should be treated using statins even if without other CV risk factors.
- △ Side-effects are *more common* in CKD. Myalgia and a small rise in creatine kinase common. ▶ More rhabdomyolysis reported. Liver function abnormalities also more common.
- Targets: in the absence of helpful evidence, these should be as for 2° prevention in the general population e.g. total cholesterol <4.0mmol/L, LDL <2.0mmol/L.

Hyperphosphataemia

(See 📖 p.176) Calcium phosphate deposition in the renal interstitium may contribute to progression of CKD, strengthening the argument for good control of the serum phosphate in these patients.

Acidosis

Acid in the nephron, experimentally at least, causes complement activation and interstitial damage. *But* there is no current evidence that administration of sodium bicarbonate slows CKD progression. Correction of acidosis is desirable for other reasons, however (📖 p.156).

Anaemia

It has been suggested that treatment with EPO (📖 p.162) may slow progression, but again, robust evidence is lacking.

Drugs, toxins, and infections

Once renal failure is established, remaining kidney function is highly susceptible to further (often irreversible) damage. Avoid:
- Hypovolaemia.
- Obstruction or recurrent urinary infection.
- Nephrotoxins:
  - Drugs (e.g. NSAIDS)
  - Radiocontrast (📖 p.132).

Smoking

As well as increasing overall CV risk, tobacco consumption → ↓GFR in CKD. Patients should be strongly encouraged to quit.

Diabetes

In patients with diabetic nephropathy, tight glycaemic control *may* minimize the rate of decline of renal function (as well as prevent other CV complications).

Dietary protein restriction

In animal models, lowering protein intake protects against the development of glomerulosclerosis. Mediators appear to be ↓intraglomerular pressure and ↓glomerular hypertrophy. Non-haemodynamic effects, such as ↓TGF-ß and ↓matrix accumulation, may also be important. In humans, the benefit of dietary protein restriction remains controversial. Although progression may be retarded, a huge investment of effort is required on the part of the patient and dietetic staff. Long term compliance is often poor. At present, optimal dietary treatment of patients with CKD is uncertain. ☛A reasonable regimen is an intake of ~0.8 to 1.0 g/kg of protein/day. Lower levels may risk malnutrition (particular in the context of either advanced CKD or nephrotic range proteinuria). Diabetic nephropathy *may* be more responsive.

Preventing progression—what's on the horizon?

The degree of tubular and interstitial damage is a better predictor of long term renal prognosis than the severity of glomerular changes. So reducing scarring may slow declining GFR in progressive CKD. Experimental tubular injury may be reduced by:

- ACEI (already shown in clinical practice to ↓proteinuria) may ↓tubular complement activation and ∴ interstitial inflammation.
- Experimentally, activation of the mineralocorticoid receptor → interstitial fibrosis and vascular changes. ACEI or ARB may provide some protection against this. Additive mineralocorticoid receptor antagonism using eplerenone or spironolactone may provide additional benefit. Hyperkalaemia would be a potentially dangerous complication of this strategy.
- Mycophenolate mofetil (MMF) may ↓proteinuria (and renal scarring).
- Pirfenidone may inhibit, or even reverse, fibrosis in the interstitium, partly by suppressing TGF-β.
- BX471, a chemokine antagonist, appears to have an anti-fibrotic effect.

Managing CKD

General advice (all stages)

- Smoking cessation.
- Weight reduction if obese.
- Encourage aerobic exercise.
- Aspirin 75mg od if 10 year cardiovascular risk >20% (🕮 p.298), as long as BP <150/90.
- Check lipids and treat according to national guidelines.
- Avoid NSAIDs and other nephrotoxic drugs.
- Limit alcohol to <3 units per day (♂) or 2 units per day (♀).
- Vaccination against influenza and pneumococcus.

CKD stages 1–3

- ► Most of these patients will not progress to ESRD, so the emphasis should be on CV risk reduction.
- Can usually be effectively managed in primary care setting.
- Suggested criteria for referral to a specialist renal service are shown opposite.
- Stages 1–2: at least annual follow up:
  - eGFR, urinalysis and PCR.
  - Meticulous BP control (🕮 p.150 for targets).
- Stage 3: at least 6 monthly follow up:
  - eGFR, urinalysis and PCR.
  - Meticulous BP control (🕮 p.150 for targets).
  - If Hb <11g/dL check ferritin (start on PO iron if <100mg/dL), B12 and folate. Refer for IV iron ± EPO according to locally agreed protocols (🕮 pp.164–6).
  - Annual check of serum calcium and phosphate.
  - Annual PTH and seek advice if >70pg/mL.

CKD stages 4–5

- Refer to a renal unit (► urgently if stage 5). Late referral of patients with advanced CKD is associated with poor outcomes.
- Full dietary assessment (🕮 p.190).
- Optimise calcium, phosphate and PTH (🕮 p.174).
- Correct acidosis (🕮 p.157).
- Hepatitis B immunization.
- Information and discussion regarding future treatments (dialysis, transplantation, or conservative/palliative treatment).

When to refer to a nephrologist

- eGFR <30mL/min/1.73m^2
- eGFR <60mL/min/1.73m^2 **and any of:**
  - Progressive fall (>10mL/min/m^2 in 2 successive years)
  - Microscopic haematuria
  - Proteinuria (PCR >100mg/mmol)
  - >15% decline in eGFR with commencement of an ACEI or ARB (?renovascular disease)
  - Possible systemic illness (e.g. SLE, myeloma)
  - Hb< 11g/dL despite correction of haematinics
  - Abnormal calcium or phosphate
  - PTH>70pg/mL
  - Refractory ↑BP (150/90 despite 3 antihypertensive agents)
- eGFR >60mL/min/1.73m^2 **and** other evidence of renal disease/damage
  - PCR >100mg/mmol (or ACR >65)
  - PCR >45 (or ACR >30) and microscopic haematuria
  - Abnormal renal imaging
  - Family history of renal disease
- Other indications
  - Suspected acute renal failure

Low clearance clinic

The transition from CKD to ESRD is a physically and psychologically demanding time. Such patients are best cared for in a multidisciplinary clinic (see ~6 weekly, more often in the latter stages), with attention to:

- Ongoing measures to minimize rate of progression.
- Dietary intervention.
- Active management of complications (anaemia, renal bone disease, acidosis, malnutrition).
- Pre-dialysis counselling: choice of dialysis modality, individualized advice and support in the decision making process.
- Preparation for transplantation—education, identify potential living donors. Pre-emptive transplantation should be a goal.
- Formation of dialysis access (referral to a surgeon at least 6 months prior to start of dialysis is preferable).
- Access to palliative services for those who elect not to undertake dialysis treatment.
- Timing initiation of dialysis—avoid symptomatic uraemia.

Composition of the low clearance clinic

- Nephrologist.
- Specialist nurses (e.g. pre-dialysis counselling, anaemia management, pre-transplant assessment, palliative care).
- Renal dietitian.
- Vascular access surgeon.
- Pharmacist.
- Social worker.
- Counsellor.

Complications of advanced CKD

Fluid overload

Salt and water overload is usual in advanced CKD. However, as tubulo-interstitial scarring progresses, loss of concentrating ability may → fixed (and often large) urine volumes and a relative salt-losing state (📖 p.408). Such patients may be chronically hypo- rather than hyper-volaemic, and require salt and water supplementation (e.g $NaHCO_3$ 0.5–1.5g tds and increased fluid intake).

Treating salt and water retention in CKD

▶ Careful clinical assessment of volume status.
● Dietary salt restriction (📖 p.191).
● Fluid intake restriction.
● Start furosemide 40mg od and titrate as necessary (max 250mg daily).
● If poor response, consider thiazide diuretic (metolazone 2.5–10mg od) for synergistic effect. ⚠ Diuresis may be brisk. Beware ↓Na^+, ↓K^+ and volume depletion (consider admission).
● Monitor:
  • Daily weight—the best day to day guide of salt and water status. Ask the patient to keep a diary of their weight at home. Weight loss should generally be ≤ 0.5-1kg/day.
  • BP (esp. postural ↓BP if over-diuresed).
  • A rise in Ur ± Cr may restrict dose escalation. If Ur >25mmol/L, consider dose reduction (or cessation), depending on clinical need.
  • Refractory volume overload may signal the need for renal replacement therapy.

Hyperkalaemia

↓Na^+ delivery to the distal convoluted tubule → ↓aldosterone-mediated Na^+/K^+ exchange and ↓K^+ excretion. ▶ ↑ K^+ is a common and potentially fatal problem in advanced CKD, particularly in those treated with ACEI or ARBs. Rapid rises in K^+ are generally more dangerous than gradual ones, as cell membrane stability is more vulnerable to acute changes.

What constitutes a worrying K^+ level...?

Depends on context and chronicity.
● 5.5–6.0mmol/L: recheck routinely. Review medications. Arrange dietary advice.
● 6.1–6.5mmol/L: recheck *urgently*. Review medications (withhold ACEI/ARB). Arrange dietary advice.
● >6.5mmol/L: ▶ admit. See 📖 p.104 for emergency management.

Measures to prevent ↑K⁺

- Dietary restriction (📖 p.191).
- Diuretics: a loop diuretic (e.g. furosemide 40–160mg od) may promote urinary K⁺ loss (thiazides may be ineffective).
- Drug withdrawal or dose reduction if taking an ACEI or ARB. Review other contributory drugs (e.g. spironolactone, beta blockers, NSAIDS).
- Correct acidosis (see below).
- Refractory ↑K⁺ may indicate the need for dialysis.

Acidosis (📖 p.557)

Systemic effects of acidosis

- *Bone:* ↑bone resorption and impaired mineralization, contributing to renal osteodystrophy (📖 p.168).
- *Metabolism:* muscle weakness, fatigue, sense of ill-health.
- *Effects of respiratory compensation* (📖 p.554): overventilation; may → symptoms of dyspnoea ± exhaustion.
- *Hyperkalaemia:* aldosterone-mediated exchange of H⁺ for K⁺ is enhanced in the collecting duct, → ↑K⁺. Acidosis also lessens K⁺ ingress via cell membrane Na⁺/K⁺ pumps.
- *Ionized calcium:* ↑ionized (free) calcium (acidosis → ↓ albumin-bound fraction). ⚠ Correction of acidosis may → ↓Ca²⁺ and provoke tetany.
- *Nutrition:* acidosis promotes catabolism by induction of proteolysis and resistance to growth hormone (→ malnutrition).

How to correct acidosis?

- Treat when venous HCO₃⁻ is <21mmol/L.
- Give NaHCO₃ 0.5–1.5g/tds (start at low dose and titrate).
- ⚠ Na⁺ load may cause or worsen fluid overload. Consider concomitant loop diuretic.
- Refractory acidosis is an indication for dialysis.

Uraemia

Uraemia is the clinical syndrome caused by a substantial fall in GFR—it is *not* a result of ↑ blood urea concentration, but rather of failure to eliminate potentially toxic small and middle molecules. This leads to chronic inflammation and oxidative stress, with accumulation of metabolic end-products, accelerated atherogenesis, disruption of the immune system, and anaemia. The retained compounds or toxins have multiple effects:

- Many remain unidentified.
- They are divided into 'low' and 'middle' molecular weight molecules, by size (<500D = low; >500D = middle).
- Ur and Cr are routinely measured, but are not directly toxic. They act as markers for other LMW substances, including guanidines such as asymmetric dimethyl arginine (ADMA)—a potent inhibitor of NO synthase.
- Retained middle molecules include:
  - β_2 microglobulin (12,000D)—a component of MHC (the cause of dialysis-related amyloid).
  - Advanced glycation end-products (AGE)—products of non-enzymatic breakdown of sugars. Also retained in normal aging and diabetes. Linked to atherogenesis and susceptibility to infection.
  - Complement Factor D—may activate the complement system and contribute to chronic inflammation in uraemia.
  - Cytokines—may maintain uraemic chronic inflammation and malnutrition (short half life suggests over-production is more important).
  - Many, many others.
- ↑Oxidant stress → ↑oxidation products with ↓anti-oxidant levels (in part due to impaired polyamine balance).
- Phosphate is retained, contributing to hyperparathyroidism, arteriosclerosis, and vessel calcification (→ ↓arterial compliance, systolic hypertension, and diastolic dysfunction). (See 📖 p.189).

See 📖 p.159 for clinical manifestations of the uraemic syndrome.

When to start dialysis

Current guidelines recommend commencing dialysis when:
- GFR <15mL/min with uraemic symptoms (persistent nausea and vomiting, anorexia, malnutrition, volume overload, restless legs).
- GFR <10mL/min whether symptomatic or not.
- Refractory hyperkalaemia, acidosis, pulmonary oedema, pericarditis, encephalopathy, and neuropathy are all (urgent) indications for dialysis (the aim should be to start dialysis *before* any of these are present).
- There is no clear evidence that an early start to dialysis confers a survival benefit.
- ▶ Pre-emptive transplantation is the treatment of choice of ESRD. Consider when GFR<20mL/min.

Anaemia of CKD

Erythropoietin (EPO) and the kidney

Red blood cell production is tightly regulated by a number of different growth factors. EPO is essential for the terminal maturation of erythrocytes, and differs from other growth factors in that it is produced by peritubular interstitial fibroblasts in the outer renal medulla and deep cortex of the kidney rather than the bone marrow. The kidney is ideally placed to regulate RBC production, as it is uniquely able to sense and control both O_2 tension *and* circulating volume (and differentiate between the two):

- Red cell mass is regulated by EPO.
- Circulating volume is regulated by salt and water excretion.
- The kidney maintains the haematocrit at 45% in normal conditions (maximizing tissue O_2 delivery).

Chronic kidney disease and renal scarring → ↓EPO synthesis, ↓RBC production, and anaemia. This occurs in most forms of advanced CKD (eGFR<35mL/min), with a few exceptions:

- Adult polycystic kidney disease.
- Benign renal cysts.
- Renal cell carcinoma.

In these instances, EPO may be overproduced.

Differential diagnosis of anaemia in CKD patients

▶ EPO deficiency is not the only cause of ↓Hb in CKD.

Patients with CKD are susceptible to *all* other causes of anaemia, so these should be actively sought in patients who appear disproportionately anaemic or EPO resistant (📖 p.163):

- Iron deficiency (📖 p.166)
- Blood loss (GI tract, haemodialysis)
- Folate deficiency
- B12 deficiency
- Haemolysis
- Myelodysplasia
- Myeloma.

EPO: mechanism of production

In states of normal O_2 tension, intracellular hypoxia-inducible factor 1 (HIF1) is inactivated by constitutive proline hydroxylation of one its two subunits. This allows the α-subunit to be targeted by von Hippel-Landau (VHL) protein for continuous proteasomal degradation. In hypoxic conditions, α-subunit degradation does not occur, permitting full activation of functional HIF1 (and other) signalling pathways → EPO transcription. The renin–angiotensin system also plays a role, with renin → ↑ EPO production (▶ an effect abolished by ACEI, hence their propensity to cause a mild fall in Hb).

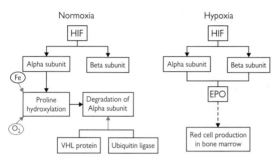

Fig. 3.2 Regulation of EPO production

Erythropoietin

Recombinant EPO is a safe and effective means of maintaining Hb for most patients with CKD. Prior to its introduction patients were almost invariably transfusion dependent, with all the attendant problems of iron overload, sensitization to foreign antigens (which had implications for future transplantation), and risk of blood-borne viral infection. EPO also has a number of beneficial non-haematological effects.

Non-haematological effects of EPO
- Enhanced quality of life scores
- Reduced fatigue
- Improved cardiorespiratory function and exercise capacity
- Reduction in LVH
- Improved cognitive function
- Improvement in sexual dysfunction
- Partial normalization of cortisol and carbohydrate metabolism
- ↓Morbidity/mortality in EPO-treated patients after starting dialysis
- Improved sleep quality

Who needs EPO?

Any anaemic CKD patient, assuming other causes are unlikely or have been ruled out. Consider EPO when Hb <11g/dL (local protocols may vary). Measuring EPO levels is expensive and rarely necessary.

Preparation for EPO therapy
- Have other causes of anaemia been excluded, especially iron deficiency (📖 p.166)?
- Is the patient likely to respond to EPO? Inflammatory cytokines associated with infection (or chronic inflammatory states) inhibit the effect of EPO. ▶ Treat these first. ↑CRP often predicts poor response.
- Is BP controlled? EPO tends to ↑BP. Severe ↑BP was not uncommon in the early days of EPO use (mechanism: vasoconstriction and enhanced adrenergic responsiveness), but has ↓ in incidence with refinement of treatment algorithms.

Which EPO?

There are three major preparations on the market:
- Epoietin-α (Eprex®, Janssen-Cilag)
- Epoietin-β (NeoRecormon®, Roche)
- Darbepoietin α (Aranesp®, Amgen)

Epoietin-α and -β are clinically indistinguishable, and usually given SC 1–3 times per week. Darbepoietin-α is a hyperglycosylated EPO derivative with a longer $t_{1/2}$, that can be administered weekly, fortnightly, or (occasionally) monthly. Prices are comparable.

EPO non-response

Arbitrarily defined as a failure to reach target Hb, or the need for ≥20,000 IU/week of EPO (or darbepoietin-α equivalent) to maintain Hb at target.

▶The most common cause is iron deficiency. Once this is excluded or treated consider the following:
- Chronic blood loss (▶ particularly GI)
- Infection/inflammation (measure CRP)
- Severe hyperparathyroidism (causes bone marrow fibrosis—check PTH)
- Aluminium toxicity (📖 p.175)
- Haemoglobinopathies (Hb variants screen)
- B12 or folate deficiency
- Occult malignancy
- Haemolysis (blood film, Coombs' test, haptoglobins, LDH)
- Inadequate dialysis (Kt/V, 📖 pp.213 and 234)
- PRCA (📖 p.165)
- Malnutrition
- Inadequate dosing
- Poor compliance?

Prescribing erythropoietin

Route of administration?

- Either SC or IV (IV often used in haemodialysis patients - given at the end of a dialysis treatment).
- SC route ↓ dose requirements by ~25% (for EPO α and β, not darbepoietin).
- Rare reports of pure red cell aplasia (PRCA) in patients treated with SC epoietin-α now appear to have been resolved (Ⅲ p.165).
- Patients can be taught to self-administer EPO at home using a range of user friendly devices (EPO should be kept in a fridge).

Starting EPO

- ▶ Ensure iron replete (Ⅲ p.166).
- EPO-α or -β as 80–120IU/kg/week in 2–3 divided doses (~2000IU 3 times per week). A single weekly dose of 30–50IU/kg/week (esp. if no urgency), is an alternative.
- Darbepoietin-α has a typical starting dose of 0.45μg/kg/wk SC.
- To convert from EPO to darbepoietin ÷ total weekly dose by 200 and give once/wk.
- Double the starting dose if there is clinical urgency and/or EPO resistance is likely.
  - Measure Hb and BP weekly at first.
  - If rapid deterioration in BP, intensify antihypertensive medications (it is rarely necessary to withhold EPO).
  - Aim for ↑Hb of 1–2g/dL/month until in target range (see box).
  - ↑ Dose monthly (~25% increments) if Hb rise is slow. Conversely, be prepared to ↓ dose if Hb rise is too rapid.
  - Iron stores are likely to rapidly deplete: ∴ monitor and replace as necessary.
  - Once in 'steady-state', monitor Hb and iron stores 1–2 monthly in pre-dialysis patients and monthly in dialysis patients.
  - Check reticulocyte count in non-responders (should ↑).

Target haemoglobin

- UK Renal Association: >10g/dL. Upper limit not specified.
- European guidelines: >11g/dL (but not >14g/dL). Aim for 11–12g/dL if risk of CCF or ischaemic heart disease.
- US K-DOQI guidelines: 11–12g/dL.

✒ Although higher targets have been sought as early fears about ↑ thrombotic risks (and loss of vascular access in haemodialysis patients) were dispelled, it is now thought that over-zealous correction (>12g/dL) → increased mortality in patients with ischaemic heart disease and heart failure. Individualized targets are the likely future direction of EPO therapy.

Pure red cell aplasia (PRCA)

PRCA presents as an abrupt decline in Hb with normal platelet and white cell counts. Bone marrow examination reveals absent erythroid precursors. There has always been a low incidence of PRCA due to viral infections (parvovirus), lymphoma and certain drugs. Acquired PRCA was first reported in the late 1990s, with ~250 patients worldwide developing anti-EPO antibodies that rendered them profoundly anaemic.

Almost all these cases occurred in dialysis patients on SC (but not IV) Epoietin-α (Eprex®). Extensive (and expensive) investigation revealed that polysorbate (in the vehicle) was able to react with compounds leaching from uncoated rubber stoppers to promote immunogenicity of the molecule.

In suspected cases, a bone marrow examination should be performed, and anti-EPO antibodies sought. EPO should be stopped (rather than switched to an alternative, as the antibody cross-reacts with other preparations). A trial of immunosuppression may be appropriate.

The risk of PRCA led many countries to abandon Epoietin-α by the SC route—however, the manufacturing process has now been changed, and Eprex® is once again licensed by the SC route. PRCA has also been reported in a handful of cases treated with epoietin-β.

Iron stores and iron therapy in CKD

▶ Giving EPO to an iron deficient patient is a waste of time and money.

Iron deficiency is found in ~40% of patients with advanced CKD and high iron availability is required to maximise response to exogenous EPO. Patients are at risk of enhanced iron loss by various routes:
- GI bleeding (often sub-clinical).
- Multiple blood tests.
- Haemodialysis itself (HD patients may lose up to 2g of iron per year).

Monitoring of iron status is not always straightforward. Use ferritin and at least one additional test:
- Ferritin:
  - Target: 150–500µg/L (i.e. well above the normal physiological range). Avoid >1000µg/L.
  - Rationale: the cellular storage protein for iron. Plasma ferritin concentration usually reflects iron status.
  - Problems with interpretation: ferritin is an acute phase protein. If inflammation is present (▶ measure CRP simultaneously), a high or normal ferritin may be misleading.
- Percentage hypochromic red cells. Target <10%.
- Transferrin saturation (TSAT) >20%
  - TSAT = (serum iron/TIBC) × 100

Iron replacement
- If GFR <50mL/min supplementation is likely to be necessary.
- Oral iron is not well tolerated (GI side effects) and compliance is generally poor.
- In many patients iron stores do not improve.
- Many units have developed policies based entirely on IV iron.

Pre-dialysis
- Give iron orally.
  - If ferritin <150µg/L, start FeSO$_4$ 200mg tds.
  - If intolerant, try Fe gluconate 300mg bd–tds.
- Warn patients about GI intolerance, and consider add-on ranitidine 150mg od as prevention. Oral iron should not be taken simultaneously with phosphate binders (📖 p.176). If oral iron is poorly tolerated (or response inadequate), give IV iron.
- Trial of oral iron for 4–6 weeks → re-check stores.

If on dialysis
- Give parenteral iron.

Monitoring
Iron stores and Hb should be measured every 1–2 months pre-dialysis and monthly in dialysis patients.

Types of IV iron

- Iron dextran:
  - Carries a risk of allergic reactions and anaphylaxis (0.6%).
  - A test dose should be given to new starters.
  - Resuscitation facilities should be available.
- Iron sucrose/saccharate (e.g. Venofer®):
  - Newer preparation.
  - Risk of anaphylaxis appears to be minimal (0.05%). Test dose unnecessary.
  - Typical dosing: pre-dialysis (or CAPD): 200mg weekly for 3 doses, then every 1-3 months. Haemodialysis: 100mg/dialysis session for 10 doses (usually into the bubble trap).
- Sodium ferric gluconate (Ferrlecit®):
  - Increasingly popular.
  - Anaphylaxis rare. Test dose unnecessary.

⚠ Iron overload should be avoided, particularly as free iron may cause oxidative tissue damage, increasing infections and cardiovascular risk. If ferritin consistently >1000µg/L consider desferrioxamine chelation.

Renal bone disease 1

Definition

- Renal bone disease (osteodystrophy) is a heterogeneous disorder leading to diminished bone strength in patients with impaired kidney function.
- Virtually ubiquitous beyond CKD stage 3, its management represents a significant challenge.
- Uraemic mineral metabolism (and its treatment) may impact on cardiovascular morbidity and mortality in CKD patients.

Classification (Fig. 3.3)

Osteodystrophy is a function of bone turnover, density, mineralization and architecture. Strictly speaking, bone biopsy with histological and histomorphometric assessment is required for diagnosis and classification. In practice biopsies are very rarely performed (invasive, considerable expertise needed to interpret) and surrogate markers of bone turnover are (over) relied on (Table 3.1).

Secondary hyperparathyroidism (SHPT): ↑PTH causes increased bone resorption and formation ('high turnover' disease). Haphazardly organized, weakened bone results (classically osteitis fibrosa cystica).

Adynamic bone disease: paucity of cells with decreased bone resorption and formation ('low turnover' disease). Pathophysiology remains poorly understood, but incidence has increased rapidly over the last two decades.

Mixed turnover disease: relatively common, as is evolution from one form to another.

Osteomalacia: refers to a defect in mineralization. Uncommon as an isolated finding and not helpful as a clinical description. Generally related to a deficiency of $1,25(OH)_2D$, but aluminium intoxication and uraemic acidosis are also risk factors.

Osteoporosis: usually defined in terms of bone mineral density (BMD) ∴ has little diagnostic meaning in the context of osteodystrophy where low BMD can coexist with low or high turnover disease. DEXA scanning does not predict fracture risk in CKD.

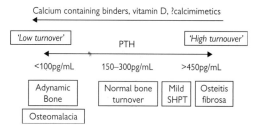

Fig. 3.3 The spectrum of renal bone disease (note pg/mL = ng/L. For pmol/L multiply by 0.11)

Table 3.1 Features of 'high' and 'low turnover' renal bone disease

	High turnover	Low turnover	
	Hyperparathyroid bone disease	Adynamic bone disease	Osteomalacia
Bone biopsy findings	↑Osteoblast and osteoclast activity	↓Osteoblast and osteoclast activity	↓Osteoblast and osteoclast activity
	Fibrosis	Thin osteoid seams	Widened osteoid seams
			Aluminium deposition
PTH	High	Low or normal	Usually low or normal
Alkaline phosphatase	Raised	Normal	Normal
Calcium	Variable	Often ↑	Normal or ↑
Phosphate	↑	Normal or ↑	Normal or ↑
DFO test*	Normal	Normal	Often elevated

*DFO test = desferrioxamine test: a non-invasive means of detecting aluminium overload.

Renal bone disease 2: physiology

Introduction

If renal function is intact, concentrations of PO_4 and Ca^{2+} are maintained through interaction between PTH, $1,25(OH)_2D$ (calcitriol) and their 3 primary targets: bone, kidney and GI tract.

Parathyroid hormone: PTH secretion (and parathyroid gland proliferation) is stimulated by $\downarrow Ca^{2+}$, $\downarrow 1,25(OH)_2D$ and $\uparrow PO_4$. In most circumstances $\downarrow Ca^{2+}$ (acting via the parathyroid calcium sensing receptor) overrides the other two. PTH acts on 3 fronts (i) mobilizing skeletal calcium; (ii) $\downarrow$urinary Ca^{2+} + $\uparrow$urinary PO_4 excretion; (iii) $\uparrow$renal production of $1,25(OH)_2D$ (in turn → $\uparrow$intestinal Ca^{2+} and PO_4 absorption).

Vitamin D: inactive vitamin D (from dietary sources and UV conversion in the skin) is metabolized in the liver to $25(OH)D$ and then converted to $1,25(OH)_2D$ by the renal 1α-hydroxylase enzyme. $1,25(OH)_2D$ alters gene expression by binding to an intracellular receptor (VDR) and exerts a number of important effects (Fig. 3.4).

Bone biology: bone is not static, it continuously adapts to mechanical and metabolic requirements by a remodelling process centred around the coupling of osteoblastic formation and osteoclastic resorption. Multiple systemic hormones (including PTH and $1,25(OH)_2D$) and local growth factors (e.g. RANK/OPG) influence this process. Bone is the most important body reservoir of Ca^{2+} and PO_4.

The effect of renal failure

- Loss of functioning renal mass →
  - Phosphate accumulation.
  - $\downarrow 1,25(OH)_2D$ (→ $\downarrow$serum Ca^{2+}).
- Secondary hyperparathyroidism.
  - $\downarrow Ca^{2+}$ + $\downarrow 1,25(OH)_2D$ + $\uparrow PO_4$ → $\uparrow$PTH synthesis and release.
  - Prolonged stimulation of parathyroid tissue → clonal proliferation of parathyroid cells (with areas of nodular hyperplasia).
  - These clones express less calcium sensing receptor (CaR) and VDR.
  - Refractoriness to treatment is inevitable (termed tertiary or autonomous HPT).
  - In addition there is relative 'skeletal resistance' to the effects of PTH (mechanism unclear).
  - Abnormal bone turnover results.
  - $\uparrow$PTH also has non-skeletal effects: LVH, cardiac fibrosis, extra-skeletal calcification, peripheral neuropathy, impotence.

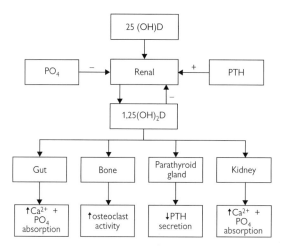

Fig. 3.4 Overview of vitamin D metabolism

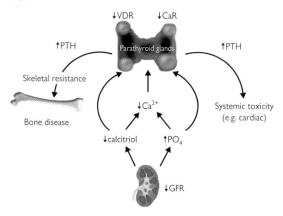

Fig. 3.5 The pathogenesis of SHPT

Renal bone disease 3: clinical features

Secondary hyperparathyroidism (SHPT)
- Usually asymptomatic.
- Clinical sequelae occur late (with significant biochemical and histological disease), including:
  - Bone pain and arthralgia
  - Muscle weakness (esp. proximal).
  - Pruritis (cutaneous calcium phosphate deposition).
  - Bony deformity (e.g. resorption of terminal phalanges).
- ↑ fracture risk (hip fracture risk ~5x in dialysis patients).
  - Mortality following fracture rises ~2.5x.
- Marrow fibrosis contributes to anaemia and poor response to EPO therapy.

Adynamic bone disorder
- Usually asymptomatic.
- Probably no ↑fracture risk ●.
- Adynamic bone buffers calcium poorly; ↑Ca^{2+} is common.
- Aluminium related low turnover bone disease is often painful.

Cardiovascular risk
- ► Poor control of serum PO_4, calcium phosphate product (CaxP) and PTH are all associated with ↑CV morbidity and mortality.
- ↑CaxP is associated with soft tissue and cardiac calcification.

Diagnosis
No one marker is perfect, so a clinical dataset is used (Table 3.1, 🕮 p.169).

Biochemical
- Check Ca^{2+}, PO_4, and PTH at least 3 monthly (more often if treatment changes are made) in CKD stages 4 and 5. Annually in stage 3.
- PTH: the ability of serum PTH to predict high and low turnover disease is actually quite poor, though improves at extremes of PTH (>450pg/mL: high turnover disease, <100pg/mL: low turnover disease).
- Calcium: ↓ in untreated SHPT (though rises with vitamin D analogue and calcium based phosphate binder treatment); often ↑ in ABD.
- Phosphate: raised.
- Alkaline phosphatase: ↑ in SHPT (a marker of bone formation—others, e.g. osteocalcin, are also elevated).

Radiology
The availability of PTH measurements means X-rays are rarely necessary.
- SHPT: subperiosteal bone resorption (distal and middle phalanges of hands and feet), osteosclerosis (→ 'rugger jersey spine' on lateral films).
- ABD: generally normal.

PTH assays

- In addition to intact PTH (PTH 1–84), which acts on its targets via the classical PTH-1 receptor, most commonly utilized assays also detect other biologically active fragments (e.g. 7–84) of the hormone.
- These N-terminally truncated peptides appear to exert an inhibitory influence on bone cells (probably via a distinct C-PTH receptor) and could be a contributory factor to skeletal PTH resistance.
- A new generation of assays, more specific for 'whole' PTH, have been developed and are likely to attract increasing attention as their clinicopathological validation progresses.

Factors contributing to adynamic bone disease

- Low PTH
- Overtreatment with vitamin D
- ↑Calcium intake
- Diabetes mellitus
- ↑Age
- Aluminium accumulation
- Acidosis
- CAPD
- Corticosteroid therapy.

Renal bone disease 4: treatment

Goals

- Keep serum Ca^{2+} and PO_4 within the normal range.
- Keep bone turnover and strength as near normal as possible.
- Keep serum PTH appropriate to the above objectives.
- Prevent the development of parathyroid hyperplasia.

The standard treatment package comprises:

- Measures to ↓ serum PO_4:
  - Dietary PO_4 restriction
  - Removal through adequate dialysis
  - Oral phosphate binders (prevent absorption).
- Measures to ↑ serum Ca^{2+} and suppress PTH synthesis and secretion:
  - Calcium salts (e.g. $CaCO_3$); also act as phosphate binders
  - Vitamin D analogues (e.g. calcitriol, alfacalcidol).
- Measures to suppress PTH synthesis and secretion directly:
  - Calcimimetic agents.

Therapeutic targets

- Guidelines developed by NKF-K/DOQI[1] reflect that renal osteodystrophy and its treatment may be associated with a modifiable increase in cardiovascular risk.
- Much more rigorous targets for calcium, phosphorus and PTH than previously are advocated (see below).
- Suggested phosphate levels at CKD stages 3 or 4 are similar to the normal physiological range, with only a minor concession at stage 5.
- The target for PTH is also close to normal in patients up to stage 3 CKD.
- In stages 4–5, target PTH is 3–6 × the upper limit of normal, reflecting observational data that suggests normal bone turnover is most likely to be achieved in uraemic bone when PTH is modestly elevated ♥.

CKD stage	GFR (mL/min)	PTH (pg/mL)	Calcium (mmol/L)	Phosphorus (mmol/L)
3	30–59	35–70	Normal	0.87–1.48
4	15–29	70–110	Normal	0.87–1.48
5	<15 or dialysis	150–300	2.1–2.37	1.13–1.78

- Data confirming that achieving these goals will have a significant impact on mortality is awaited.
- Currently practice falls well short of meeting these targets.

1 National Kidney Foundation (2003) K-DOQI™ clinical practice guidelines for bone metabolism and disease in chronic kidney disease *Am J Kid Dis* **42**, S1–201.

Aluminium toxicity

History: in the 1970–80s, clusters of dialysis units reported patients with aluminium toxicity. Investigation found high geographic concentrations in dialysate water to be responsible and improved purification techniques eliminated this route of exposure. Aluminium containing phosphate binders were left as the main source.

Presentation: aluminium toxicity (→ ↓PTH secretion, ↓mineralization, and ↓osteoblastic activity) previously accounted for the majority of low turnover pathology. Also: EPO-resistant anaemia, encephalopathy, neurotoxicity.

Current practice: aluminium containing phosphate binders should be avoided (use for <4 weeks and in those with limited life expectancy are possible exceptions). If extended use is necessary, aluminium levels should be monitored. Serum aluminium should be <20µg/L (0.7µmol/L) in dialysis patients. Levels >60µg/L (2.2µmol/L) suggest aluminium overload. Sequential levels may detect the development of overload in at risk patients. However, serum aluminium is not a reliable indicator of overall body content and a desferrioxamine (DFO) stimulation test may be required (→ rise in aluminium level after IV DFO). Symptomatic patients may benefit from regular DFO chelation treatment.

Hyperphosphataemia

Control of phosphate

Phosphate control is the weak link in the therapeutic approach to SHPT.

Dietary restriction (📖 p.191)

- Phosphate is contained in almost all foods (esp. meats, milk, eggs, and cereals).
- It is difficult to balance dietary phosphate restriction against adequate protein intake (recommended levels of daily dietary protein provide 30–40mmol of phosphate).

Phosphate binders

- Taken a few minutes before a meal to bind phosphate in the gut. The amount taken is proportional to size of meal and serum PO_4 (usually 1–3 tablets).
- None are particularly potent and ∴ large amounts are needed.
- The most effective binder is one that the patient will take—demanding regime + unpalatable tablets = poor compliance (>50% dialysis patients do not take their binders regularly).
- Should not be taken at the same time as iron supplements.
- Aluminium hydroxide is the prototype binder and remains the most effective. ⚠ Aluminium toxicity (skeletal and neurological) restricts use (<4 weeks).
- Calcium containing phosphate binders (CCPB) have been the mainstay.
  - Not only bind PO_4, but help correct ↓Ca^{2+} (and suppress PTH).
  - ☞ Patients receiving CCPBs are in +ve calcium balance. CCPBs have ∴ been implicated as a cause of vascular calcification (and adverse CV outcome).
  - CCPBs should ideally be restricted to 1500mg elemental calcium/day.
  - Avoid if low turnover disease (PTH <150pg/mL).
- Non-calcium, non-aluminium containing binders; e.g. sevelamer hydrochloride (Renagel®) and lanthanum carbonate (Fosrenol®) allow calcium and aluminium to be avoided.
  - Both are extremely expensive. Others are likely to be developed.
  - No more effective than CCPBs.
  - Efficacy in preventing CV morbidity and mortality unproven.
  - Sevelamer may lead to less hypercalcaemia and is associated with slower progression of coronary calcification.
  - Sevelamer lowers LDL cholesterol and may provide additional CV risk modification.

Adequate dialysis

- Dietary intake of phosphate exceeds daily removal by dialysis.
- A significant amount of phosphate is in the intracellular compartment, so significant rebound occurs post HD treatment. CAPD is more efficient at PO_4 removal than haemodialysis.
- Poor PO_4 control may be an indication for more frequent dialysis.
- Daily dialysis regimens can control phosphate with no binder requirement (supplementation may be necessary!).

Table 3.3 Phosphate binders

Binder	Advantages	Disadvantages	Examples
Calcium based binders	Inexpensive Help correct Ca^{2+} and suppress PTH Calcium acetate has a smaller calcium load per equivalent phosphate binding dose.	Calcium load may predispose to vascular and soft tissue calcification	• Calcium carbonate • Titralac® (168mg calcium) • Calcichew® (500mg calcium) • Calcium 500® (500mg calcium) • Adcal® (600mg calcium) • Calcium acetate Phosex® (250mg calcium)
Aluminium based	Cheap Very effective	• Risk of aluminium toxicity • Need to monitor levels • Short term use only	• Alucaps® • Al(OH)₃ 475mg • Aludrox® (liquid)
Sevelamer HCl	Avoids calcium and aluminium	• Expensive • GI intolerance • Large doses needed • Long-term outcome data not yet available • Causes a mild metabolic acidosis	• Sevelamer hydrochloride (Renagel®) • 1–3 800mg tablets with each meal
Lanthanum	Avoids calcium and aluminium	• Expensive • Long term consequences of administration unknown (no toxicity in short term studies) • Role in clinical practice not yet established	• Lanthanum carbonate (Fosrenol®) • 750–3000mg/d in divided doses

One strategy is to use multiple binding agents to achieve a normal phosphate, with each binder used at a different meal. This avoids excessive calcium administration and ameliorates the cost of newer binders

Vitamin D analogues

The other mainstay of SHPT treatment. Vitamin D requires 1α-hydroxylation at the level of the kidney for activity. This is pharmacologically bypassed by using the 1α hydroxylated vitamin D analogues calcitriol or alfacalcidol (1α-calcidol).

Nutritional vitamin D deficiency

In CKD stages 3–4 screening for nutritional vitamin D deficiency is recommended when PTH >70pg/mL (serum 25-hydroxyvitamin D <80nmol/L or <30µg/L). If necessary treatment with ergocalciferol (800U/day orally) or colecalciferol (800U/day orally or 10,000U/monthly IM) can be given. There will be sufficient remaining functioning renal tissue for this substrate to be converted to active 1,25(OH)$_2$D (calcitriol) that will then suppress PTH.

Treatment

- ▶ *Control serum phosphate first.*
- Start with a low dose (0.25µg/d alfacalcidol orally) and increase as necessary over several weeks (rarely >0.5–1.0µg/d).
  - CKD stage 3: treat elevated PTH to target of 35–70pg/mL
  - CKD stage 4: treat to target 70–110pg/mL
  - CKD stage 5: treat to target 150–300pg/mL
- Pulsed oral and IV therapy (usually 0.5–2.0µg x3/wk) are an alternative to daily regimens and appear equally efficacious.

Monitoring: monitor serum Ca^{2+}, PO$_4$, and PTH (monthly initially). Avoid ↑Ca^{2+} and PTH over-suppression.

Side effects and toxicity: ↑Ca^{2+} and ↑CaxP frequently complicate treatment. More than just a therapeutic inconvenience, this has implications for bone turnover (↑adynamic bone disease), soft tissue/vascular calcification, and CV morbidity/mortality.

Newer vitamin D analogues

- Much attention has been given to the development of vitamin D analogues with less propensity to hypercalcaemia.
- Many have shown potential in the experimental setting and a few are available for clinical use (e.g. paricalcitol in the UK).
- Advantages over calcitriol and alfacalcidol remain unproven, though there may be marginal benefits.
- ✒ One large cohort study has suggested a possible survival advantage for those patients treated with paricalcitol.
- A therapeutic trial may be warranted in patients prone to ↑Ca^{2+}.
- Paricalcitol is given IV on dialysis (0.04–0.1µg/kg). An oral formulation is under development.
- Further randomized, prospective studies are awaited.

Vascular calcification

- There has been increasing recent appreciation that vascular calcification, hitherto considered relatively benign, might predict, or even contribute to, uraemic CV risk.
- Identification and quantification has been facilitated by advances in radiological techniques, particularly electron-beam CT (EBCT).
- Two types:
  - Intimal (within atherosclerotic plaques).
  - Medial (medial wall—'Mönckeberg's sclerosis').
- Both occur in CKD patients:
  - Calcium content of atherosclerotic plaques from HD patients is greater than age matched controls.
  - Medial calcification causes arterial stiffness (→ diastolic dysfunction → ↑ morbidity and mortality).
- An association between calcification and oral calcium intake has called into question the future role of both calcium containing phosphate binders and vitamin D analogues ♠.
- This may be simplistic; a new paradigm that departs from the traditional view of ↑CaxP promoting passive soft tissue calcification is emerging:
  - Evidence: (i) spontaneous vascular calcification in mice carrying specific gene deletions, (ii) recognition of certain hitherto 'bone-specific' regulatory proteins in calcified arteries, (iii) ability of several stimuli (including inorganic phosphate and uraemic serum) to provoke calcification in vascular smooth muscle cells.
  - Hyperparathyroidism, phosphate loading, ↑BP, abnormal glucose metabolism, ↑lipids, and natural inhibitor deficiencies are all likely to play a role in addition to calcium and vitamin D intake.
- This integration of bone and vascular biology is yielding novel treatments; e.g. the bone morphogenetic protein BMP-7 has been shown to be efficacious effects in animal models of vascular calcification and bone disease.
- Some advocate routine screening for vascular calcification with quantification if possible (e.g. aortic calcification on AXR, pulse wave velocity studies, EBCT).

Calcimimetics

The calcium sensing receptor (CaR)

First cloned in 1993, the CaR is constitutively expressed across multiple cell types and credited with roles in many aspects of cell function. Its main purpose is the control of extracellular Ca^{2+} concentration and regulation of steady state PTH secretion.

Calcimimetic agents

- Small molecules that bind to the parathyroid CaR and mimic the effect of ↑extra-cellular Ca^{2+}:
    - Type I: include Ca^{2+} itself and other cationic compounds. Directly activate the CaR.
    - Type II: not strictly agonists, but allosteric modulators that ↑CaR sensitivity to ambient Ca^{2+}.
- Calcimimetics ↓PTH with a simultaneous ↓ in serum Ca^{2+}.
- Parallel reductions in PO_4 and CaxP are also seen. In this respect they differ importantly from other available treatments (Table 3.4).
- Side effects: upper GI intolerance (10–15%), mild ↓Ca^{2+} frequent (though rarely problematic). Despite the ubiquitous distribution of the CaR, CNS, cardiac and other side effects have not been noted.
- Evidence for clinical efficacy in HD patients has increased (and data is emerging for pre-dialysis and CAPD). It is hoped they will facilitate improved compliance with national Ca^{2+}, PO_4 and PTH targets.
But
- Extremely expensive. Uptake in many countries likely to be limited (use restricted by a NICE guideline in the UK).

Role

More data is needed to decide where need is greatest.

- From the biochemical standpoint, therapy (vitamin D sterol or calcimimetic) can be chosen according to the clinical phenotype of the patient (Table 3.5).
    - The 'vitamin D phenotype': the SHPT patient in whom serum Ca^{2+}, PO_4 and CaxP product are all low-normal or subnormal. Vitamin D therapy is usually effective in bringing biochemical parameters to target. Risk of ↑Ca^{2+} or ↑PO_4 is relatively low.
    - The 'calcimimetic phenotype': potentially more difficult to treat. Here SHPT is accompanied by a high-normal or frankly elevated Ca^{2+}, often with ↑PO_4 and CaxP product. Treatment with vitamin D will ↓PTH, but aggravate ↑Ca^{2+} and ↑PO_4.
- Vitamin D and calcimimetics work well together. Their modes of action at the level of the parathyroid are different and effects on PTH suppression appear additive. Calcimimetics may ↓ serum Ca^{2+}, 'making room' for the use of vitamin D analogues.

Dosing: cinacalcet (Mimpara® in the UK, Sensipar® in the USA)

Oral: Initial: 30 mg od, increased incrementally (60mg, 90mg, 120mg, 180mg) as necessary to maintain target PTH. Hypocalcaemia may require dose reduction.

Table 3.4 Relative actions of current treatments on calcium, phosphorus, CaxP and PTH concentrations.

	Calcium-based binder	Calcium-free binder	Vitamin D sterols	Calcimimetics
PTH	↓↓	↓	↓↓↓	↓↓↓
Calcium	↑↑	↔ or ↑	↑	↓
Phosphorus	↓↓	↓↓	↑	↓
CaxP	↓ or ↑	↓	↑	↓

Table 3.5 The two clinical phenotypes frequently encountered in CKD patients.

	Calcium	Phosphorus	CaxP
'Vitamin D phenotype'	Low-normal or low	In target	In target
'Calcimimetic phenotype'	High normal or high	Above target	High

Parathyroidectomy

▶ An elevated PTH alone is not an indication for parathyroidectomy.

Indications

- Tertiary or autonomous hyperparathyroidism: failure of hyperplasic, overactive glands to suppress adequately in response to optimal medical therapy.
- Manifests clinically as ↑PTH (usually >500pg/nL) with persistent ↑Ca^{2+}.
- PO_4 and alkaline phosphatase usually raised.
- If calcium is low or normal, ↑PTH indicates SHPT and further medical treatment is necessary.
- Calcimimetic therapy (🕮 p.180) may prove to have a role in reducing the need for parathyroidectomy and may be an alternative in those in whom surgery has failed, is refused or is deemed too high risk.
- Inappropriate parathyroidectomy may have deleterious consequences for the skeleton (→ low turnover disease).

Pre-op considerations

Imaging: isotope scans (e.g. MIBI) allow localization of the parathyroid glands prior to surgery and identify ectopic (e.g. retrosternal) tissue.

ENT: all patients should have their vocal cords visualized pre-op—there is a risk of damage to the recurrent laryngeal nerve during surgery so pre-existing problems need documentation.

Prevention of 'hungry bone syndrome': high dose vitamin D for a few days pre-op (e.g. alfacalcidol 4µg daily for five days) may help prevent rapid and severe falls in Ca^{2+} post-op (calcium influx into bone).

Post-op considerations

Haemorrhage: rare, but may cause tracheal compression. Monitor drains carefully.

Hypocalcaemia: may be profound in the days following surgery. Check Ca^{2+} 2-4h post-op, then 12h for 2-3 days. Give calcitriol or alfacalcidol 0.5–2.0µg/d with oral calcium (1–3g in divided doses. If serum Ca^{2+} falls below 1.8mmol/L or tetany develops, administer IV calcium (see 🕮 p.540 for regimen) and continue oral vitamin D.

PTH: measured post-op to ensure success.

Parathyroidectomy technique

The amount of parathyroid tissue removed at operation can be varied.

Partial parathyroidectomy: parathyroid tissue is deliberately left behind in an attempt to avoid the consequences of absent PTH (principally ABD). Unfortunately, further autonomous PTH secretion often necessitates repeat (and technically more difficult) surgery.

Total parathyroidectomy with re-implantation: parathyroid tissue is implanted into an extra-parathyroid site (usually the arm). This tissue is then more easily accessible if recurrent hyperparathyroidism develops. Unfortunately parathyroid re-growth in the neck remains common.

Total parathyroidectomy: attempted removal of all parathyroid tissue. Currently the favoured technique. Serum calcium is subsequently maintained with calcitriol or alfacalcidol. Regrowth of islands of parathyroid cells is not uncommon. Serum PTH will ↑ with time.

Radiological ablation: Ultrasound localization and ablation through ethanol injection has met with variable success.

Calciphylaxis

Definition

Calciphylaxis (calcific uraemic arteriolopathy) is a small vessel vasculopathy involving mural calcification with intimal proliferation, fibrosis, and thrombosis. It occurs predominantly in individuals with renal failure and results in ischaemia and necrosis of skin, soft tissue, visceral organs, and skeletal muscle.

Incidence

First described in 1962 and considered rare until recently. On an ESRD programme: incidence 1%, prevalence 4%. Mortality 80% at one year (almost always due to sepsis).

Presentation

- *Painful* erythematous livedo reticularis-like skin patches which ulcerate. Panniculitis and secondary infection follow.
- Two patterns recognized: (i) ulcers on the trunk, buttocks or thighs (over adipose tissue), and (ii) ulceration on the extremities.
- Not just the skin is affected—may also occur in arterioles supplying other organs (lung calcification on the CXR is common).
- Bone scans show ↑uptake over lesions.
- Skin biopsy is characteristic.

Risk factors

- Uraemia (though also seen post-transplantation, and in primary HPT)
- ↑ Calcium phosphate product
- ↑ PTH
- Vitamin D analogue use
- Race (Caucasian)
- ♀ > ♂
- Obesity (BMI >30)
- Warfarin use
- Protein C or S deficiency
- Diabetes mellitus
- Malnutrition.

Treatment

⚠ No treatment is of proven benefit.
- Scrupulous wound care.
- Aggressive treatment of sepsis.
- Lower CaxP: avoid calcium based binders, daily haemodialysis, lower dialysate Ca^{2+}.
- Parathyroidectomy *may* help if ↑PTH and ↑CaxP.
- Stop warfarin.
- Bisphosphonates, hyperbaric oxygen, sodium thiosulphate under study.
- Steroids probably of no benefit (⚠ sepsis).

Renal bone disease management summary

SHPT

- Check calcium, phosphate and PTH at least 3 monthly (more often if treatment changes made) in CKD 4 and 5. Annually in stage 3.
- In CKD stages 3 and 4, if PTH >70pg/mL measure serum 25-hydroxyvitamin D and consider replacement if <80nmol/L (<30µg/L).
- Control serum phosphate with combination of diet, phosphate binders and adequate dialysis.
- Once phosphate controlled, add alfacalcidol or calcitriol, titrating the dose up aiming for a target PTH according to CKD stage and a serum calcium in lower half of normal range.
- Uncontrolled SHPT: review diet, intensify phosphate binder and vitamin D therapy if possible. Consider paricalcitol and cinacalcet if high calcium limits further vitamin D treatment.
- If $\uparrow Ca^{2+}$, switch to non-calcium containing binder and consider lowering dialysate Ca^{2+}.
- Parathyroidectomy: last resort if medical management unsuccessful.

ABD

- Aim to increase PTH driven bone turnover.
  - Reduce or stop calcium containing binders and vitamin D analogues (aim for serum Ca^{2+} in the low normal range).
- Lowering the dialysate calcium concentration (HD and CAPD: 1.0mmol/L) may help $\downarrow Ca^{2+}$ and $\uparrow PTH$.
- Excluded significant aluminium deposition, if applicable.
- Exogenous PTH (pulsatile administration) and calcimimetics may prove to have an anabolic role in ABD as circadian PTH release is thought necessary for normal bone formation.

Cardiovascular disease in CKD

Patients with early CKD are at increased risk of CV disease — most will die a CV death before progressing to ESRD. Those starting RRT often do so with a high CV disease burden—dialysis patients are ~20x more likely to die a CV death than the general population. A cardiac cause of death is implicated in >40% of all deaths at ESRD. Several factors contribute.

Traditional cardiovascular risk factors more common in CKD

- Hypertension (almost always present) and LVH
- Diabetes (common cause of CKD)
- Dyslipidaemia
- Physical inactivity.

Risk factors common in (or unique to) uraemia

- Arteriosclerosis and diastolic dysfunction
- Albuminuria
- Volume overload
- Oxidant stress and inflammation
- Malnutrition
- Accumulation of advanced glycation end-products
- Left ventricular hypertrophy
- Hyperparathyoidism, calcium overload, and metastatic calcification
- Anaemia
- Myocardial fibrosis and possible abnormal myocyte function
- Nitric oxide/endothelin derangement
- Carnitine deficiency
- Hyperhomocysteinaemia.

Take 100 patients with an eGFR<60mL/min. ~ 1% will progress to ESRD each year. However, there is a 10% death rate (mainly CV disease), so after 10 years, 8 patients will require RRT, 27 will have 'smoldering' CKD and 65 will be dead.

▶ An estimated 8,000,000 people in the USA have an eGFR<60mL/min.

Managing risk factors

All CKD patients are at high risk of CV events. Microalbuminuria itself is an independent risk factor for cardiovascular outcomes, possibly because it is a marker of generalized endothelial dysfunction. Interventions should include:
- Lifestyle advice re: smoking, diet, obesity, exercise.
- Meticulous BP control.
- Management of lipids, usually with a statin (□ p.298).
- Glycaemic control (if diabetic).
- ☞ Good evidence for the benefit of such interventions in CKD patients is lacking—advice is currently based on extrapolation from the non-renal population.

Acute coronary syndrome (ACS) in CKD

▶ CKD is a significant predictor of mortality in ACS patients. ACS may present atypically (silent ischaemia, hypotension, collapse) in patients with advanced CKD. Typical chest pain and ST elevation are uncommon in dialysis patients. CKD patients with an ACS should receive standard management, but with some provisos:

- LVH (and strain) can complicate ECG interpretation.
- Cardiac enzymes:
  - CK may be non-specifically elevated in CKD.
  - Troponin levels may not be helpful. Troponin T, and to a lesser extent troponin I, are often elevated in CKD (and may be independent markers of CV risk). ▶ A significant ↑ level in the right context is likely to be a true positive (especially if rising).
- CKD and dialysis do not contraindicate thrombolysis. Recent renal biopsy, line insertion (especially if accidental arterial puncture), uncontrolled ↑BP (>200/110) or uraemic pericarditis might. Percutaneous coronary intervention may be preferable in these circumstances.
- Platelet function is deranged in uraemia: aspirin and clopidogrel carry a greater bleeding risk than in the general population. Studies on these agents have generally excluded patients with renal disease. Consensus is to administer them, unless bleeding risk is particularly high.
- Glycoprotein IIb/IIIa inhibitors require dose reduction.
- Low molecular weight heparins require dose adjustment if eGFR <30mL/min (→ 50% standard dose). Preliminary evidence suggests less bleeding risk with fondaparinux. Unfractionated heparin may be safer.
- Fluid status should be optimized: overloaded patients should be diuresed or dialysed.
- Correct anaemia. Tranfuse if necessary (on dialysis if fluid overload or hyperkalaemia). Aim for Hb 11–12g/dL.
- Beta blockers (⚠ may need dose reduction), statins, calcium channel blockers, and nitrates can be administered as usual.
- Hypotension peri-MI or ACS may cause ↑Cr in the CKD patient (→ temporary or permanent dialysis dependence).
- Haemodialysis in the context of an ongoing ACS may be dangerous (⚠ haemodynamic instability, arrhythmia). Treat in a high dependency environment. CRRT (📖 p.121) may be preferable.

Coronary angiography in the renal patient

✦ Angiography and emergency angioplasty may be the treatment of choice in the renal patient with ACS. However:
- Ensure adequate hydration and give NAC if time permits (📖 p.133).
- Minimize contrast dose if possible.
- These renoprotective measures apply equally to dialysis patients who retain significant residual renal function.
- Re-stenosis rates *may* be higher in CKD patients.
- Even with these attempts at renoprotection, a decline in renal function may follow intervention. ▶ Measure daily U+E until stable, and optimize fluid balance.

Pre-transplant work-up

CKD patients considered fit for potential transplantation merit cardiovascular work-up, as early post-transplant mortality is 50% cardiac. Prior to listing any potential recipient:

Recommended screening tests
- No test is ideal. Coronary angiography is sensitive and specific, but invasive and carries the risk of contrast nephropathy (📖 p.132).
- Less invasive screening tests (exercise stress test, thallium/sestamibi radionuclide imaging, dobutamine stress echocardiography) are relatively insensitive in this population (high pre-test probability of significant disease).

Screen according to risk
- Coronary angiography for all 'high risk' patients, defined as any patient with significant CKD who has one or more of:
  - History of ischaemic heart disease.
  - ECG compatible with ischaemic heart disease.
  - Diabetes mellitus.
  - Peripheral vascular disease.
- Duplex USS assessment of iliac and carotid arteries is also desirable.
- 'Medium risk' patients (age >50, smokers, history of hypertension or dyslipidaemia) should have non-invasive assessment followed by angiography if the results are positive or inconclusive (sensitivity of these tests is low, so threshold for angiography should also be low).
- 'Low risk' patients (non-smokers, age <50, non-diabetic, no clinically overt CV disease) do not require cardiac screening.

Intervention
Revascularization for clinically significant coronary lesions. Early studies suggested that angioplasty was less effective than bypass grafting. However, the introduction of stents (and more recently drug-eluting stents) is likely to have changed the risk/benefit ratio—further studies are awaited.

Uraemic cardiomyopathy

Probably not the result of one specific uraemic toxin, but of a combination of factors:

- ↑*Arterial stiffness:* ↑phosphate → vascular smooth muscle cell trans-differentiation into osteoblast-like cells, causing vascular medial calcification. This leads to arteriosclerosis, ↓arterial compliance, and ↑pulse pressure. This is analogous to the arterial changes seen in the elderly, but premature. The result is ↑cardiac workload and worsening LVH and diastolic dysfunction.
- *Cardiac fibrosis:* local and systemic angiotensin II and PTH → ↑cardiac stiffness, myocyte injury, and diastolic and systolic dysfunction.
- *Anaemia:* → ↑LVH and ↑cardiac work.
- *Myocyte dysfunction:* myocyte contractility is reduced, possibly as a result of changes in intracellular bioenergetics.

Table 3.6 Pre-transplant investigations

Age <50 non-diabetic	Age 50–60 non-diabetic	Age >60 non-diabetic	Diabetic
History	History	History	History
Examination	Examination	Examination	Examination
ECG	ECG	ECG	ECG
CXR	CXR	CXR	CXR
Tissue typing	Tissue typing	Tissue typing	Tissue typing
Virology*	Virology*	Virology*	Virology*
Patient information	Patient information	Patient information	Patient information
Surgical assessment	Non invasive cardiac testing	Non invasive cardiac testing	Non invasive cardiac testing (possible angiography)
	Leg arterial dopplers	Carotid dopplers	Carotid dopplers
	Surgical assessment	Leg arterial dopplers	Leg arterial dopplers
		Surgical assessment	Post-micturition bladder USS
			Surgical assessment

*Virology: hepatitis B & C, HIV, CMV, EBV, varicella-zoster (± HTLV 1 & 2)

Diet and nutrition in CKD

Dietary advice is extremely important in the management of CKD and the maintenance of broader health in CKD patients.

Measurement of nutritional status

▶ No single parameter should be considered in isolation.

Assessment should include:

- History and examination to identify ongoing medical problems which may limit nutritional intake—psychosocial issues may be important.
- *Dietary interview or diary:* quantitative intake of nutrients.
- *Subjective global assessment (SGA):* is a simple scoring (subjective and objective) made on history and examination. It is well-validated in CKD, and powerful enough to predict outcome.
- *Anthropometric measurements:* body mass index, skin-fold thickness, estimated percent weight loss, and mid-arm muscle circumference.
- *Serum albumin:* reflects not only protein intake, but susceptible to changes with inflammation or infection. A strong predictor of future mortality in new starters on dialysis.
- *Adequacy of dialysis:* inadequate dialysis is a common contributing factor to malnutrition (uraemic toxins are anorectic and pro-inflammatory). Dialysis adequacy (🕮 pp.213 and 234) should be assessed in conjunction with the normalized protein catabolic rate (nPCR), which is a measure of the rate of urea formation(🕮 p.211). When any patient is in steady state, urea formation correlates with protein intake and protein breakdown.

Fluid restriction

- CKD stages 4–5: fluid and salt restriction is often important to prevent volume overload.
- On dialysis: when the urine output drops, fluid restriction is vital to minimize weight gains. Aim for weight gains of 1–1.5 kg or less/day. In an anuric patient, this means a fluid restriction of 750–1000ml. This must be combined with salt restriction.

Protein intake

- Intake averages ~80g/day in the developed world, although requirements may be only 50g.
- A low protein diet has been shown to slow the progression of renal failure in patients with CKD (🕮 p.153). Set against this is the danger of patients reaching dialysis with significant malnutrition. Most units advocate no more than *moderate* protein restriction. Daily protein targets:
  - 0.8g/kg per day for CKD stages 3–5.
  - 1.2g/kg per day when on dialysis.
- Protein sources include meat, fish, eggs, milk, nuts, pulses, and beans.

Carbohydrate intake
- Adequate energy intake is essential for patient with CKD, especially those undergoing protein restriction.
- Target 30–35kcal/kg per day.
- Source: mainly complex carbohydrates, some from mono- or poly-unsaturated fats. Dovetailing a diabetic diet with a renal diet can be difficult.
- Examples: sugar, jams, marmalade, specialist high energy renal drinks.

Phosphate restriction (see also 📖 p.176)
- The kidney is the main route of phosphate excretion. Current guidelines suggest a restriction of dietary phosphate of 0.8–1g/day if:
  - Serum phosphate >1.5mmol/L in CKD stages 3–4 *or*
  - Serum phosphate >1.8mmol/L in CKD stage 5 *or*
  - ↑PTH
- Prescribe phosphate binders if dietary restriction alone fails (📖 p.176).
- Phosphate-rich foods include all protein-containing foods, making phosphate restriction difficult to achieve. Examples: milk, cheese, custard, yogurt, ice cream, cola, chocolate drinks, beer, liver, baked beans, dried peas, and beans (e.g. chick peas), nuts, whole grain products, bran cereals, many convenience foods.

Potassium restriction
- Typical UK intake ~50–120mmol/day. With failing renal function, potassium excretion falls making potassium restriction necessary (esp. in patients taking ACEI or ARBs).
- K^+-rich foods include dairy products, potatoes (baked, chips, and crisps), some fruits (bananas, grapes, dried fruit, fresh pineapple), fresh fruit juice, tomatoes, sweet corn, mushrooms, chocolate, and coffee.

Salt restriction
- Typical UK intake ~150–200mmol/day (or 9–12g).
- This is a vast excess over physiological needs.
- Salt restriction is helpful if ↑BP ± volume overload (helps reduce thirst and hence fluid intake). Aim for an intake of <5–6g/day.
- Na^+-rich foods include cheese, salted butter/margarine, salted meat (bacon, ham), tinned meat, vegetables and soups, packaged meals.

There are several resources on the internet that can help patients and their families understand and adjust to these dietary restrictions. The nutrition section of the National Kidney Foundation (US) website is a good starting point (www.kidney.org)—even containing a complete cookbook.

Malnutrition in CKD

Malnutrition is common in CKD (affecting up to 50% of dialysis patients), and a powerful predictor of survival. Contributors include:
- Anorectic uraemic toxins (leptin)
- Chronic low-grade inflammation
- Dietary restriction (low protein diet)
- Medication (phosphate binders, iron)
- Dialysis itself (esp. CAPD, where protein losses into the dialysate may be 1–2g/L, or ~10g/day: this would be considered nephrotic range if lost in the urine!).

Managing malnutrition in the CKD patient
- Assess the severity of malnutrition (📖 p.190).
- Measure current nutritional intake.
- Address correctable factors:
  - ► Correct under-dialysis (e.g. change modality, improve access).
  - Seek and treat occult infection.
  - Investigate and treat gut problems or gastroparesis.
  - Define and intervene if psychosocial problems.
- Consider dietary supplements. A wide range are available. Renal-specific oral supplements are low in potassium/phosphate and are concentrated (limiting the volume of fluid given).
- Overnight naso-enteral (or PEG) feeding may be beneficial in more severe cases of malnutrition when adequate oral intake cannot be maintained.
- IDPN = intra-dialytic parenteral nutrition. Given on dialysis, it provides amino acids, glucose and lipids. It is not a substitute for oral supplements, but can deliver ~1500kcal/session (of which ~500kcal is lost in dialysate!). Can be a useful adjunct if the patient is able to manage 50% of the desired daily intake by mouth.
- Amino acid containing PD solutions (Nutrineal®) may offer benefit in malnourished PD patients ●※
- Total parenteral nutrition (TPN) should be reserved for those who cannot be fed enterally. Electrolyte quantities (particularly potassium, phosphate and magnesium) should be reduced and monitored daily.
- ●※ Appetite stimulants/anabolic agents are of uncertain benefit:
  - Growth hormone (costly).
  - Nandrolone (an androgen) by weekly IMI (100 mg ♂, 50mg ♀).
  - Ghrelin offers some promise in CAPD patients.

Inflammation in CRF

Patients with CKD have ongoing low-grade inflammation, with ↑acute phase proteins (CRP, ferritin), ↑inflammatory cytokines, hypoalbuminaemia and hypercholesterolaemia. Contributors include:
- Repeated infections
- Oxidant stress (decreased levels of anti-oxidants, increased oxidative and carbonyl stress)
- Accumulation of AGE products
- Arteriosclerosis and abnormal endothelial function
- Malnutrition (both a cause and an effect of chronic inflammation).

Protein–energy malnutrition may co-exist—there is increasing evidence that chronic inflammation and oxidant stress increase metabolic demands and predispose to malnutrition. The triad of malnutrition, inflammation, and accelerated atherosclerosis has been labelled the *MIA syndrome*. A vicious cycle may commence, often culminating in death from cardiac disease. This may account for the apparent paradox that patients on dialysis with a higher body mass index tend to survive longer.

Endocrine problems in CKD

Thyroid function

Tests may be difficult to interpret as thyroid binding globulin is lost in the urine if heavy proteinuria, causing a ↓ measured T4. Clinical assessment and measurement of T3 and TSH may be necessary for correct interpretation.

Adrenal axis function

Addison's disease is difficult to diagnose in the context of CKD, especially in dialysis patients, as the characteristic electrolyte changes may be masked by renal dysfunction and dialysis. Suspect if persistent hypotension (or postural hypotension). Many renal patients have received corticosteroid therapy, with consequent steroid-related side-effects (📖 p.372).

Sexual dysfunction (♀)

Reduced libido frequent. Comorbidity (vascular disease, diabetes) and concomitant drug treatment may be relevant. Altered body image and self-perception may also play a role, as may depression and anxiety. Offer counseling. ► Anaemia contributes to reduced libido and should be corrected. Disturbances in menstruation and fertility are common. Amenorrhoea is virtually ubiquitous at ESRD. Gynaecological assessment is often helpful. Pregnancy in CKD and dialysis is discussed in Chapter 10.

Sexual dysfunction (♂)

Erectile dysfunction is common. It may be multifactorial (arterial disease, neuropathy, psychological factors, side-effects of drug treatment). Where possible, treat the underlying cause. Testosterone deficiency is not uncommon in dialysis patients and should be corrected with replacement therapy. Sildenafil (Viagra®) is effective, but should be avoided in patients on nitrates, with significant coronary artery disease or hypotension. Vacuum devices or penile implants may be useful, esp. if physical cause for impotence.

Hyperprolactinaemia

Elevated circulating prolactin concentrations, 2° to increased secretion and decreased clearance, are common in advanced CKD. Causes galactorrhea (♀) and gynaecomastia (♂). Bromocriptine may normalize levels. The contribution of ↑prolactin to sexual dysfunction in both sexes is unclear.

Early menopause

Not associated with CKD per se, but may occur in patients treated with cyclophosphamide or other cytotoxic agents.

Growth retardation

Resistance to growth hormone (GH) is an important consequence of advanced CKD. Although circulating GH levels are normal (or elevated), resistance to its action causes growth retardation in children and muscle wasting in adults. This resistance is the consequence of multiple defects in the GH/IGF-1 axis: GH receptor expression is down-regulated as is activity of the downstream JAK/STAT signal transduction pathway. IGF-1 (a major mediator of GH action) expression and activity is also significantly reduced. Growth delay can now be treated with recombinant GH. Other contributors to growth retardation are steroid therapy, malnutrition, and renal osteodystrophy.

Palliative treatment of advanced CKD

The decision not to have dialysis

- Patients who start dialysis with significant co-morbidity and functional dependence typically only survive a few months—months which may be filled with hospital admissions, painful illnesses, and unpleasant procedures.
- For such patients, continuing supportive care without commencing dialysis, may allow a better quality of life with little or no reduction in life expectancy.
- The decision whether to commence dialysis at ESRD is ultimately made by the patient (assuming the patient has capacity). The renal team has a duty to ensure that this decision is as informed as possible, by explaining the implications of withholding dialysis and the pros and cons of commencing it. Family members should also be involved.
  - The process cannot be rushed. A decision not to accept dialysis should be made over time, and be consistently held.
  - Patients may (and often do) change their minds (in either direction).
  - If severely uraemic, a patient may be unable to be involved in the decision making process.
  - It can often be difficult to determine whether debility is uraemic in origin (and ∴ potentially reversible), or 2° pre-existing comorbidity.
  - Patients referred late have no time to go through the pre-dialysis counseling process and may be denied the opportunity to make informed decisions about their care.

Symptomatic management of ESRD

As uraemia advances, so do uraemic symptoms (📖 Chapter 1). However, with prompt symptomatic treatment, patients can feel reasonably well and remain active until the very end of life. Many units now run a service specifically for such patients, concentrating resources and care to include:

- Physical and social support—patients may become increasingly reliant on family members ± other carers. District nurses, social workers, home care teams, physiotherapists, and occupational therapists can be involved as required.
- Diet: anorexia is common. Medroxyprogesterone 100–200mg daily may stimulate appetite. Check for oral candida and if present, treat with fluconazole 50–100mg daily. Harsh dietary restrictions may be inappropriate and can be relaxed.
- Taste disturbance: try zinc 220mg qds.
- Nausea and vomiting: consider conventional anti-emetics (e.g. cyclizine 25–50mg tds, metoclopromide 5mg tds, haloperidol 0.5–2.0mg od). If dyspeptic symptoms: PPI (e.g. lansoprazole 30mg od). Constipation may be contributory: use laxatives early.
- Confusion (usually a late development): check for reversible causes (e.g. ↓Na^+, ↑Ca^{2+}, constipation, drug toxicity).
- Seizures are rare: manage acutely with benzodiazepines.
- Skin: dry skin, pruritis and excoriation are common. Control ↑PO_4 and SHPT (often the cause), use emollients (e.g. aqueous cream, E45®, Diprobase®), Oilatum® in bath water, antihistamines may give some

relief (e.g. cetirizine 5mg od), if localized try capsaisin 0.025% cream (SE: burning sensation). Thalidomide 100mg nocte if intractable (SE: neuropathy).
- Acidosis: may cause dypnoea and exhaustion. Consider $NaHCO_3$.
- Dyspnoea: if pulmonary oedema consider diuretics, bronchodilators, ?O_2: give advice on sleeping position.
- Anaemia: transfusion, IV iron, EPO.
- Anxiety and depression (▶ common and should be actively sought): lorazepam 0.5-1mg orally, opiates, SSRIs (e.g. citalopram 20mg od).
- Restless legs: correct anaemia and iron deficiency. Clonazepam 250–500µg nocte. Co-careldopa 12.5/50mg nocte (may give short term relief, but worsen symptoms over time), pergolide 25µg nocte (SE: nausea).
- Pain control: as in all palliative care, the WHO 'analgesic ladder' should be used with gradual escalation of drug potency.
    - Paracetamol in therapeutic doses is safe and effective in uraemia.
    - NSAIDs are usually contra-indicated (worsen remaining renal function).
    - Opioids are often required in the terminal stages (see box, p.198).
- Psychological support: this is a terminal illness, and patients need appropriate support.

Withdrawal of dialysis
- As with the decision not to start dialysis, the decision to withdraw should be made by the patient with the help and support of the multidisciplinary team.
- Withdrawal means that death will probably occur within a few days if the patient has no significant residual renal function. The decision to withdraw may be prompted by a catastrophic medical event (e.g. a CVA, loss of vascular access). Less often, it is the culmination of a number of smaller events which has, in the view of the patient, had unacceptable consequences for their quality of life.
- ⚠ Depression should be looked for and treated as it may be influencing the decision.
- The decision to withdraw should be made over a period of time, and be held consistently.

Care of the dying patient
- The patient should be able to die peacefully and with dignity, in a place of his or her choosing, surrounded by loved ones. This requires planning, so that care at home, in a hospice, or in hospital can be arranged at short notice.
- Care pathways (e.g. Liverpool Care Pathway for the Dying) may facilitate the management of the last few days of life.
- Family support: before death family members may be involved in the physical care of the patient, and need support and help. At the time of death and afterwards, help should be available to cope with the grieving process (this will need to be culturally appropriate).

Prescribing opioids in renal failure

Effective, but use with caution. Opiates accumulate and may cause significant side-effects (e.g. drowsiness, confusion, respiratory depression, twitching and seizures). Consider:

- Tramadol (50mg tds po) for mild-to-moderate pain not controlled by non-opioids.
- Hydromorphone 1.3mg 4 hourly + 1.3mg prn for more severe pain (titrate dose up daily if necessary).
- Fentanyl transdermal patch (25mcg/hr) for stable severe pain. Equivalent to 8–16mg hydromorphone or 60–120mg morphine. Increase dose when oral opiate dose reaches this level.
- Avoid morphine if possible as breakdown products more likely to accumulate and cause unwanted side effects .

Renal replacement therapy

RRT: a brief history

In the last 40 years it has become possible to keep ESRD patients alive.

1861	Term 'dialysis' first coined
1913	First 'artificial kidney' built and used in animals
1923	First human PD
1924	First human HD
1933	First (unsuccessful) cadaveric kidney transplant
1946	First dialysis in UK
1946	PD used to treat ARF
1947	First cadaveric kidney transplant. Patient had pregnancy related ARF. Graft placed externally (on arm) and lasted 6 days (and ARF had resolved)
1948	Kolff–Brigham dialyser developed—a major technological advance
1948	HD used to treat ARF in the Korean war
Early 1950s	Cadaveric transplants for CRF (into thigh with ureterostomy); no immunosuppression—all rejected within 6 months.
1954	First successful monozygotic twin transplant[*]
1959	Non-monozygotic twin transplant (with whole body irradiation as immunosuppression)
1959	Intermittent PD, with repeated abdominal puncture, described
1960	Peter Medawar and Franc Burnet receive Nobel Prize for describing principles of immunologic rejection
1960	Scribner shunt—the first access device enabling repetitive use
1960	First long term HD patients (Seattle USA)
1962	6-mercaptopurine used successfully for immunosuppression
1963	Steroids and azathioprine used with greater success
1964	First home HD patients
1966	Cross-matching introduced
1966	Forearm AVF developed
1967	First successful liver and heart transplants
1968	Tenckhoff PD catheter introduced
1975	Haemofiltration introduced
1976	Introduction of ciclosporin—1 year graft survival dramatically improves
1977	Continuous AV haemofiltration described
1976	Continuous ambulatory peritoneal dialysis (CAPD) introduced
1982	First kidney pancreas transplant
1990	[*]Joseph Murray awarded Nobel Prize for his pioneering transplant work.

Introduction

Normal functioning kidneys:
- Remove excess salt, water and acid.
- Remove or regulate other electrolytes (e.g. K^+, Ca^{2+}, Mg^{2+}, PO_4).
- Remove waste products of metabolism (Ur and Cr measured routinely, but many others).
- Make EPO.
- 1 α hydroxylate ($\therefore$ activate) vitamin D.

Dialysis acts as surrogate for all but the last two of these (which can be achieved pharmacologically). Even at best, it is only partially effective. Transplantation completely replaces normal kidney function and should be regarded as the optimum treatment of ESRD. Transplanted patients survive longer and have a better quality of life. However, not everyone is fit for transplantation—ESRD patients are often frail with appreciable co-morbidity, especially vascular disease.

Facts and figures

The number of people receiving RRT is expected to ~double over the next 10 years. Eventually it will reach 'steady state'—number of patients starting dialysis = those leaving through transplantation, withdrawal or death.

The current UK acceptance rate for RRT is 104pmp (~6,000 patients annually). This is lower than most developed countries (Table 4.1). There are wide regional variations explained (partly) by demographic factors (ethnic populations → ↑incidence of CKD).

2003 UK Renal registry data showed:
- The established RRT modality after 3 months was HD in 67.5%, PD in 19.2%, and transplant in 3.3%.
- Of those patients initially established on HD after 3 years: 42% remained on this modality, 3% had switched to PD, 12% had received transplants and 40% had died.
- Of patients initially established on PD after 3 years: 29% remained on this modality, 23% had switched to HD, 21% had been transplanted and 25% had died.

In the UK 22% of new RRT patients and 12% of prevalent RRT patients are ≥ age 75.

Resources

- Current cost of RRT is estimated at 1–2% of the total NHS budget (whilst affecting only 0.05% of the population).
- Average cost of HD in a satellite unit is ~£21,000 per annum.
- Transplantation is the most cost effective form of RRT.

Morbidity and mortality

In the UK, 35% of RRT patients die from cardiac disease, 20% from infection, 13% from withdrawal of dialysis, 9% from malignancy, and 7% from cerebrovascular disease

Table 4.1 RRT treatment rates by country. From the UK National
Service Framework for renal services, part 1[1]

Country	New patients starting treatment (pmp)	Overall number of patients (pmp)
United States	336	1403
Germany	184	919
Greece	163	812
Belgium (Dutch speaking)	160	855
Spain (Catalonia)	146	1022
Denmark	138	679
Italy	136	835
Austria	136	750
Sweden	124	735
New Zealand	119	655
Wales	105*	641*
Scotland	101	644
Netherlands	100	639
Australia	97	633
Norway	94	606
England	91*	547*

* Estimate from partial coverage of UK Renal Registry

1 Available at www.doh.gov.uk/NSF/renal

Data sources: US Renal Data Service, ERA-EDTA Registry, UK Renal Registry, ANZ Data, QuaSi-Niere, Italian Registry of Dialysis and Transplantation (RIDT)

Haemodialysis (HD)

What is HD?

- During dialysis blood is exposed to dialysate (a solution containing physiological concentrations of electrolytes) across a semi-permeable membrane.
- Pores in the membrane allow small molecules (e.g. Ur [MW=60 Da], Cr [113 Da]) and electrolytes, but not larger ones (e.g. plasma proteins [albumin 60,000 Da, IgG 140,000 Da]), or blood cells to pass through.
- Concentration differences across the membrane allow molecules to diffuse down a gradient. This allows waste products to be removed and desirable molecules or ions (e.g. HCO_3) to be replaced.
- Water can be driven through the membrane by hydrostatic force (ultrafiltration or UF).
  - By varying the pressure gradient across the membrane (trans-membrane pressure or TMP) the amount of water removed can be controlled.
  - In addition to a means to remove water (~1–4L) that has accumulated between dialysis sessions (ingestion of fluid, foods and by-product of metabolism) UF can also be used as a means of solute clearance by convection (see haemofiltration below).

Haemofiltration (HF)

- In addition to *diffusion*, fluid shifts across the dialysis membrane also allow solutes to cross by *convection* (termed 'solute drag'). This underlies the technique of haemofiltration.
- Because large volumes of fluid must cross the membrane to enable significant solute removal, physiological fluid *replacement* is mandatory to avoid hypovolaemia.
- During routine haemodialysis, HF is used only as a means of removing fluid that has accumulated between sessions ∴ no fluid replacement is necessary.
- In continuous techniques (📖 p.121), as used on ITU, HF plays a more prominent role. It may also be combined with diffusion in *haemodiafiltration* (see box opposite).

What is required for haemodialysis?

- Vascular access (indwelling venous catheter, arteriovenous fistula, or arteriovenous graft 📖 p.214): large volumes of blood must be removed from the patient, exposed to a dialysis membrane, and then returned.
- Anti-coagulation (📖 p.212): prevents blood clotting in the extra-corporeal circuit (usually with heparin).
- Dialysis membrane (📖 p.208): as biocompatible as possible, with an adequate surface area and permeability to facilitate solute clearance and ultrafiltration.
- Dialysate (📖 p.206): of sufficient purity and containing the required concentration of electrolytes.
- Effective control and safety mechanisms (📖 p.206): blood and dialysate flow, TMP, temperature, detection of blood leaks or air.

Haemodialysis and haemofiltration

Haemodialysis

- Solute clearance by diffusion (mainly).
- Dialysate is required.
- Diffusion is maximized by maintaining high flow rates of blood and dialysate and by pumping the two through the dialyser in countercurrent directions.
- Larger MW (>20KDa) molecules are generally poorly removed.
- Usually administered intermittently (e.g. 4h, 3×/week).

Haemofiltration

- Solute clearance by convection (mainly).
- Achieved by generating a TMP across the membrane.
- No dialysate required.
- Large volumes need to be filtered to achieve adequate solute clearance. This would cause hypovolaemia unless replacement fluid administered (usually pre-prepared 5–10L bags).
- Removes larger MW (30–50KDa) molecules (e.g. vitamin B12 and β_2-microglobulin) more efficiently than dialysis.
- Continuous (24h) HF is associated with greater haemodynamic stability and often favoured for RRT in an ITU setting (📖 p.118).

Haemodiafiltration

- Combines HD and HF to get the best of both modalities.
- Use is growing in many outpatient dialysis facilities.
- Set up as for HD, but with a higher TMP to produce a significant filtration.
- Both dialysate and replacement fluid are required.
- 'On-line' generation of replacement fluid is now available in some centres—fluid is produced from ultra-pure water and dialysate within the dialysis machine itself. This ↓cost and dispenses with the need for unwieldy bags of fluid in the dialysis unit.

HD apparatus

Principle
Blood is removed from the patient, anti-coagulated, pumped through a dialyser, and then returned to the patient (Fig. 4.1). Within the dialyser blood and dialysate (flowing in opposite directions) are separated by a semipermeable dialysis membrane.

Dialysate
- A solution of purified water, Na^+ (132–150mmol/L), K^+ (usually 1.0–3.0mmol/L), Ca^{2+} (1.0–1.25mmol/L), Mg^{2+}, Cl^-, dextrose, and buffer.
- Purified water is generated in a treatment plant (involves microfilters, activated carbon, deionization, and reverse osmosis).
- UK Renal Association standards for water purity are <0.25IU/mL endotoxin, <100cfu/mL microbial count.
- H^+ ions have a low plasma concentration and are not removed by dialysis. Buffer (alkali equivalent) is ∴ added to dialysate.
- Bicarbonate is now preferred to acetate as a buffer.
- HD machines either mix dialysate concentrate, buffer, and water for the individual patient or this is done centrally before distribution around several machines.

Alarms and monitors
These will stop the blood pump and clamp lines if the situation demands.
- Air detectors: located distally in the venous circuit, prevent air emboli.
- Pressure monitors:
  - Arterial → detect ↓pressure 2° to poor access flow and line disconnections.
  - Venous →: detect ↑pressure 2° to resistance to venous return (usually represents an access problem).
  - Dialysate outflow pressure → monitor TMP (to vary UF rate).
- Dialyser integrity.
- Temperature.
- Conductivity:
  - Electrical conductivity is used to monitor proportioning of dialysate to water.
  - Many machines use conductivity to enable changes to Na^+ concentration ('Na^+ profiling') (📖 p.218).

Newer machines
- Blood volume monitoring: haematocrit (Hct) in the arterial line is used as a surrogate for blood volume (↓plasma H_2O → ↑Hct). Used to fine tune UF and BP control.
- Access recirculation measurements: ensures the same small volume of blood is not dialysed repetitively.
- Delivered Kt/V: Ur concentration in the dialysate outflow line or dialysate conductivity used to calculate delivered dialysis dose.

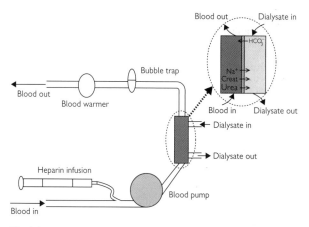

Fig. 4.1 The HD circuit

Apparatus

- Blood pump: usually a roller 'peristaltic' pump.
- Bubble trap: traps air → ↓risk of air embolism.
- Heparin (📖 p.212): the HD machine is primed with heparinized saline and further heparin is administered as an infusion or intermittent bolus into the arterial side of the extracorporeal circulation.
- Blood flow rate: usually 200–500mL/min
- Dialysate flow rate: usually 500mL/min
- Heaters: dialysate and blood are kept at 37°C.
- Dialyser: a rigid polyurethrane shell (~30cm long) containing hollow fibres (capillaries) of dialysate membrane. This arrangement maximizes the available surface area for dialysis (0.5–2.1m^2). Two ports each allow blood and dialysate to enter and exit. Priming volume ~50–100mL. To reduce cost dialysers are often re-sterilized and used again (rare in UK, common in USA and several other countries).
- Dialyser efficiency: depends on membrane thickness, pore size and dialyser structure. Efficiency of solute clearance is measured as KoA (mass transfer urea coefficient), provided for each dialyser by the manufacturer. KoA varies from 300 to 1100 (>600 = high efficiency dialyser, requiring higher blood and dialysate flows).

Dialysers and membranes

Biocompatibility
- Dialysis membranes are not inert. They can activate complement and inflammatory cascades (→ short and long-term complications).
- A biocompatible membrane is one that elicits the minimum inflammatory response in patients exposed to it.
- Improved biocompatibility may →
  - ↓hypersensitivity reactions
  - Less intradialytic ↓BP
  - Slower loss of residual renal function
  - Improved nutrition
  - ↓amyloid deposition
  - ↓morbidity and mortality (✻).

Cellulose membranes (e.g. Cuprophan®)
- The original membrane and least biocompatible.
- Largely superseded by synthetic membranes.

Modified cellulose (e.g. Hemophan®, Diaphan®)
More biocompatible.

Synthetic membranes (e.g. Polysulfone®, polyamide, polyacrylnitrile)
- Recently developed.
- Most biocompatible.
- More permeable than cellulose membranes:
  - Solute clearance similar to cellulose membranes.
  - ↑β_2-microglobulin clearance.

High vs. low flux
High flux membranes are usually synthetic membranes with a large pore size → enhanced clearance of middle and large molecules. ✻ May lead to better outcomes.

Surface area
↑Dialyser surface area (usually 0.5–2.1m^2) → ↑delivered dialysis.

HD prescription

Introduction

Intermittent HD places exacting demands on a patient. As it only partially replaces renal function, fluid and dietary restrictions remain of paramount importance.

Dialysis can be considered adequate if it provides relief of uraemic symptoms and controls acidosis, fluid balance, and serum K^+. It should also allow a feeling of physical and psychological well being.

Aspects of dialysis adequacy

- *Solute clearance.* Small molecule clearance is relatively easy to measure (see box opposite). Aim to achieve a target Kt/V of >1.2 or URR >65%.
- *Blood pressure and fluid balance.* As a general rule, ↑BP in a dialysis patient should be treated by ↓'dry weight' (i.e. post dialysis weight). This should be the weight at which salt and water balance are optimal. Oligo-anuric patients (majority of chronic HD patients) need to restrict their inter-dialytic salt and fluid intake in order to achieve this, aiming for weight gains of 1–2.5kg (maximum) between sessions. Targets:
  - Pre-dialysis BP <140/90
  - Post-dialysis BP <130/80
  - Preferably without anti-hypertensive agents.
- *Nutrition.* Blood Ur levels depend on rate of production as well as rate of excretion. ⚠ A low pre-dialysis Ur may reflect poor nutrition rather than good dialysis. Targets:
  - Serum albumin >35g/L
  - nPCR >1.0 g/kg/day (see box opposite)
  - Acceptable anthropometric measures.
- *Clearance of other molecules*:
  - 'Middle' molecule clearance thought to be important to prevent the long-term complications of dialysis. β_2 microglobulin is the most used marker.
  - Phosphate clearance is also important, and appears to correlate more with hours of dialysis than rate of small molecule clearance.
- *Quality of life and life expectancy.* There is a trade off to be made between the number of hours spent on the machine (∴↑dialysis dose) and quality of life. For patients with a limited life expectancy, the latter may be a more important consideration.

Measuring dialysis adequacy

In the 1980s The National Cooperative Dialysis Study (NCDS) established timed average Ur concentration as a determinant of morbidity and mortality on HD. Subsequent mathematical analysis of this data has led to the development of urea kinetic modelling (UKM) as the accepted method of measuring small solute clearance.

Kt/V is a measure of Ur clearance where:
- K = dialyser urea clearance
- t = time on dialysis
- V = volume of distribution of Ur (estimated from patient size).

The *single-pool Kt/V* assumes that at the end of dialysis the concentrations of intracellular and extracellular Ur are equal:

$spKt/V = -\ln[Upost/Upre-0.008t]+[4-3.5Upost/Upre] \times UFvol/wt\ post$

Upre = urea pre-dialysis; Upost = urea post-dialysis: UFvol = volume removed on dialysis

The *two compartment model* acknowledges that in reality it takes time for Ur to be redistributed post-dialysis and that the extracellular Ur concentration is lower than intracellular. An equilibrated Kt/V or eKt/V can be calculated from the spKt/V.

A simpler measurement of Ur clearance is the *urea reduction ratio* (URR), which does not take account of the amount of fluid removed by ultrafiltration. It is thus less accurate, but has been shown to correlate with outcome:

$URR = (1- Upre/Upost) \times 100$

Normalized protein catabolic rate (nPCR)

A measure of Ur generation, which reflects nutritional status. It can only be reliably used in patients who are 'stable' when Ur generation will broadly reflect protein intake. It is felt that patients require an nPCR >1.0g/kg/day. nPCR of <0.8g/kg/day is associated with higher mortality.

Residual function

When HD is first commenced, residual renal function may contribute greatly to the total amount of solute clearance (Kru). This is usually calculated with a 24h urine collections. Residual function tends to diminish quickly on HD ($\rightarrow$ repetitive ↓BP ± bio-incompatibility) (📖 p.208).

Variables in the dialysis prescription

- *Number of sessions per week.* Less than three usually means inadequate dialysis (unless there is significant residual renal function). Daily (or nocturnal) dialysis delivers excellent biochemistry and quality of life scores, but is only practical in a few enthusiastic (and well resourced) centers with equally enthusiastic patients. Most patients dialyse three times per week.
- *Number of hours per session.* As above, the more the better, though there are diminishing returns as the number of hours is increased. Control of BP, phosphate, and middle molecule clearance are easier to achieve with longer hours.
- *Blood flow.* Higher blood flow rates = more dialysis if all else equal. A blood flow rate of <250ml/min is suboptimal. Thus inadequate access = inadequate dialysis.
- *Dialyser size and type.* The larger the surface area of the dialyser, the greater the delivered dose of dialysis per unit time. High flux dialysers have larger pore sizes, and are able to deliver enhanced middle molecule clearance per unit time if blood flows are adequate. Studies have yet to show long term benefits.
- *Haemodiafiltration.* May deliver enhanced middle molecule clearance, phosphate clearance, haemodyamic stability, and ($\bullet$) life expectancy.
- *Dialysate composition and flow rate.* The concentrations of Na^+, K^+, Ca^{2+} and HCO_3^- may be altered in the dialysate. Higher flows may enhance clearance.

Anticoagulation

The extra-corporeal circuit will usually clot without anticoagulation.

Aim: Minimize risk of dialyser clotting the blood, whilst minimizing risk of bleeding complications in the patient.

Heparin is usually used, with a bolus of 1000–5000 units (~50U/kg) at the start of dialysis given into the 'arterial' side of the extracorporeal circuit followed by an infusion of 1000–1500 units/h, stopping 15–60 min before the end of the session. Usually monitored by measurement of activated clotting time (ACT) on the dialysis unit. Normal: 90–140s, target 200–250s (baseline +80%). Intermittent boluses according to ACT can also be given.

Patients at ↑bleeding risk are given 'tight reduced' or no heparin, accepting the increased risk of clotting. Heparin induced thrombocytopenia (HIT) is a rare complication associated with long term heparin use. LMW heparin can also be used an anticoagulation for dialysis. It is usually given as a single dose pre-treatment, but is much more expensive than unfractionated heparin. Prostacyclin (infused IV at 4–8ng/15g/min) and citrate (complex administration protocol!) are alternatives, especially if bleeding risk is high.

Ensuring adequate small solute clearance is delivered

Kt/V

UK and US guidelines suggest a single pool Kt/V >1.2 for patients dialysed x3/week, equating to a URR of ~65%. The landmark HEMO study compared two target Kt/V levels. Patients with a target Kt/V of 1.2 had no difference in mortality or cardiac events compared to those with a Kt/V of 1.6.

Residual renal function should always be taken into account.

Prescribed versus delivered Kt/V

Most guidelines suggest monthly measurement of Kt/V. On-line methods of measuring Kt/V are provided on modern dialysis machines (often using Na^+ clearance to estimate urea clearance).

If Kt/V fails to meet target, options are to:
- Improve vascular access: if flows are poor, or if there is access recirculation, it will be hard to improve clearances.
- Increase blood flow/ larger needles—beneficial if access reasonable.
- Increase dialyser size—modest impact.
- Increase dialysate flow.
- Increase dialysis time/frequency—major benefit.

Computer modelling software can help decide which elements of the prescription require modification to improve Kt/V.

⚠ HD adequacy is multi-faceted. Achieving a desired Kt/V does not necessarily equate to optimal dialysis.

Vascular access

Introduction

Reliable vascular access is the cornerstone of HD therapy and timely planning of access creation is a major facet of CKD care. ~25% of all admissions in the dialysis population relate to access failure or other complication and remain an important source of morbidity and mortality.

- *AV fistula.* The optimal form of vascular access. Requires the surgical anastamosis of an artery and a vein (under LA or GA), either at the wrist (radiocephalic) or elbow (brachiocephalic, brachiobasilic). If suitability of veins is in doubt then vascular mapping with USS is desirable. Maturation for 6–8 weeks (minimum) is required prior to needling (∴ advance planning crucial).
- *PTFE graft.* Second best. A synthetic graft is interposed between an artery and a vein. A larger operation than AVF creation. Necessary if veins inadequate to fashion an AVF (e.g. DM, previous phlebotomy/ cannulation). Lower limb (femoral loop) sites possible in addition to upper limb. Useable within days, but thrombosis and infection (usually necessitating removal) are problematic. Half-life shorter than AVF.
- *Tunnelled (and cuffed) dialysis catheter.* A dual lumen (or two single lumen) venous catheter is placed in a central vein (internal jugular or subclavian; femoral less common). Available for immediate use and usually left in situ for 1–3 months (occasionally longer). A useful bridge until an AVF matures. Blood flows (300–450mL/min) lower than AVF or graft.
- *Temporary dialysis catheter* (📖 p.634). For immediate use (ARF). Internal jugular, subclavian, or femoral should ideally be left in situ ≤2 weeks (femoral: <5 days). Much higher infection risk than other forms of access.

Principles of vascular access monitoring

- Poor access flow: inadequate arterial inflow, venous stenosis, intra-access thrombosis, poor needle positioning.
- Normal blood flow is 800–2000mL/min (graft >AVF). Poor flow → poor dialysis and ↑risk of thrombosis.
- Measuring flow:
  - Venous pressures: measured whilst on dialysis. High (or rising) pressures (>150mmHg at 200mL/min pump speed) may indicate venous obstruction (examine for evidence of collateral venous enlargement).
  - Serial measurements of flow can be made with USS dilution techniques. Flow <600mL/min or 25% decrease from baseline predicts significant stenoses and impending thrombosis.
  - Further investigations: doppler USS, fistulography (± balloon angioplasty).

Fistula care: what every doctor and patient should know

- Dialysis access is extremely precious.
- Arm veins should be preserved in pre-dialysis patients (no IV cannulae between elbow and wrist).
- Needling should only be carried out by a trained operator (usually a dialysis nurse, ideally the patient).
- Technique: avoid using the same site repetitively (→ false aneurysm formation).
- Never put a tourniquet or BP cuff on a fistula arm.
- Do not use a fistula to take blood.
- Hypotension → ↑thrombosis risk.
- ↑Hct (too much EPO) predisposes to thrombosis. Keep within recommended guidelines, and at the lower end of these if at risk.
- A clotted fistula or graft requires immediate attention (time to declotting is a major determinant of success).

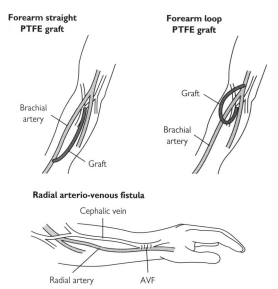

Forearm straight PTFE graft

Brachial artery

Graft

Forearm loop PTFE graft

Graft

Brachial artery

Radial arterio-venous fistula

Cephalic vein

Radial artery   AVF

Fig. 4.2 Permanent vascular access for haemodialysis

Reproduced with permission from Levy J, Morgan J, and Brown E (2004). *Oxford Handbook of Dialysis*, 2nd edn. Oxford: Oxford University Press

Complications of vascular access

Lines

▶ *Infection*
- Mortality 2° sepsis is 100–300 fold higher in dialysis patients compared to the general population.
- Fever in a HD patient with a line = line sepsis until proven otherwise.
- Infection of temporary lines is extremely common (15–60% insertions) Risk ↑ with duration of use. For tunneled lines: 3–4 episodes per 1000 catheter days (0.7–1.5 episodes/yr).
- Causes: ~70% → *Staph. aureus* (⚠MRSA) or *Staph. epidermidis*. Gram–ve organisms more common with femoral catheters.
- Sterile insertion technique (📖 p.634) and meticulous nursing care mandatory.
- Eradication of *Staph.* carriage may ↓ incidence (e.g. nasal Mupirocin cream).

Clinical features
- Usually presents with fever, rigors, ± ↓BP whilst on dialysis. Also N+V, diarrhoea, confusion.
- Examination and investigation:
  - The line: often appears innocent, but check for erythmatous or purulent exit site (→ swab for C+S). Is there a tunnel infection?
  - General exam: stigmata of endocarditis, chest signs, other sources of infection.
  - Blood cultures: from line and peripheral vein.
  - CRP.
  - CXR if chest signs.

Treatment
- Start antibiotics empirically if fever >38°C, rigors, or ↓BP.
  - Give vancomycin 10–20mg/kg (usually 1g) + gentamicin 1–2mg/kg IV and measure levels daily (↓ quicker in patients with significant residual function). Third generation cephalosporins are an alternative to gentamicin. Tailor therapy to culture results. Vancomycin is not removed by HD, gentamicin is.
  - Continue for at least 2–4 weeks.
- If fever still present after 12–24h → remove line, earlier if ↓BP (some advocate immediate removal in all cases).
- If persistent fever or ↑CRP, consider metastatic infection: infective endocarditis, arthritis, osteomyelitis, epidural abscess.
- Avoid inserting new lines until sepsis cleared ('in-out' femoral lines for each dialysis session may be necessary).

Other line complications
- Thrombosis. Instill thrombolytic agent tPA 1mg/mL to the internal lumen and leave for 4–24h.
- Catheters may → central venous stenosis, preventing subsequent catheter placement and compromising AVF maturation and flow. May lead to SVC obstruction with swollen arms, chest wall, and face. Multiple collateral veins may be visible. Balloon angioplasty ± stent insertion may be successful, but recurrence common.

▶ **Clotted fistulae or grafts**
- No thrill or buzz = thrombosis (ensure the patient knows this).
- Admit and arrange urgent declotting. This may be radiological (physical declotting or local thrombolysis) or surgical in the first instance (local policies differ).
- Check U+E. Insert a temporary line if dialysis required.
- The longer time between thrombosis and declotting, the less chance of success (especially for AVF)
- Prevention.
  - Grafts: Some evidence for dipyridamole ± aspirin. Warfarin may have a limited role in selected patients.
  - AVF: no evidence of benefit for any agent.

Other complications of fistulae and grafts
- Infection: fistulae rarely become infected beyond a superficial cellulitis. PTFE infection is not uncommon. May be occult causing weight loss, EPO resistance, and failure to thrive. Antimicrobials rarely successful and management usually involves surgical removal.
- Aneurysm or pseudo-aneurysm formation: may occur at needling sites, especially if sites not rotated. Surgery may be necessary.
  - Bleeding from an infected or aneurysmal AVF or graft is a much feared complication (proceeds under arterial pressure!).
  - ▶ Wear a gown, gloves, and goggles. Seal the bleeding site with the lid of a universal container and secure with a tight bandage. Establish wide bore IV access, check clotting, cross-match blood and inform a surgeon.
- Distal ischaemia or steal syndrome: flow through the fistula or graft may compromise distal blood supply. Cold or numb peripheries are common, but may → infarction or ischaemic pain. AVF ligation or graft removal may be necessary.
- Excess flow: may → large ↑ in cardiac output with cardiac decompensation. 'Banding' an AVF may ↓flow.
- Extravasation: blood leakage into the soft tissues. Can cause rapid limb swelling, haemodynamic compromise, compartment syndromes, 2° infection, access thrombosis.

Acute HD complications

Intradialytic hypotension

- ↓BP requiring intervention occurs during 10–30% of treatments.
- Pathogenesis is complex, but in essence: fluid removal on dialysis → contraction of the intravascular compartment, compensatory vasoconstriction and compartmental fluid shifts.
- Patients at risk:
  - Large fluid gains (removal of >1.5L/h)
  - Poor LV function
  - Anti-hypertensive therapy
  - DM
  - Autonomic dysfunction
  - Sepsis
  - Hypoalbuminaemia.

Management

- Place head down, stop UF, give 100mL bolus of saline.
- Exclude cardiac cause (ischaemia, arrhythmia, pericardial effusion)
- Education re: importance of salt and water restriction.
- Reassess post dialysis ('dry') weight—is it too low?
- Omit anti-hypertensive agents on the day of dialysis.
- Longer dialysis hours, enabling slower fluid removal, or daily dialysis (often impractical).
- Bicarbonate not lactate dialysis buffer.
- ↓dialysate temperature.
- UF profiling: isolated UF before dialysis.
- Na^+ profiling—start with high dialysate Na^+ and gradually reduce.
- Drugs: midodrine, a peripherally acting vasoconstrictor (α_1 agonist) appears to be of benefit in selected patients. Given orally pre-dialysis.
- Blood volume monitoring (📖 p.206).

Table 4.2 Acute HD complications

Complication	Cause	Management
Air embolism	Air in dialysis circuit	Clamp lines. Give O_2 Place head down in L lateral pos[n]
Arrhythmias	Multifactorial	Check electrolytes, cardiac investigation
Blood loss	Bleeding tendency, heparin	↓heparin
Chest pain	Angina, ↓BP, air embolism	Address cause
Cramps	Volume contraction ±↓ osmolality, ↓Mg, ↓ carnitine	↑osmolality (e.g. 25mL 50% dextrose). Stop dialysis
Haemolysis	Dialysate contaminated or too warm	Run safety checks
Hypoxaemia	Bioincompatibilty (📖 p.208), lactate buffer	Synthetic dialyser, HCO_3 buffer
Nausea, vomiting, and headache	Unknown (?minor disequilibrium syndrome 📖 p.121)	Analgesia Coffee (caffeine)

Chronic HD complications

Dialysis falls well short of providing the clearance of native kidneys. As the number of years on dialysis ('dialysis vintage') increases, the consequences of this shortfall become more apparent:

- Loss of access sites.
- Renal bone disease (□ p.168).
- Dialysis arthropathy: accumulated β_2 microglobulin deposits in joints, causing pain and carpal tunnel syndrome. HDF and other methods which improve middle molecule clearance may be of benefit.
- Chronic inflammation: HD is associated with chronic activation of inflammatory cascades (→ membrane bioincompatibilty, repeated episodes of clinical/subclinical infection, ↑advanced glycation end-products, ↑oxidative stress and malnutrition). Effects may be:
  - Malnutrition (a vicious cycle develops)
  - Poor EPO response
  - Accelerated vascular and cardiac disease (□ p.186)
  - ↑Susceptibility to infection
  - ↑Mortality.
- Quality of life: transplanted dialysis patients report greatly improved QOL scores. HD makes great physical and psychological demands on both patients (and their carers).

Peritoneal dialysis (PD)

Introduction

PD is the dialysis modality of approximately 100,000 patients worldwide. It is generally accepted that patient survival on PD compared to HD is similar: in fact, these modalities should be seen as complementary, offering different advantages that individuals may benefit from at different times in their dialysis history—the so-called 'Integrated Dialysis Care' approach.

Physiology and concepts

The semi-permeable dialysis membrane of the peritoneum comprises the capillary endothelium, supporting matrix, and the peritoneal mesothelium. Fluid and solute move between the fluid-filled peritoneum and blood through what is known as the 'three-pore model' of PD.

- *Large pores (20–40nm)*: allow macromolecules such as proteins to be filtered between compartments (effectively via venular or lymphatic absorption)
- *Small pores (4–6nm)*: responsible for the transport of small solutes such as sodium, potassium, urea and creatinine.
- *Ultrasmall pores (<0.8nm)*: transport water alone, and are likely to be aquaporins.

The net movement of solutes such as urea then depends on:
- Net diffusion through small and convection through large pores
- Total volume of dialysate infused
- Net fluid ultrafiltration (or absorption).

Effective peritoneal surface area

Peritoneal capillary endothelium is the predominant barrier to peritoneal solute transport. However, at any one time, not all capillaries are equally perfused and not all are close enough to the mesothelium (and thus dialysate) for effective dialysis. The 'effective peritoneal surface area' then varies (e.g. with peritonitis, or changing dialysate volumes). Increasing the effective peritoneal surface area allows faster rates of small solute transfer, but not necessarily better dialysis—by increasing dissipation of glucose, UF might ↓ (📖 p.226).

Ultrafiltration (UF)

The net movement of water (UF) relies on the presence of a high intraperitoneal osmotic gradient (generated by glucose) or oncotic gradient (generated by glucose polymers such as icodextrin). Opposing fluid movement into the peritoneum is any absorption of dialysate via lymphatics (esp. if ↑intraperitoneal hydrostatic pressure from patient posture or high instilled PD volumes).

The osmotic gradient is usually generated by glucose and depends on:
• The glucose concentration of the dialysate.
• A patient's blood glucose.
• The rate of absorption of glucose itself from PD fluid.

UF is optimized by:
• Ensuring normoglycaemia (relevant for diabetics).
• Adjusting the tonicity of the PD solution (glucose concentration).
• Altering the duration of each dialysis dwell.
• Adjusting dwell volumes; an ↑ often (but not always) leads to ↑UF.

As an alternative to glucose-based solutions, glucose polymers (such as icodextrin) are poorly absorbed and metabolized slowly—these PD solutions provide a sustained *oncotic* gradient over longer dwells and permit ↑UF particularly for high transporters (📖 p.226).

   ↑dwell volumes of dialysate may maintain the glucose gradient for longer, but ↑intraperitoneal pressure may ↑lymphatic return. Also, ↑volume might increase effective peritoneal surface area, with more rapid absorption of glucose, lessening the glucose gradient.

Types of PD

Intermittent PD was originally developed for the treatment of ARF where HD facilities are not available (📖 p.122). Rapid exchanges over a 24-hour period are repeated 2 or more times a week. For cost reasons, the peritoneal catheters used for treatment of ARF are often different from those used for patients with ESRF.

Continuous ambulatory PD (CAPD) consists of 3 to 5 exchanges with dwell times of 4—10 hours in 24 hours. Usually performed by the patient connecting and disconnecting the PD catheter to dialysate bags. A night-time exchange can be performed by machines (such as Quantum®). Advantages include simplicity and flexibility—the timing of the exchanges can be adjusted to times convenient for patients although dwells less than 3 hours are generally discouraged.

Automated PD (APD) uses an automated machine to perform exchanges at night whilst the patient is sleeping. The machine is usually programmed to perform at least 4 exchanges over 8 hours (can be more depending on individual tolerance). At the end of the overnight exchanges, the machine can be programmed to leave the patient 'dry' during the day (night-time intermittent peritoneal dialysis; NIPD). Alternatively, the machine can perform a 'last fill', leaving PD fluid in the peritoneum. Patients may then perform a further exchange during the day (either manually or using the APD machine—continuous cycling peritoneal dialysis (CCPD)).

Tidal APD has the machine programmed to only partially drain out PD fluid at the end of any dwell during the nightly cycles ('75% tidal' indicates that the machine will stop draining fluid out when 75% of the expected drain has been extracted). Although efficiency of dialysis is reduced, it is useful for patients whose sleep is disturbed through discomfort experienced when 'dry'.

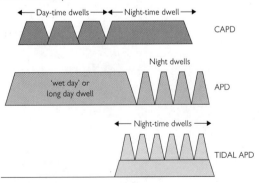

Fig. 4.3 Types of PD

Reproduced with permission from Levy J, Morgan J, and Brown E (2004). *Oxford Handbook of Dialysis*, 2nd edn. Oxford: Oxford University Press

CAPD technique

Disconnect, flush-before-fill Y-systems are now the norm. The connectology has been refined over the years to minimize peritonitis through touch-contamination. At the time of an exchange, the patient connects a Y-shaped set with a sterile drain bag and a fresh dialysate bag. Patients are taught to make this connection using sterile techniques although various assist devices are available to aid patients with dexterity or visual problems (e.g. UV Flash Compact®). After the waste dialysate is drained into the empty bag, the Y-connector is flushed (theoretically flushing away any contaminating bacteria in this portion of the giving set) using a small volume of fresh dialysate. The remaining dialysate is infused into the patient's abdomen.

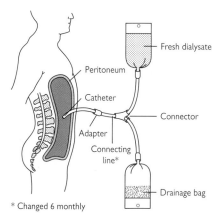

* Changed 6 monthly

Fig. 4.4 'Disconnect' PD system

Reproduced with permission from Levy J, Morgan J, Brown E (2004). *Oxford Handbook of Dialysis*, 2nd edn. Oxford: Oxford University Press.

PD fluids

Peritoneal dialysate needs to remove uraemic toxins and fluid, normalize electrolytes, and correct acidosis. Ideally, fluid should be compatible with long-term peritoneal health. Each CAPD bag has a volume of usually 2L. The contents of each dialysis bag is designed with the above in mind:

- Volume: usually 2L, but 1.5, 2.5 or 3L also available.
- Glucose concentration: three standard concentrations, usually about 1.5, 2.5 and 4.0% (roughly 25g, 50g and 75g glucose per bag)
- Sodium: Na^+ 135mmol/L (although lower concentrations may improve salt and thus water removal)
- Electrolytes: calcium ranges from 1.25–1.75mmol/L and 0.25mmol/L of magnesium.
- Buffer: lactate is widely used at 36mmol/L (rapidly converted in the liver to bicarbonate).

Newer solutions may contain:
- Bicarbonate rather than lactate as the buffer.
- Icodextrin rather than glucose as colloid to achieve UF.
- Amino acids as nutritional supplement that also lacks the toxicity of glucose (see below).

Biocompatible solutions

PD fluid is sterilized through heat treatment. During this process, at the pH of lactate-based glucose solutions, glucose-degradation products (GDP) and advanced glycation end products (AGE) are formed. These are believed to damage the peritoneal membrane: AGE exposure correlates with fibrotic changes. Thus, more 'biocompatible' solutions have been developed with this in mind.

One solution depends on a twin-bag system; heat sterilization of the compartment containing glucose (at very low pH) generates very low levels of GDP and advanced glycation end products (AGE). The second compartment contains the acid-buffer—e.g. predominately bicarbonate in the case of Physioneal® or lactate in the case of Balance®. Definitive evidence that use of these solutions lead to improved clinical outcome is awaited although retrospective analysis of registry data suggested patient survival was better in the group treated with biocompatible solutions.

Other solutions that rely on molecules other than glucose to provide the osmotic gradient have no GDP or AGE. In this respect, they can be considered biocompatible

Commercially available solutions in the UK

- Baxter
  - Dianeal®—glucose/lactate containing (see Table 4.3).
  - Physioneal®—glucose/bicarbonate containing.
  - Nutrineal®—contains amino acids. Osmotically equivalent to 1.36% glucose solutions.
  - Extraneal®—(7.5%).
- Fresenius
  - Staysafe®—glucose/lactate in single compartment (see Table 4.3).
  - Staysafe Balance®—glucose/lactate in twin Bag system.
- Gambro
  - Gambrosol trio 10®.

Table 4.3 Range of glucose concentrations commercially available in the UK

	Baxter	Fresenius
'Light'	1.36%	1.5%
'Medium'	2.27%	2.5%
'Heavy'	3.36%	4.25%

Prescribing PD

Aim for 'adequate' dialysis with as little impact on the patient's social or psychological well-being. Dialysis adequacy (📖 p.234) and UF failure (📖 p.236) are discussed elsewhere.

The concept of 'transporter' status

High concentrations of glucose generate an osmotic gradient across the peritoneal membrane. During the dialysis dwell, glucose is absorbed → ↓glucose concentration and dialysate osmolality within the peritoneum. The rate of glucose dissipation correlates with the rate at which creatinine equilibrates across the peritoneal membrane and can change over time (termed the 'transport' status of the patient) and can be measured during a peritoneal equilibration test (PET, 📖 p.235).

'High' transporters allow rapid movement of urea and other small molecules across the peritoneal membrane (through small pores, 📖 p.220). But glucose is also rapidly absorbed, ↓ the gradient: thus UF at the end of a CAPD dwell is likely to be low. So a high transporter often has difficulty achieving adequate small solute clearance.

- High transporters are particularly suitable for APD (frequent short dwells maximize UF and total solute removal).
- Low transporters benefit less from very short dwells on APD. Introducing a 5th PD exchange may be preferable (either manually or using an automated machine to deliver a single exchange at night, 📖 p.222).

Most patients start CAPD on 4 'light' (1.36–1.5% dextrose) PD bags. If this fails to provide adequate UF, one exchange is changed to a higher glucose concentration bag or Extraneal®. Further increases in glucose concentration may be necessary to achieve adequate dialysis and UF.

Avoiding glucose exposure

High peritoneal glucose exposure over time (often years) predicts the development of UF failure, and causality has been suggested. An alternative to glucose in the dialysate is icodextrin (Extraneal®).
- Icodextrin is a 20-glucose polymer with potent colloidal effects.
- Usually used for the longest dwell (overnight in CAPD, day-time dwell in APD).

Particularly suited to high transporters. Icodextrin is absorbed into the lymphatics, so the osmotic gradient is maintained even in high transporters (reflection of rate of movement across small pores).

⚠ Increasing the volume of each exchange can increase intraperitoneal pressure and adversely affect UF.

Based on individuals' membrane transport characteristics (PET 📖 p.235), computer software can be used to predict small solute clearance and UF. These can be particularly useful when responding to falling UF or solute clearance.

Peritonitis

Peritonitis is (one of) the major complication(s) of PD, leading to significant morbidity and mortality. Repeated episodes of peritonitis might also accelerate peritoneal membrane failure, requiring transfer to haemodialysis. The incidence of peritonitis has declined from about 3 episodes/patient/year in the 1980s to 0.6–0.7 episodes/patient/year (or roughly 1 episode every 18 months), attributed to improved patient education and better catheter technology. The disconnect 'flush-before-fill' system has also been an important advance.

Clinical feures

Abdominal pain, nausea and vomiting. 'Cloudy' PD effluent is highly suggestive. High fever and being systemically unwell with signs of an ileus, and peritonism can also occur. Diagnosis:

- PD fluid for microscopy and Gram stain. Should have dwell-time of 4h or more. >100wbc/mm^3 (>50% neutrophils).
- Culture PD fluid (discuss with microbiology) and blood.
- FBC (↑WCC).

Patients should be taught to report cloudy effluent as soon as seen. Abdominal pain can be very severe. Rapid peritoneal flushing can improve symptoms, but samples from the original cloudy bag should be sent for microscopy, Gram-stain and culture.

▶ Always consider other causes of peritonitis (e.g. perforation, strangulated hernia).

Bacteriology

- Gram +ve cocci, 45–75% (coagulase negative staphylococci, *S. aureus*) Often introduced after touch contamination of the connections, or catheter exit site infections. Colonization of catheter biofilms can lead to recurrence of peritonitis and necessitate catheter exchange.
- Gram –ve organisms, 15–25% (*Pseudomonas*, coliforms). Usually of bowel origin. Air in the peritoneum is common, and may not indicate bowel perforation. Suspect perforation if mixed Gram –ve organisms on culture.
- Culture negative or 'no growth' (ideally, positive cultures in >85%).
- Mycobacterial infections, 1% (TB) should be considered in patients with culture negative peritonitis not responding to empiric antibiotic therapy. Smears of PD effluent are rarely positive for acid-fast bacilli and diagnosis is usually made on culture (6-weeks) or at laparoscopy/otomy with confirmation on peritoneal biopsy.
- Fungal, 3% (usually *Candida* sp) peritonitis is infrequent, but has a poor prognosis. It often follows recent antibiotic therapy in at risk patients.

Allergic peritonitis is well described, often found with newly prescribed icodextrin solutions (although it can occur with glucose-based solutions). In general, the elevation of WCC is modest and the proportion of eosinophils in PD effluent can be high (>10%). Does not respond to antibiotics. Withdrawal of icodextrin usually helps.

Complications of peritonitis

- *Relapsing peritonitis*. A second episode of peritonitis with the same organism within 4 weeks of completing antibiotic therapy. It is our practice to consider a second episode of culture negative peritonitis as a relapse if it fulfils the temporal relationship. Prolonged antibiotics (particularly for relapses secondary to staphylococcus) are required.
- *Antibiotic treatment failure*. Need to exclude abscess formation if no response to protocol antibiotic therapy. PD catheters should be removed and laparotomy considered especially if other intra-abdominal pathology is suspected. CT abdomen is useful for diagnosis and drainage of infected encysted fluid.
- *Acute and chronic UF failure*. Vasodilatation as a result of inflammation may lead to ↑ glucose absorption, reduced glucose gradient, and impaired UF. Repeated bouts of peritonitis can lead to long-term changes in peritoneal membrane structure and function causing chronic UF failure.
- *Malnutrition*. Peritoneal protein loss through the inflamed peritoneum can be very high. Anorexia and prolonged ileus can exacerbate nutritional status further.

Treatment

Empiric antibiotic therapy should be initiated in cases of definite peritonitis without awaiting results of culture. Many protocols exist, and are influenced by local experience—contact your microbiologist. The International Society of Peritoneal Dialysis recommends:
- Gram +ve cover with vancomycin or a cephalosporin +
- Gram –ve cover with an aminoglycoside or third generation cephalosporin.

In the UK, despite concerns over the development of vancomycin-resistance, most units use vancomycin-based regimens. Protocols differ from unit to unit but as an example:
- Vancomycin 2g IP on day 1, with a further dose on days 5–7 depending on trough vancomycin levels +
- Either gentamicin 0.6 mg/kg IP daily (adjusted against trough gentamicin levels on days 3–5) or, alternatively, to spare residual renal function (defined in terms of UO) from aminoglycoside nephrotoxicity, ceftazidime 1g IP daily.

Once culture result and sensitivities known:
- If Gram +ve: continue weekly vancomycin. If *S. aureus*, add in rifampicin 300mg po bd. Stop gentamicin/ceftazidime.
- If Gram –ve: continue ceftazidime or gentamicin. Although concerns about aminoglycosides affecting residual renal function exist, this is not borne out by evidence. It is our practice to administer ceftazidime if UO >100 mL/day, and gentamicin if functionally anuric (<100 mL/day). Stop vancomycin.
- If culture negative: continue both, doses adjusted according to trough drug levels.

- If mixed Gram−ve growth: add in metronidazole and consider laparotomy (suspect bowel perforation).
- Treat for 14–21 days.

▶ Mupirocin ointment administered to the catheter exit site can prevent, not only exit site infection, but also *S. aureus* peritonitis. Gentamicin cream may be as effective against *S. aureus*, and prevent pseudomonal peritonitis as well.

Special considerations for APD

Even in the absence of peritonitis, long day dwells may be 'misty'. However, because cycling times may be short, cloudy overnight dialysate is less common than with CAPD. Moreover, in some cases, PD effluent is directly drained into a sink. Thus, it is important for APD patients to recognize potential symptoms of peritonitis and to perform a dwell of at least 2 hours (for inspection and sampling of fluid for M, C+S) when such a diagnosis is in doubt. Treatment also requires some technique modifications. One option is to convert patients to CAPD for the duration of the episode. Alternatively (and we believe, preferably), give antibiotics as above into the last dwell on the machine (1st ambulatory dwell).

Catheter exit site infection

A purulent and/or bloody discharge from an exit site, often associated with erythema, or pain. Crusting alone is not indicative of an acute exit site infection.

Causes: usually S. aureus, pseudomonas

The use of prophylactic topical exit site ointment (with mupirocin or gentamicin) reduces such infections. Reducing nasal carriage of S. aureus also reduces exit site infections.

Treatment:

- Swab for culture and confirm PD fluid is clear.
- Adjust therapy once culture result and sensitivities known.
- Topical antibiotics are not appropriate.
- Empiric therapy: start flucloxacillin 500mg qds or cefuroxime 500mg bd.
- Gram +ve organisms: continue flucloxacillin or cefuroxime depending on sensitivities. Treat for 14d. If S. aureus confirmed, add in rifampicin 300mg bd.
- Gram −ve organisms: ciprofloxacin 500mg po bd for 14 days.
  If pseudomonas, treat with IP ceftazidime as for PD peritonitis.

Trauma to the exit site increases the likelihood of infections. Increasing the frequency of exit site care (to daily or twice daily dressings) is often advocated during infections. Crusts or scabs should not be forcibly removed and the exit site in general should be protected from trauma (that includes dressings that immobilize the catheter thereby preventing pulling on the exit site).

A tunnel infection is defined as erythema and/or tenderness over the subcutaneous catheter pathway, ± intermittent discharge from the exit site. Diagnosis of tunnel infection can be confirmed by ultrasound examination. Treatment usually involves removing the catheter, as peritonitis is a common complication.

Other complications

Drainage problems

This should be differentiated from UF failure. Catheter flow problems can present with either slow drainage (drainage takes >15–20 minutes under gravity) or incomplete drainage; high residual volume measured on PET or when the drain volume is less than the infused volume of a 'rapid' exchange. Causes include:

- Constipation.
- Catheter occlusions (external kinking, thrombus and omental wrapping).
- Fluid leaks into subcutaneous tissue from herniae or insertion site.

Inflow problems can also occur, for many of the same reasons. In addition, if the catheter tip is trapped in a small area of intra-abdominal adhesions, inflow can be limited. Careful history and examination should sufficient to determine the majority of causes. Plain KUB can be performed to exclude catheter malposition and constipation.

The majority of drain problems can be improved without surgery:

- Laxatives (regular senna and lactulose, or sodium picosulphate).
- Intra-catheter heparin locks. (e.g. 500 units as a lock, or 500 units/L in exchanges).
- Thrombolytics such as urokinase infused down the catheter.
- Endoluminal brushes.

If surgical re-positioning required, it is often useful to perform an omentectomy (and adhesolysis if appropriate).

Peritoneal leaks

Dialysate may leak down the catheter tunnel into the subcutaneous tissues or externally via the exit site. A patent processus vaginalis may allow PD fluid to track into the scrotum mimicking a hernia or hydrocele. Small diaphragmatic herniae may permit PD fluid to enter the pleural space.

Clinically, local oedema ± skin peau d'orange appearance may signify a subcutaneous leak. Fluid leaking from the exit site can be dipsticked for glucose to confirm it is glucose-rich dialysate. Similarly, pleural taps or aspirates from hydroceles can be tested for glucose. If in doubt, perform CT peritoneogram. Our protocol is to infuse 100mL of non-ionic contrast into a 2L PD bag and drain in 1L. Perform CT 1–2 hours thereafter.

Leaks around the catheter often heal with temporary (2–4 weeks) discontinuation of PD (may require temporary HD). We re-start PD using smaller volumes to reduce intra-abdominal pressure. If leaks recur, the PD catheter can be repositioned with a new insertion site. Hernias should be repaired in a standard manner. APD with a dry day (NIPD) can be particularly successful to minimize recurrence.

Sclerosing encapsulating peritonitis (SEP)

A feared complication of long-term PD therapy with very poor prognosis. The incidence is about 0.9%, usually in PD patients at an average of 65 months from the initiation of PD. The peritoneal cavity becomes encased in fibrous tissue, with bowel wall thickening and peritoneal calcification. It is thought to be multifactorial in origin, with prior severe peritonitis, foreign body reactions to plasticizers on catheters and long-term PD using less biocompatible solutions all suggested to be pathogenic.

Clinically:
- Symptoms of intermittent bowel obstruction.
- Poor UF or UF failure.
- Malnutrition is frequent.

Symptoms may occur after peritonitis, or even after stopping PD.

Investigation of choice is CT abdomen, demonstrating peritoneal thickening and calcification with entrapped bowel loops. Peritoneal biopsy is diagnostic.

Treatment is limited and based on anecdotal evidence:
- Stop PD.
- Renal transplantation if possible.
- Trial of immunosuppression (e.g. rapamycin) is a therapeutic option.
- Tamoxifen has also been suggested to be effective in case reports.
- Surgery may is associated with a high risk of perforating bowel.

PD adequacy

The absence of uraemic symptoms and volume overload does not imply dialysis adequacy. Other imprecise criteria for adequacy include:
- Patient quality of life (e.g. by subjective global assessment scoring).
- Improved biochemistry and correction of anaemia.
- Adequate nutrition.

Formally, delivered dose can be measured by calculating weekly clearance for urea (Kt/V (p.211) and creatinine (CCr).

Although there is a minimum threshold of dialysis clearance to maintain good health, increasing dialysis dose beyond this does not appear to improve survival. The most powerful predictor of patient survival on PD is not dialysis adequacy, but the presence of residual renal function.

With these provisos, the current US and UK PD adequacy guidelines are:
- US K/DOQI®:
    - CAPD: weekly Kt/V > 2.0 and CCr 50–60 L/wk per 1.73m^2 (depending on transport status).
    - APD: weekly Kt/V > 2.1 and CCr 63L/wk per 1.73m^2.
- UK Renal Association:
    - CAPD: Kt/V > 1.7 and CCr 50 L/wk per 1.73m^2.
    - Recommends aiming for higher targets for high average and high transporters (p.226) and APD patients.

How to improve a low Kt/V / CCr

CAPD
Review transport status (p.226):
- If high or high average transporter, consider converting to APD.
- If low or low average transporter, ?↑dwell volume or add 5th exchange.
- Increasing dialysate osmolality to increase drain volume will also improve total clearance

APD
- Consider introducing daytime dwell(s).
- Optimize cycle duration in accordance to patient transport status (short cycles for high transporter). This might necessitate increasing total duration of APD.

Increasingly, preserving residual renal function and controlling salt and water balance in PD patients is seen as a vital measure of technique success. If meaningful UO, consider:
- ACE inhibitors as reno-protective agents.
- Avoid nephrotoxins (NSAIDs, *perhaps* aminoglycosides).
- Diuretics to better achieve salt and water balance.

The peritoneal equilibration test (PET)

This is an assessment of peritoneal membrane transport function; the ratio of dialysate and plasma creatinine concentrations (D_{cr}/P_{cr} ratio) after a 4 hour dwell is a measure of solute equilibration. High and low transporters are defined to be $D_{cr}/P_{cr} > 0.8$ or < 0.5 ($\pm$ 1 SD) respectively.

Since glucose absorbed from the dialysate is very quickly metabolized, D/P ratio for glucose is meaningless. Instead, the fraction of glucose absorbed from the dialysate at 4 hours is compared with the initial dialysis solution (D/D_0). This is also a useful indicator of transport status.

A PET is also a useful objective assessment of ultrafiltration. However a UF volume <400mL after modified PET utilizing a 4.24% or 3.86% glucose dwell is more specific for UF failure.

Ultrafiltration failure

PD patients with fluid overload are either non-compliant with a realistic fluid restriction, or have inadequate UF. Inadequate UF might be the result of inappropriate dialysis prescription, or the failure of an appropriate prescription to drain adequate volumes: the latter is *UF failure*.

Patients are asked to achieve a dry weight through fluid restriction and use of hyperosmolar PD bags. However, setting accurate dry weights is difficult in PD, so aim to adjust the dialysis prescription for adequate fluid removal (sum of urine output and net UF). As a general rule, aim for a target of 1L/day. If anuric (UO <100mL/day), minimum daily UF should be 750mL.

General rules for better fluid removal:
- Consider modified PET to differentiate UF failure from other cases of fluid overload. Calculating D_{cr}/P_{cr} ratio can also help diagnose the cause of UF failure (🕮 p.235).
- Evaluate the residual volume during PET: a 'normal' residual volume is up to 200–250mL. Higher volumes might suggest catheter related drainage problems (also check drain time for the PET test).
- Exclude mechanical problems (🕮 p.232).
- Avoid long dwells (>4h) with low glucose concentrations.
- Use icodextrin instead of glucose for the longest dwell.
- If on APD, consider additional short day exchange.

Causes
- High transporter status (often seen in longstanding PD patients).
- If not high transporter, consider:
  - Leaks.
  - Reduced effective peritoneal surface area from peritoneal adhesions.
  - Increased lymphatic absorption.
  - Aquaporin deficiency or failure (indicated by loss of sodium sieving during modified PET).

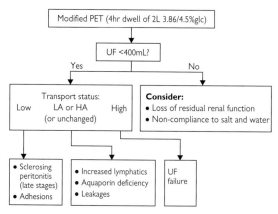

Fig. 4.5 Diagnosing causes for hypervolaemia in PD

The well PD patient

Introduction

Adequate dialysis: maintain residual renal and peritoneal membrane function.

- Dialysis adequacy should be measured in terms of clearance of small solute clearance (including Kt/V and CCr) and nutritional parameters.
- Aim for normotension by good salt and water removal—generally achieving minimum daily fluid removal of 750mL.
- Preserving residual renal function (basically, UO) makes the above goals easier to achieve, and may improve outcomes (argument for use of ACE inhibitors, avoiding NSAIDs).

Increments in patients' transport status (📖 p.226) makes maintaining good UF and small solute clearance difficult without onerous dialysis regimens. High intra-peritoneal glucose concentrations and exposure to GDP or AGE are suggested to hasten peritoneal membrane changes, so use of solutions low in GDPs such as twin bag 'physiological' solutions or icodextrin and amino acid solutions *may* be desirable (◆).

Complications

Minimize peritonitis and exit site infections through education about good technique. This includes teaching the patients to identify and present themselves for early treatment. Monitor nutritional status closely. Early stages of sclerosing peritonitis may be reversible and early diagnosis relies on high index of suspicion.

Social rehabilitation

Rehabilitation is also extremely important for individual PD patients, and should encompass adapting the timing of PD exchanges or APD to the working environment (perhaps negotiating a dedicated area at the work place, or delivery of solutions to the workplace). Travel (either within the same country or abroad) improves patients' sense of well-being and should be supported. Support for the other family members including children and spouse should not be overlooked.

Basic transplantation

Practical transplant immunology

Histocompatibility and allorecognition

The immune response to a transplanted kidney is determined by an array of cell surface proteins, encoded by a group of histocompatibility genes known as the major histocompatibility complex (MHC). The MHC presents fragments of 'non-self' proteins to T lymphocytes to initiate an immune response.

In humans the MHC genes encode a polymorphic group of proteins called the human leucocyte antigens (HLA).

- Class I HLA includes HLA-A, HLA-B, and HLA-C present on most cell surfaces. Antigens associated with class I molecules are recognized by cytotoxic CD8+ T lymphocytes which become activated.
- Class II HLA consists of HLA-DR, HLA-DQ, and HLA-DP and are generally only present on antigen presenting cells (APCs) such as macrophages, renal mesangial, and dendritic cells. Class II antigens are recognised by CD4+ T lymphocytes leading to their clonal expansion. Activated CD4+ cells release cytokines that activate CD8+ cells.

Each individual inherits an allele from each parent (a haplotype).

The recognition of transplanted antigens by recipient T cells is by *direct* and *indirect* pathways (Fig. 4.6).

- Direct pathway: donor APCs present foreign peptides to recipient cytotoxic CD8+ T lymphocytes leading to their activation. This pathway is largely responsible for early rejection. Donor APC can also present proteins to recipient CD4+ T helper lymphocytes leading to their activation.
- Indirect pathway: donor proteins shed from cell surfaces or donor cells engulfed by recipient APCs are presented to recipient CD4+ helper T lymphocytes.

The binding of a T cell to an APC leads to the initiation of the immune reaction. This process requires 3 distinct steps or 'signals'.

- Signal 1: binding of APC MHC molecule to the T cell receptor (TCR) leads ↑ intracellular calcium → activation of calcineurin. Calcineurin activates NFAT → release of IL-2 but only in the presence of signal 2.
- Signal 2: binding of complementary co-stimulatory pathway molecules present on APC and T lymphocytes (e.g. B7:CTLA4, ICAM:LFA1 etc.) → activation of tyrosine kinase, which together with signal 1 leads to induction of IL-2 and other T cell activation genes.
- Signal 3: signals 1 + 2 → induction of cytokine and cell activation genes (principally IL-2) which bind their receptors → clonal proliferation.

If signal 1 occurs without the subsequent signal 2 then activation of the T cell does not occur and instead *apoptosis* may occur. This process may lead to donor specific tolerance and is the subject of intensive research.

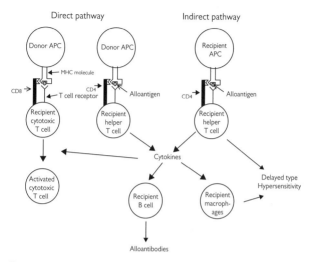

Fig. 4.6 Direct and indirect recognition

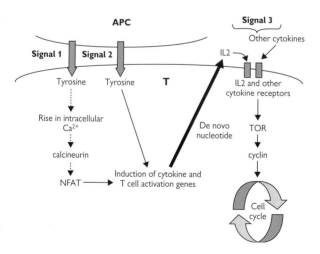

Fig. 4.7 T-cell activation (TOR = Target of rapamycin)

Compatibility

Matching donor to recipient

Four areas need to be considered:

- Blood group
- Tissue type (HLA)
- Antibodies
- Donor: recipient characteristics.

Blood group

ABO antigens are expressed on endothelial cells in the kidney and naturally occurring anti-blood group antibodies develop at 6 months of age.

▶ The same rules apply for transplantation and blood transfusions, i.e. group 'O' are universal donors and 'AB' universal recipients. ABO incompatible transplants are generally avoided.

Tissue typing

The most clinically relevant HLA antigens are HLA-A and -B (Class I) and HLA-DR (Class II). The degree of mismatch between the donor and recipient is usually quoted at these 3 loci i.e. HLA identical donors have a 0,0,0 mismatch, whereas those pairs which share 1 HLA-A, 1 HLA-B, and 1 HLA-DR have a 1,1,1 mismatch. Minor HLA antigens exist, but their clinical impact is small. Benefits of a well matched graft include:

- Lower acute rejection rates .
- Better long term graft survival.
- Fewer subsequent anti HLA antibodies.
- Lower incidence of delayed graft function.

The effect of matching on acute rejection is less evident in the modern era of immunosuppression. The impact of matching on long term survival however is still relevant (Fig. 4.8).

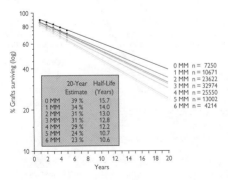

Fig. 4.8 % survival HLA A+B+DR mismatches: first cadaver kidney transplants 1985–2003. From the Collaborative Transplant Study (www.ctstransplant.org). Used with permission.

Each mismatched HLA antigen is likely to initiate an immune response, which is especially important if repeat transplantation is ever required Recipients may develop anti-HLA antibodies or memory T cells against mismatched antigens, 'forbidding' organs with these antigens being used in a given recipient.

Panel reactive antibodies (PRA)

PRA is the individual response to a notional pool of antigens in a local population (i.e. all the antigens weighted for frequency). Patient sera is incubated with lymphocytes from a panel of representative donors and complement: PRA is expressed as the percentage of donor wells with cell lysis (45% PRA should imply recipient antibodies against 45% of the most commonly occurring antigens in that population). The higher a patient's PRA, the more likely a +ve crossmatch (📖 p.245) at the time of transplantation.

Anti-HLA antibodies

Patients are 'sensitized' to develop anti-HLA antibodies when previously exposed to non-self HLA antigens. Both direct and indirect pathways → B cell activation and anti HLA antibody production.

Sensitization events

- Previous transplant (degree of mismatching important: '0,0,0' less likely to be sensitized).
- Pregnancy.
- Blood transfusion.

▶ The presence of circulating donor specific anti-HLA antibodies at the time of transplantation → hyperacute rejection.

Anti-HLA antibodies may disappear with time, and desensitization protocols aim to remove preformed antibodies prior to transplantation (📖 p.274).

Donor: recipient characteristics

Donor and recipient should be as closely 'biologically' matched as possible: for instance, kidneys from elderly donors do not, on average, last as long as those from younger donors, and may sensitize younger recipients to subsequent (better matched) grafts. Unfavourable donor characteristics include (not absolute—use of marginal kidneys is one means of expanding the overall donor pool):

- ↑BP or DM.
- Prior donor viral hepatitis or IVDU.
- Donors with systemic sepsis or certain malignancies at brain death.
- 'Non-heart beating' donors have an increased incidence of delayed graft function (itself a predictor of poor outcome).

Recipient characteristics:

- May be technically difficult to implant a kidney from a large donor into a small recipient
- Small donor (e.g. paediatric) → large recipient may not transplant enough nephron mass.
- Large recipient polycystic kidneys may limit placement of new organ (native nephrectomies may be necessary).
- Patients failing to thrive on dialysis (particularly through lack of access) are sometimes prioritized.

Pre-transplant assessment

Medical (See 📖 p.188)

Potential recipients should be fit to undergo surgery and long-term immunosuppression.

- Cardiac: ischaemic heart disease should be treated. High risk patients (e.g. DM) are usually screened with thallium scans or angiography (📖 p.188).
- Vascular: ?peripheral vascular disease.
- Malignancy: at least 2, preferably 5, years disease-free.
- ♂: PSA (age >50), ♀: cervical smear, mammography.
- No evidence of occult infection (?CRP).
- Obesity (BMI >30 at ↑surgical risk).
- Thrombosis history: exclude thrombophilia (→ ↑risk of graft loss).
- Bladder: LUTS or recurrent UTIs require urological assessment.
- HIV and hepatitis B + C are not necessarily contraindications to transplantation.
- Compliance.
- Reassess fitness every 1–2 years if on transplant waiting list.

Immunological

- Tissue type for HLA matching.
- Regular determination of PRA and anti-HLA antibody status.
- Crossmatch:
  - On the day of transplant.
  - Detects pre-formed anti-donor HLA and non-HLA antibodies that predict hyperacute rejection.
  - Either cell dependent cytotoxicity assay (CDC—recipient sera incubated with donor lymphocytes + complement) or flow cytometry.
  - +ve crossmatch → abandon transplant.
- Patients at high immunological risk usually require heavier immunosuppression.

High immunological risk

- Patients receiving their 2nd or subsequent transplant.
- Patients having lost a previous transplant to rejection.
- Black recipients.
- Patients with historic donor specific anti HLA antibodies.
- Patients with a high PRA.

Cross-matching

Prior to successful transplantation, any anti-donor antibodies need to be identified to exclude hyperacute humoral rejection and immediate graft failure. This is done by mixing recipient serum (containing potential anti-donor antibody) with donor cells (expressing HLA). A number of tests can be used to detect antibody/antigen interactions:

The complement-dependent crossmatch (CDC)

- Once recipient serum and donor T cells are combined in a multi-well tray, complement is added (with dye, see below).
- Sensitivity can be increased by adding goat anti-human light chain antibody (binds recipient antibody → improved antibody cross-linkage and fuller complement activation).
- Cell death (by complement-dependent killing) is identified by adding a dye that binds exposed DNA (ie loss of membrane integrity) under fluorescence.
- Transplanting across a positive CDC predicts hyperacute rejection.

Flow cytometry

- More sensitive than CDC. A flow cytometer mixture is prepared of:
  - Donor lymphocytes
  - Anti-CD antibodies (e.g. CD3 identifies T cells, CD19 B cells)
  - Recipient serum
  - Anti-Fc antibodies (directed against the Fc component of Ig) tagged with a fluorescent dye.
- Flow cytometry read-outs allow specific cells to be grouped (eg, all T cells), and the intensity of the dye fluorescence (i.e. binding of anti-Fc to antibodies bound in turn to HLA on cells) qualifies positivity.
- A positive T cell crossmatch (but not necessarily B cell) → rejection.

Donor specific antibodies (DSA)

- A powerful and sensitive tool for detecting anti-donor antibodies (DSA).
- Donor tissue type is described conventionally.
- Latex beads containing commercially prepared implanted specific HLA antigens when mixed with recipient serum allow detection of recipient antibodies (often at very low titre) to specific antigens.

Living donor transplantation

Introduction
▶ Living donor transplantation is the treatment of choice for ESRD.

Advantages
- Better graft and patient survival than cadaveric transplantation—regardless of genetic relationship and HLA mismatch.
- ▶ Pre-emptive transplantation (prior to dialysis) → best outcome of all.
- Avoidance of prolonged dialysis whilst waiting for transplantation (median wait for a cadaveric donor kidney in the UK: 589 days blood group A, 1370 days group B). Time on dialysis may be a risk factor for poorer transplant outcome.
- Closer HLA matching might be possible.
- Expands overall donor pool.
- Surgery can be scheduled electively.
- Minimal ischaemic damage to graft (∴ ↓delayed graft function).
- Less potent immunosuppression (possibly).
- Psychological benefits (better compliance, sense of well-being, etc.).

Disadvantages
- Stress to donor (and family).
- Perioperative donor morbidity (wound problems, DVT) and mortality (~1 in 3000).
- ☙ Later development of donor ↑BP, proteinuria or CKD (mean donor CrCl at 25 years ~72% of that prior to nephrectomy).
- Difficult to guarantee 'freely given' consent. ?coercion. Potential donors should be assessed in isolation from recipients and allowed to withdraw (without explanation) at any stage.

Assessment of a potential live donor
1. Willing to donate? → information & discussion.
2. ABO compatibility.
3. HLA typing and crossmatching (recipient against donor).
4. Medical evaluation:
    - History, clinical exam
    - Urine: dipstick, MSU & ACR
    - U+E, Cr, eGFR
    - FBC, clotting, LFTs, bone ± Hb electrophoresis (?sickle cell trait).
    - Fasting glucose ± glucose tolerance test (if fasting value 6–7mmol/L, ↑BMI, or family Hx T2DM)
    - PSA (♂ >60).
    - ECG, CXR.
    - Isotope GFR.
    - HIV, hep serology, CMV, EBV.
5. Donor anatomy: IVU, CTA/MRA ± angiography (?multiple renal arteries).
6. Informed consent.
7. Donor nephrectomy: laparoscopic techniques (→ less invasive, smaller scar, ↓hospital stay, more appealing to donors) increasingly popular.
8. Donors should be followed-up (and outcome data collected).

Absolute and relative contraindications to live donation
- Age <18 or >75 years.
- Hypertension (BP >140/90 or on antihypertensive medication).
  - Donation may still be possible if BP well-controlled and estimates of overall CV risk are low.
- BMI >30–35kg/m^2.
- T2DM, abnormal glucose tolerance, previous gestational DM.
- Malignancy.
- Other significant comorbidity.
- Microalbuminuria or overt proteinuria.
- Recurrent renal stone disease.
- Other significant renal disease.
  - Microscopic haematuria: donation may still be possible (need urology work up (📖 p.53) and renal biopsy).
- ↓GFR (<70mL/min, though some age-related flexibilty).
- Transmissible infection (HIV, hepatitis).

Pre-transplant management

Types of donors

Cadaveric (CAD): commonest transplant in the UK. Organs retrieved from donors certified as brainstem dead. After consent (either as an advance directive from a donor, or from the family) is confirmed, organs are perfused and harvested, and cold-stored for transport.

Requires an organ distribution network (UKT in the UK) that selects potential recipients from differing centres according to tissue type. The best immunological match is usually offered the kidney. The kidney is then transported from harvesting to transplanting centre. However, there is a significant and growing organ shortfall: the transplant waiting list is increasing rather than decreasing, and waits for organs lengthening.

Non-heart beating (NHB): organs retrieved following circulatory arrest. The inevitable delay between circulatory arrest and perfusion results in a period of warm ischaemia (📖 p.250). Delayed graft function common and long-term graft survival may be less good.

Living donors (LD) (📖 p.246): *commonest donor type in many countries.* May be related or unrelated, though there is generally an established emotional relationship between the pair (spouse or good friend). Altruistic ('good Samaritan') donation refers to the allocation of a live donor kidney to an appropriate patient on the cadaveric waiting list (with donor/recipient anonymity). ☛ The purchase of organs is generally illegal.

Before surgery

- NBM with insulin sliding scale if diabetic
- Document full donor details, including:
  - Age, gender, and cause of death
  - Associated co-morbidity and complications on ITU
  - Haemodynamic stability
  - Renal function (Cr) at harvesting ('perfusion')
  - Whether L or R kidney, and any anatomical anomalies or surgical damage.
- Full history and examination of potential recipient, including:
  - Any recent ill-health.
  - Current effort tolerance, and date of last cardiac assessment.
  - Quality of peripheral (groin and distal) pulses.
  - Any thrombotic events or risk.
  - Estimate native UO.
- Document tissue type and mismatch.
- CMV status of donor and recipient (📖 p.268).
- Discuss the surgery with the patient.
- Plan immunosuppression:
  - Stratify risk (immunological, and non-immunological, 📖 p.244).
  - Document current and historical PRA (📖 p.243).
  - Prescribe immunosuppression to local protocols.
- Ensure adequately dialysed pre-operatively (and limit anticoagulation if haemodialysis).

The transplant operation

Cadaveric donor issues

Meticulous management of brain dead potential donors is critical for the viability of harvested organs. Usually undertaken by ITU in liaison with a regional transplant coordinator. Important issues:

- Respiratory: adequate ventilatory support and treatment (often prophylactic) of infection.
- Haemodynamic: volume resuscitation ± inotropes/pressor agents.
- Endocrine: diabetes insipidus (↓vasopressin secretion), adrenal insufficiency, thyroid dysfunction all common (an empirical cocktail of steroids, vasopressin and tri-iodothyronine is often administered).

Retrieval

- Takes place in theatre. Several retrieval teams (heart–lung, liver, renal) often present.
- Both kidneys are harvested with each (usually) sent to a different centre.
- Along with the kidney, the renal artery (on a cuff of aorta), the renal veins (with a cuff of IVC), and the ureter (with peri-ureteral tissue) are removed.
- The kidneys are perfused with a physiological solution (e.g. Marshall's or University of Wisconsin) and placed on ice for transport.

Warm ischaemic time: period between circulatory arrest and start of cold storage (should be close to zero).
Cold ischaemic time: period of cold storage before transplantation.

Recipient operation

- The kidney is examined 'on the bench', paying particular attention to the arterial anatomy (accessory arteries cannot be sacrificed as there is no collateral supply).
- Graft implantation is heterotopic, usually into the right iliac fossa.
- Native kidneys are not removed.
- Vascular anastomoses are end-to-side to the iliac vessels (usually external iliac).
- An implantation biopsy may be taken (esp. if marginal donor).
- The ureter is joined to the recipient bladder. A sub-mucosal tunnel or oversew of bladder muscle prevents reflux. A JJ stent is often placed (removed cystoscopically at ~12 weeks).
- A drain is usually left in the peri-renal space.

Intra-operative CVP is maintained at >10cmH$_2$O with saline (± albumin). Mannitol (or frusemide) is often given as the vascular clamps are released.

Post-transplant management

After surgery

▶ Talk to the surgeon and review the intra-operative notes: any technical or anaesthetic complications? BP and fluid balance in theatre, induction immunosuppression given as prescribed? Immediate urine output?

Fluid balance

- CVP line (⚠CXR) and urinary catheter (→ protects the ureteric anastamosis; leave in situ for 5 days) usual.
- Maintain accurate fluid input/output charts. Daily weights.
- UO is a good indicator of adequate graft function (⚠ beware confusion with residual renal function).
- Drain volumes: if excessive send fluid for electrolytes and Cr to exclude urinary leak.
- Minimal evidence for routine use of 'renal' dopamine (📖 p.116).
- Immediate transplant function may result in brisk diuresis—nevertheless, significant fluid weight gain occurs
- Keep volume replete with IV saline. Typical regime:

CVP (cmH₂O)	IV fluid replacement
<5	UO + 100 ml
6–10	UO + 60 ml
11–15	UO + 30 ml
>16	UO only + reassess clinically

Analgesia

- Avoid NSAIDs.
- Patient controlled analgesia (PCA) favoured (⚠ opiate accumulation, especially if anuric).

Graft assessment

- Immediate (⚠ post-op ↑K⁺ especially if UO poor).
- Examine patient and ensure blood supply to feet good and symmetrical.
- Assess graft perfusion as soon as feasible:
  - DTPA/MAG-3 perfusion scan .
  - Doppler USS.
  - ▶ Particularly important with delayed graft function, or if abrupt tail off in UO to exclude a vascular event. In those passing good quantities of urine, and clearing biochemically, not as pressing.
- Daily U&E, FBC, LFT, bone.
  - ↓phosphate is often an early sign of tubular function, and may precede a fall in Cr.
  - Expect a fall in Hb (blood loss, haemodilution).
- Daily blood glucose (steroids and CNIs may → hyperglycaemia).
- Therapeutic levels: ciclosporin, tacrolimus, rapamycin.
- Lymphocyte subsets in those receiving anti-T cell antibody induction.
- Protocol transplant biopsy? (some centres).

General measures

- NBM until advised by surgical team.
- Chest physiotherapy.
- DVT prophylaxis—TED stockings, LMW heparin.
- Consider osteoporosis prophylaxis (steroid-induced bone loss occurs early—good evidence for beneficial effect of bisphosphonates):
  - IV pamidronate 1mg/kg rounded up or down to 60mg or 90mg within 48 hours and repeated on 30 day.
  - Oral weekly alendronate or risedronate.
- CMV prophylaxis (🕮 p.268), especially if CMV– recipient/ CMV+ donor.
- Pneumocystitis prophylaxis (co-trimoxazole 480mg bd).
- 🖢 Tuberculosis prophylaxis if previous infection or high risk population—evidence poor (isoniazid 100mg od + pyridoxine 10mg od).
- Nystatin or amphoteracin lozenges for prophylaxis against oral candida whilst on high-dose corticosteroids.

Principles of recipient management

Early: discharge–12 weeks

- See frequently (3 times a week).
- FBC, U+E, Cr, bone, LFT.
- ANY rise in creatinine needs further attention and perhaps investigation (p.260).
- Immunosuppression—optimize levels: too low → rejection; too high → graft dysfunction (calcineurin inhibitors).
- If at risk for CMV infection (p.268)—weekly CMV viral load.
- BP, PCR, and urine culture.
- Blood glucose (*de novo* post transplant diabetes).

Intermediate: 3 months–1 year

Less frequent clinic visits: weekly → biweekly → monthly. During this period the focus is on:

- Monitoring graft function (⚠ CNI toxicity, rejection, obstruction).
- Monitoring immunosuppression.
- Surveillance for infections.
- Modifying long-term CV risk (BP, lipids).

Late: beyond 1 year

Clinic visits monthly eventually reduced to every 3–4 months. The main focus during this period is:

- Monitoring graft function (⚠ chronic allograft nephropathy).
- Cardiovascular health.
- Skin malignancies.
- Post transplant lymphoma (PTLD).
- Osteoporosis.
- If applicable: managing complications of chronic graft dysfunction (anaemia, calcium, phosphate and hyperparathyroidism, nutrition).

Immunosuppression

Calcineurin inhibitors: ciclosporin, tacrolimus (FK506)

Disrupt T cell signal 1 (📖 p.240). Narrow therapeutic window ∴ monitor levels (trough). Available oral and IV (one-third of oral dose). Toxicity:

- Renal vasoconstriction → ↓GFR.
- Aggravate delayed graft function (📖 p.260).
- Renal fibrosis and scarring (→ CAN ✦ 📖 p.264).
- ↑BP.
- ↑K^+, ↓Mg^{2+}, ↑urate.
- Thrombotic microangiopathy.
- Post transplant DM (esp. tacrolimus).
- Cosmetic—virilization, hirsuitism, gum hypertrophy (esp. ciclosporin).
- Others: ↑LFTs, dyslipidaemia, coarse tremor.

⚠ Inducers (rifampicin, phenytoin) and inhibitors (erythromycin, fluconazole) of cytochrome P450 → altered drug levels → rejection or toxicity. Rapamycin should be used with caution with calcineurin inhibitors (↑ levels 2–3 fold).

Anti-proliferatives

Rapamycin (sirolimus): inhibits TOR (target of rapamycin), a regulatory kinase involved in cytokine-dependent cell proliferation. Given orally with long half-life (no IV preparation). Toxicity: delayed graft function, myelosuppression, thrombotic microangiopathy, delayed wound healing, pneumonitis, proteinuria.

Mycophenolate mofetil (MMF): prodrug; rapidly converted to active mycophenolic acid (MPA) to inhibit *de novo* purine nucleotide synthesis (→ ↓ lymphocyte proliferation). Given po or IV. Toxicity: nausea, bloating, diarrhea, mouth and oesophageal ulceration, myelosuppression. Both tacrolimus and rapamycin ↑ active MPA levels.

Azathioprine: metabolized to a purine analogue which competitively inhibits purine synthesis → ↓T cell activation. Given po and IV (half oral dose). Toxicity: myelosuppression, hepatitis. ⚠ *Allopurinol* should be used with great caution with azathioprine. Consider transfer to MMF.

Corticosteroids: inhibit cytokine-regulated lymphocyte signaling, and chemokine-driven lymphocyte homing to areas of inflammation. Given po or IVI. Toxicity: DM, osteoporosis, ↑BP. Used to prevent and TREAT rejection.

Antibodies

- Monoclonal (OKT3) and polyclonal (ATG) antibody therapy directed against CD3 are used to deplete T cells in high immunological risk patients in the peri-transplant period (📖 p.244) and to treat severe rejection. Profound immunosuppressive effect.
- Monoclonal antibodies directed at CD25, the IL2 receptor expressed on activated T cells (dacluzimab, basiliximab). Prevent activation and clonal expansion. Well tolerated and replacing T cell depleting agents as induction therapy.

- IV immunoglobulin (IVIg) is occasionally used to treat rejection and increasingly in desensitization regimens (📖 p.274).
- Alemtuzumab (Campath-1H® is a humanized anti-CD52 lymphocytic (both T and B cells) monoclonal antibody increasingly used in induction protocols. Administration may allow a reduction in maintenance immunosuppression, but long-term outlook data is awaited.

Dosing recommendations and target levels

- These are *not* absolute, and practice varies widely between centres.
- Ciclosporin (Neoral®): 7.5–10mg/kg/day in 2 divided doses against trough levels. Depends on centre, immunological risk, and nephrotoxicity. No absolutes, however, as guidance:
  - 150–200ng/mL <3 months
  - 125–175ng/mL 3–12 months
  - 75–150ng/mL >12 months
- Tacrolimus (Prograf®): load as 0.15mg/kg/day in 2 divided doses, aiming as guidance for:
  - 7–15ng/mL <3 months
  - 5–10ng/mL >3 months
- Azathioprine:
  - 1.5mg/kg/day in single dose
- Mycophenolate mofetil:
  - CellCept® 1g bd or 500mg qds (↑1.5g bd if high risk)
  - Myfortic® 720mg bd
  - ↓starting dose by 50% if on tacrolimus or sirolimus
  - Mycophenolate acid levels are measurable and be useful as there is much interindividual variation in pharmacokinetics
- Sirolimus (rapamycin, Rapamune®)
  - 6mg daily ↓ to 2–4mg of trough levels of 8–10ng/mL

If converting po to IVI, ciclosporin and tacrolimus dose should be divided by 3, (ie 33% oral). Dose equivalence for MMF or azathioprine.

Biologicals

- Anti-CD25 antibodies:
  - Basiliximab 20 mg IVI on day 0 and day 4
  - Daclizumab 1mg/kg/dose IVI on day 0, and then for 1–4 further at fortnightly interval doses
- Anti-thymocyte globulin (ATG) or OKT3 as per local protocol— they differ widely. Such agents are directed against CD3 , and → profound T cell depletion. Usually given with hydrocortisone and chlorpheniramine to minimize side-effects (fever, arthralgia, myalgia). Monitor lymphocyte subsets (number of CD3+ cells) for response to therapy.

Surgical complications

Early

Anastomotic leak

Presents abruptly after transplant as evolving haemorrhagic shock (hypotension, tachycardia, poor perfusion, oliguria and ↓Hb). Urgent re-exploration is usually indicated.

Renal arterial and venous thrombosis/occlusion

Occurs in 0.5–2% of transplants. Risk factors:

- Complex vascular anastomoses.
- Donor vascular disease.
- Recipient thrombophilia (▶ polycythaemia, anti-phospholipid antibodies).
- Recipient sickle cell disease (→ pre-transplant exchange transfusion to ↓sickle Hb + graft warmed prior to reperfusion).

Present (usually) within first week. Suspect if sudden ↓UO, macroscopic haematuria, pain (often severe), graft tenderness or swelling.

Investigations: urgent Doppler USS, isotope perfusion scan.

Management: surgical exploration (disappointingly, rarely successful).

Urinary leak

May occur (in 1–3%) anywhere along the transplant urinary tract, but most commonly at the fresh vesico-ureteric anastamosis. May occur as a complication of transplant biopsy.

Often silent, but may be painful (as the collection of irritant urine expands) ± scrotal/labial swelling. UO may taper off, or drain sites drain (or leak) ↑volumes of fluid.

Investigation: ↑serum Cr (resorbed urinary creatinine), biochemical analysis of fluid (which will differentiate the collection from a lymphocoele, which resembles serum).

Management: Isotope scanning will prove urinary extravasation. Catheterise bladder. Generally require re-implantation (though short term drainage may offer benefits in distal leaks.

Lymphocoele

Graft implantation interrupts the pelvic lymphatics. This may result in a collection of lymph around the transplant (~10% of transplants).

- Usually small and uncomplicated.
- May become large enough to obstruct the kidney or iliac veins.
- May become 2° infected.
- May cause DVT.
- More common in those treated with sirolimus.
- Diagnosis is on USS.

Indications for drainage include discomfort, obstruction or infection. Drainage is usually carried out percutaneously. Recurrent lymphocoeles may need surgical intraperitoneal 'marsupialization' for long-term drainage.

Wound infection
Contributing factors include uraemia, corticosteroid use, sirolimus use, diabetes and obesity. Causative organisms are usually Gram +ve.

Late
Renal artery stenosis
Transplant renal artery stenosis may occur early with a poor anastamosis, or later with atheromatous build-up at the origin of the transplant renal artery.

Presents with ↓GFR, poor BP control, salt and water retention ± ACEI-related transplant dysfunction. Suspect with progressive transplant dysfunction and worsening scarring on biopsy in the right clinical setting.
Investigation: Doppler USS, angiography (± angioplasty and stenting).

Ureteric stenosis
Occurs in 1–5% of transplants. Arises in the distal ureter, usually including the vesico-ureteric anastamosis. Causes include:
- Marginal blood supply (common, the ureter is supplied from some distance by the transplant renal artery ∴ ↓ blood supply
  → ureteric ischaemia and fibrosis).
- BK virus (📖 p.270) is increasingly recognised as an important cause.
- Rarely 2° urothelial tumours.

Investigation: USS will show a hydronephrosis, and allows siting of a nephrostomy to decompress the system. Once sited, antegrade examination using contrast can be performed.
Management: ureteroplasty, JJ stenting, surgical reimplantation. Occasionally a native ureter is mobilized and anastamosed to transplant pelvis as surgical reconstruction.

Bladder dysfunction
Transplantation may reveal bladder outflow obstruction, or bladder nerve, or muscle failure. Examine for a palpable bladder, consider urodynamic studies and arrange pre-/post-micturition USS bladder.

Graft dysfunction

Classification

- Delayed graft function: occurs in the immediate post-transplant period. It is unusual with living donors, but is affects ~30% of cadaveric grafts:
  - Of these, 50% will recover by day 10.
  - 33% will recover between day 10–20.
  - 10–15% after this.
  - 2–15% will not function: primary non-function.
- Early graft dysfunction: in the first 3 months post-transplant
- Late graft dysfunction: after 3 months

Delayed graft function (DGF)

- Definition:
  - Need for more than one post-transplant dialysis *or*
  - Cr > 400µmol/L after 1 week.
- Importance:
  - Impacts on long term graft survival.
  - Associated with acute rejection.
- Usually ATN histologically (📖 p.96), as hyperacute rejection is rare in the contemporary immunosuppressant era. Once early surgical complications have been excluded (📖 p.258), the differential includes:
  - ATN.
  - Early rejection.
  - Thrombotic microangiopathy.
  - Recurrent glomerulonephritis (▶ FSGS).

Table 4.4 Risk factors for delayed graft function

Donor	Recipient
Non-heart beating donor	Black race
Inadequate perfusion/cold storage	Vascular disease
Long cold ischaemia time (>24h)	Intra-op/post-op ↓BP
Pre-harvest ATN	Highly sensitised (PRA>50)
↑BP, vascular disease	Calcineurin inhibitors
Older donor (>55)	
Marginal donors[1]	

[1] Marginal donors include those with ↑BP or diabetes

- Investigations: U+E, Hb, Plt count, blood film and LDH. Drug levels. Donor specific antibodies. Isotope perfusion scan, USS → transplant biopsy (usually day 3–5 if high immunological risk or day 7 if not).
- Management: depends on the cause.

Calcineurin inhibitors and early ATN

Only reduce dose if consistent with clinical findings— otherwise repeat. If ciclosporin or tacrolimus trough levels are beyond target, suggest:
- Reduce by 10–25% total daily dose.
- If ongoing DGF, biopsy to exclude other causes.

Early graft dysfunction
- Initial graft function, but ↑Cr within the first 3 months.
- Major causes:
  - ▶ acute rejection (￼ p.262)
  - CNI nephrotoxicity
  - Thrombotic microangiopathy
  - Obstruction
  - Recurrent disease (?proteinuria, nephritic urine sediment)
  - Infection (￼ p.266).
- Investigation: USS, drug levels, transplant biopsy.

Late graft dysfunction
- Pre- and post-renal causes must be excluded.
- Chronic allograft nephropathy and recurrent disease (￼ p.264).

Thrombotic microangiopathy
- Associated with both ciclosporin and tacrolimus.
- Pathogenesis unclear: involves direct endothelial toxicity, ↓prostacyclin synthesis, vasoconstriction, platelet aggregation and thrombosis.
- May occur <1 week to >5 years.
- Often unexpected finding on transplant biopsy following ↑Cr.
- Occasionally: ↓Plt, red cell fragmentation, ↑LDH.
- Exclude antiphospholipid syndrome and CMV disease.

Optimum management unclear: ↓ or stop CNI. Conversion to rapamycin *may* be desirable. Plasma exchange uncertain.

Acute rejection

▶ Treat suspected rejection immediately.

Introduction

Acute rejection is defined as a sudden deterioration in graft function associated with specific immunopathological changes as categorized according to histological criteria (▶ Banff classification, Table 4.5).

- Modern immunosuppressive regimes have reduced the incidence of early acute rejection to 10–20%.
- <10% of patients experience rejection after 1 year (often associated with non-compliance).
- Kidneys which recover still have a 10% ↓ in 1 yr survival. Rejection also has a negative impact on long term graft survival.
- Classical presentation of fever, painful graft and oligo-anuria is now rare. Usually presents with asymptomatic ↑Cr.

Hyperacute rejection

Virtually eradicated by ABO- and cross-matching. Circulating pre-formed donor specific anti-class I HLA antibodies bind to endothelial cells, activating complement and clotting cascades → vascular thrombosis within 3 days of transplant. Graft loss is inevitable.

Acute cell-mediated rejection

- Most common form of rejection (~90%).
- Typically 1–12 weeks post-transplantation.
- Asymptomatic—may be fever, graft tenderness, and ↓UO.
- Histologically, tubulo-interstitial and vascular infiltration cause distinguished (prognostic implications):
  - Cellular: a mature lymphocytic (but usually not neutrophilic) infiltrate of the parenchyma, with interstitial oedema. Tubular architecture may be disrupted and infiltrated by lymphocytes (tubulitis).
  - Vascular: ± above findings, lymphocytic infiltration under the arterial endothelium, with endothelial cell injury (± stromal haemorrhage).
- First line treatment consists of IV methylprednisolone (0.5 or 1g/day IVI in 100mL 0.9% NaCl for 3 days).
- Maintenance immunosuppression should be increased, ± switched to more potent agents.
- Response expected within 5 days. ± 75% response rate.
- If refractory or severe (→ vascular involvement), ATG, or OKT3.

Humoral or antibody-mediated rejection

Occurs within 1–3 weeks. Anti-HLA antibodies fix complement within the graft → endothelial injury. May also occur as a late event.
- ✒ May contribute in part to ~4–20% of all acute rejection
- Histology:
  - Neutrophils marginating in peritubular capillaries, arterial inflammation → fibrinoid necrosis of arterioles.
  - C4d is diagnostic (a complement degradation product derived from classical pathway activation). Stains positive in peritubular capillaries.
- Measure circulating donor specific anti-HLA antibodies (DSA) by ELISA. Positive titres are highly suggestive in the right clinical context.
- ✒ Treatment is controversial:
  - Plasma exchange (remove anti-donor antibodies) and IVIg (anti-idiotypic effect) is increasingly reported as successful.
  - Many still advocate anti-CD3 antibodies if concurrent cell-mediated rejection (as is often the case).
  - Some recommend rituximab (anti-CD20 antibody).
- High risk of graft loss (~40%) if C4d +ve.

The revised Banff criteria

Rejection is usually classified by the Banff criteria.

Borderline		↑immunosuppression
IA	Moderate tubulitis (>4 MC in >25% of sample)	Optimize immunosuppression levels
IB	Severe tubulitis (>10 MC in >25% of sample)	Switch to more potent drug (→ Tacro, MMF, sirolimus)
		Pulse corticosteroids
IIA	Mild → moderate arteritis in one or more vessel	If unresponsive, consider anti-T cell therapy
IIB	Severe arteritis (>25% ↓ in luminal area)	
III	Transmural arteritis with fibrinoid necrosis and perivascular inflammation	Switch to tacrolimus
		Anti-T cell therapy
Antibody-mediated		Switch to tacrolimus
		Anti-lymphocyte therapy
		Consider IV immunoglobulin ± plasma exchange

MC, mononuclear cells

Chronic allograft nephropathy (CAN)

Both immunological and non-immunological factors play a role in graft dysfunction and loss beyond the first 3 months. CAN is a histological term used to describe the appearances found with progressively declining graft function. At 2 years post-transplant, 70–90% of grafts will show features of CAN.

Table 4.6 Contributors to chronic graft failure

Alloantigen dependent	Alloantigen independent
▶ Chronic rejection	▶ CNI toxicity
● Poor HLA matching	● Delayed graft function
● Prior sensitization	
● Donor specific antibodies	● Prolonged cold ischaemia
● Inadequate immunosuppression	● Reduced nephron number
	● ↑Donor age, ↑BP, ↑lipids
	● CMV disease, BK nephropathy

Histology

Characteristic histological changes include focal tubular atrophy, interstitial fibrosis and arterial narrowing. Some have tried to distinguish CNI toxicity from rejection (in practice often difficult):

● Rejection more likely (under-immunosuppressed):
  • Cellular infiltrates → subclinical rejection (i.e. unchanged Cr).
  • Presence of a chronic transplant glomerulopathy (capillary wall double contours, mesangial widening, mesangiolysis, 2° FSGS).
  • C4d staining ± donor specific antibodies.
● CNI toxicity more likely (over-exposure to CNI):
  • Nodular hyalinosis within arterial walls.
  • Stripe fibrosis.

Clinically

Usually, deteriorating eGFR (months → years) accompanied by ↑BP and proteinuria. It is analogous to CKD in native kidneys.

Prevention and treatment

● The optimal treatment remains unclear. Data from centres performing protocol biopsies suggests subclinical rejection to be a frequent early finding, and to predict subsequent CAN. ● This suggests using more potent early immunosuppression may limit the development of CAN—however, this may come at the price of more infection and gnancies.
● CNI toxicity should be remediable, by one of the following:
  • CNI avoidance immunosuppression.
  • Early CNI withdrawal.
● MMF may have anti-fibrotic effects independent of immunosuppression. Regimes using low/no CNI and MMF may offer advantages
● Similarly for sirolimus, with CNI avoidance or early withdrawal

- ❦ Using MMF or sirolimus may slow progression of CAN (i.e. treatment and not just prevention).
- Control BP with ACEI ± ARB.
- Treat hyperlipidaemia.

Recurrent and de novo glomerulonephritis (GN)

Recurrence of original disease following transplantation affects ~10–20% of patients and accounts for up to 8% of graft failures at 10 years.

	Recurrence rate	Graft loss
1° FSGS	~40%	>50%
IgAN	~40%	~20%
Membranous	<10%	~25%
MCGN I	~20%	~33%
MCGN II	>90%	~30%
Diabetic Nephropathy	~100%	<5%

- 1°FSGS may recur within days of transplantation, with torrential nephrotic syndrome and graft dysfunction (from ATN). Plasma exchange has been used with variable success.
- The commonest *de novo* form of GN post transplant is membranous nephropathy.

Transplanted Alport's patients may rarely develop *de novo* anti-GBM antibodies and a rapidly progressive crescentic glomerulonephritis as donor α5 type IV collagen is recognized as non-self.

Post-transplant infections

Introduction

Transplant recipients are immunosuppressed, and as such, susceptible to a wide variety of infectious pathogens. Generally, the aim is to prevent predictable infections (that occur at often predictable times post-transplant) if possible. Such strategies might include:
- Peri-operative broad spectrum antibiotics.
- Co-trimoxazole (PCP, UTI).
- ☞ Isoniazid (TB in high risk recipients).
- Valganciclovir/ganciclovir (CMV in at risk recipients).

Timing of infection

Infections in the first month
- Standard post-operative infections related to the procedure itself—see surgical complications, (📖 p.258).
- Urinary tract infection: common. Anuric dialysis patients often have small capacity dysfunctional bladders, and indwelling urinary catheters or ureteric stents contribute further. If recurrent, USS transplant + bladder pre- and post micturition. Plain AXR may detect a retained stent or calculi (transplant or native kidneys).
- Other bacterial infections: chest, wound and lymphocoele infections, *C. difficile*.
- Donor → recipient bacterial infections (usually *S. aureus* or Gram –ves)

One to six months
- Viral infections: CMV, HSV, shingles, EBV.
- Opportunistic infections: *Listeria, Aspergillus, Pnemocystis carinii*

Beyond six months
- Chronic viral infection: BK nephropathy, EBV-driven PTLD

General management issues

▶ When treating:
- Dose reductions for GFR: watch Cr carefully.
- Drug interactions, particularly antimicrobials that may induce/inhibit cytochrome P450 and thus modify immunosuppressant levels: watch CNI trough levels carefully.

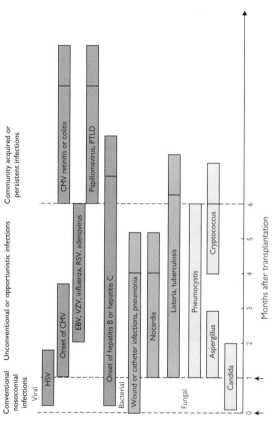

Fig. 4.9 Sequence of post-transplant infection. Adapted with permission from Davidson AMA, Cameron JS, Grunfeld J-P, et al. (eds) (2005). *Oxford Textbook of Clinical Nephrology*, 3rd edn. Oxford: Oxford University Press.

Cytomegalovirus (CMV)

▶ The most important infectious complication of renal transplantation.

Introduction

CMV is a DNA (herpes type) virus that infects about 40–50% of the normal population. Previous exposure is reflected by anti-CMV IgM positivity (measured routinely in all donors and recipients: CMV naïve patients who receive a kidney from a CMV +ve donor are most at risk).

Clinical features

- Can be asymptomatic (*CMV viraemia*).
- Fever, malaise, neutropenia, ↓Plt (*CMV disease*).
- Hepatitis, pancreatitis, pneumonitis, chorioretinitis, invasive GI disease (oesophagitis, gastritis, colitis, perforations), graft dysfunction (*tissue invasive disease*).
- Usually 1–4 months post transplant.
- ⚠ CMV causes further host immunosuppression (predisposing to 2° invasion—PCP and fungi).
- ☛ CMV may be a risk factor for rejection.
- Detection is by PCR for viral DNA:
  - Quantitative PCR >500copies/mL implies viraemia (laboratory assays vary).
  - Most will be symptomatic >3000copies/mL.
- May also identify cytopathic viral inclusions on tissue samples (colon, kidney, oesophagus, etc.).

Treatment

- If tissue invasive disease: IV ganciclovir for 10–14 days. If WCC low, stop MMF or azathioprine. Relapses not infrequent. Dose as:
  - eGFR >70   5mg/kg bd
  - eGFR 50–69   2.5mg/kg bd
  - eGFR 25–49   2.5mg/kg daily
  - eGFR 10–24   1.25mg/kg daily
  - eGFR <10, dialysis   1.25mg/kg 3×/week (after HD)
- An alternative, particularly if viraemia without tissue invasive disease, is to use oral valganciclovir:
  - eGFR >60   900mg od
  - eGFR 40–59   450mg od
  - eGFR 25–39   450mg alt. days
  - eGFR 10–24   450mg twice weekly
  - eGFR <10, dialysis   Use IVI ganciclovir
- Monitor quantitative CMV PCR weekly.

Prophylaxis

Two strategies:
- Universal prophylaxis for all 'at risk' patients immediately post-transplant.
- Pre-emptive therapy—quantitative PCR is used for surveillance to detect early disease.

If detected, consider reduction in immunosuppression. Valganciclovir (dose as above) is used for effective prophylaxis in the post transplant period (for 6 months).

Table 4.7 Risk of CMV according to serological status

Donor CMV status	Recipient CMV status	Risk
– ve	– ve	Low
+ ve	– ve	High
– ve	+ ve	Medium
+ ve	+ ve	Medium
Either donor and/or recipient CMV +ve and treatment with ATG/OKT3		High

BK virus nephropathy

Or polyoma virus-associated nephropathy. BK virus is a polyoma virus (with a prevalence of ~ 70% in adults) recently recognized as a significant pathogen in renal transplantation. First described in the late 1990s, allograft disease 2° infection with BK species affects between 3–5% of transplant recipients. The virus achieves latency in tubular cells, and infection may → graft failure (although most cases are asymptomatic). BK virus nephropathy appears to be related to the intensity of immuno-suppression.

Clinically

Presents as:
- Sterile pyuria ± haematuria.
- ↑Cr 2° lymphocytic infiltration of the allograft (⚠ difficult to distinguish from cellular rejection).
- Ureteric ulceration or stenosis → strictures, transplant hydronephrosis.
- Haemorrhagic cystitis.

Diagnosis

Urine cytology: infected tubular cells are shed into the urine—so-called 'decoy cells' are present in 90% of infected patients (>10 decoy cells/hpf suggestive of disease). Blood PCR for BKV is the most specific technique available, though not necessarily an indication to treat—*a renal biopsy is required*.
▶ The characteristic finding is a tubulo-interstitial nephritis with a mono-nuclear cell infiltrates, and viral inclusion in tubular cells. Confirm BKV using immunohistochemistry.

Treatment

- Is unsatisfactory, and many will lose their grafts.
- Generally, aim for reduction of immunosuppression.
- No clear evidence for the use of antivirals, but cidofovir 0.25–1 mg/kg/dose (fortnightly) for 1–4 doses may be of benefit. Cidofovir is nephrotoxic.

BK investigation and treatment algorithim

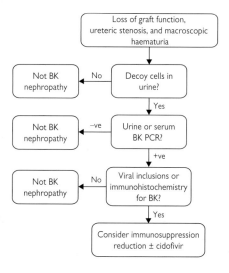

Post-transplant malignancy

Skin

~50% of transplant recipients 20yrs on have (or have had) a skin cancer, usually squamous cell carcinomas (SCC) but also basal cell carcinomas. Skin type, human papilloma virus, and sun exposure appear to be risk factors for the development of SCC.

▶ Advocate sun protection at all times, and seek regular skin review.

Kaposi sarcoma occurs more frequently in recipients from endemic areas, with human herpes virus 8 implicated.

Post-transplant lymphoproliferative disorders

The PTLDs include:
- Non-Hodgkin's lymphomas (90%), of recipient B cell origin
- Myeloma (4%)
- Hodgkin's disease (2.5%).

PTLD occurs in 1–5% of renal transplant recipients, occurring more frequently in those more heavily immunosuppressed. Diagnosis occurs at 2 peaks: 12–18 months post-transplant, and then again at > 5 years out. Primary infection with Epstein–Barr virus (EBV) infection is often implicated—EBV becomes immortalized in B cells, and may → unregulated proliferation and resistance to apoptosis.

▶ 1° EBV infection after transplantation ↑risk for PTLD by 10–76-fold. Early PTLD tends to be EBV positive and later PTLD less so.

Presentation is variable ranging from a viral-type illness to specific evidence of organ dysfunction:
- PTLD occurs in unusual sites, and is often extranodal.
- Fever is common, as is malaise.
- The transplant itself may be infiltrated.
- GI: pain, bleeding, diarrhea, obstruction.
- Hepatitis, meningeal involvement, retroperitoneal disease.
- May be ↑lymphocyte count and LDH.

There is a strong correlation between histological appearance and the response to treatment: polyclonal polymorphic types respond to treatment much better than monotypic monoclonal PTLD.

With EBV-positive B cell PTLD, patients may respond to gradual reduction of immunosuppression without the need for chemotherapy. This process can be tailored by measuring EBV-specific T cell subsets (their appearance with reduction of immunosuppression may herald regression of tumour). ✒ From this observation, there is now interest in infusing EBV directed cytotoxic T lymphocytes (CTL) as treatment for PTLD. Rituximab is being used in tumours that express CD20.

Cervical and vulval carcinoma

Post-transplant ♀ are more likely to develop these, and should be screened regularly using cervical smear screening and examination.

Solid tumours

There is a slight ↑risk of many solid tumours in transplant recipients, but specific screening programs for recipients are not merited. Tumours of the native kidneys or ano-genital region are much more common in the transplant compared to the general population.

Expanding the donor pool

Sensitized patients (those with pre-formed antibodies against a variety of common antigens) may wait for prolonged periods to be offered a well-matched cadaveric transplant, and may find living donation contra-indicated by a positive cross-match. As a result, there has been a resurgence of interest in anti-HLA antibody removal prior to transplantation, as well as other schemes that may increase available organs.

Transplanting across a positive cross-match

Once a suitable living donor is identified, the aim is to remove antibodies prior to transplant:
- Plasma exchange removes circulating antibodies (including anti-HLA).
  - Antibody removal is often a temporary phenomenon.
  - Transplantation occurs once a recipient is 'anti-donor antibody' –ve.
- IV immunoglobulin has a more sustained effect on antibody levels.
  - May be used successfully on patients waiting for a cadaveric transplant.
  - High dose IVIg is given against serial DSA (📖 p.245).
  - Mechanism of action is not fully elucidated: probably involves anti-idiotype along with immunomodulatory type actions.
- Patients receiving such treatments are at ↑risk of humoral rejection post transplant (📖 p.263).

Transplanting across blood groups

Blood group O are universal donors, and AB universal recipients. Until fairly recently, transplantation was only carried out in blood group matched pairs or according to 'transfusion rules'. This is no longer the case. Blood group A patients can be grouped as A1 and A2: those with A2 express much lower amounts of A antigen on cell surfaces and can be considered blood group O if the recipients have no/low levels of circulating anti-A antibodies. Anti-blood group antibody removal is also being increasingly performed. Using techniques such as plasma exchange or immunoabsorption these antibodies can be removed prior to transplantation. Again, rejection rates are higher.

Live donor exchange schemes

Such schemes are gaining in popularity: if a patient has a live donor, but for ABO or immunological reasons the transplant cannot go ahead, donors and recipients agree to swap pairs (see Fig. 4.11). Donor nephrectomies are carried out simultaneously in order to prevent a particular donor 'backing out' after their relative has received a kidney.

Xenotransplantation

Research continues in this area. Natural antibodies responsible for hyper-acute rejection have been identified. Concern remains regarding the possible transmission of viral pathogens to humans.

Example of live donor exchange scheme

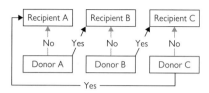

Fig. 4.11 Donor A is unable to donate to recipient A for immunological reasons. The same is true of the pairs B and C. Using and exchange scheme donor A donates to recipient B, donor B to recipient C and donor C to recipient A

Kidney–pancreas transplantation

Introduction

Transplantation is the treatment of choice for diabetic patients with ESRD. In addition to kidney transplantation alone, options are:
- Combined kidney–pancreas transplantation (80%).
- Pancreas (cadaveric) after kidney (living donor) transplantation (20%).
- Islet cell transplantation (see box opposite).

Benefits

- Pancreas transplantation corrects the glycaemic state (HbA1c falls to normal), leading to improved quality of life (freedom from both insulin and dialysis).
- Prevention of progression of diabetic complications (and possibly partial reversal ♠️).
- Beneficial effect on lipids.
- Comparable survival to live kidney transplant alone.

Selection criteria

- Type 1 DM with stage 5 CKD.
- Age <50 years (usually).
- Sufficient CV reserve (ejection fraction>50%, no uncorrected IHD).
- Established diabetic complications.

Surgical technique

Two options:
- Bladder drainage. Kidney is transplanted into the left iliac fossa and exocrine secretions of the pancreas routed into the bladder via a duodenal cystotomy. Metabolic complications:
  - Acidosis (HCO_3 depletion) and Na^+ loss (→relative hypotension requires sodium bicarbonate administration (e.g. 2g qds).
  - Calcium bladder stones (alkaline urine).
  - Chemical cystitis/urethritis.
  - Reflux pancreatitis.
- Enteric drainage: exocrine secretions drains into bowel. Fewer metabolic complications and now generally preferred.
- Pancreatic venous drainage; 2 options:
  - Into systemic circulation (→ no 1st pass metabolism ∴ hyperinsulinaemia → ?↑risk of atherosclerosis).
  - Into portal circulation (more physiological, no hyperinsulinaemia).
- Immunosuppression. Steroids, tacrolimus and MMF.
- Rejection rates are low and can be detected by renal dysfunction (and biopsy of the renal allograft).
- More morbidity in the first year (length of hospital stay doubles compared to kidney alone).
- 20–30% chance of laparotomy during post-transplant period.

- Fungal infection more common than after kidney alone.
- 85% and 70% 1 and 5 year pancreas survival after SPK (higher kidney survival).
- Post-transplant hyperglycaemia: caused by graft dysfunction, de novo T2DM (steroids), recurrent autoimmune injury.

Barriers to successful islet cell transplantation

Islet cell transplantation shows promise, but early excellent results have proved difficult to sustain. Reasons include:

- Immune mediated destruction (highly immunogenic).
- Insufficient islet cell mass (more than one donor needed).
- Drug toxicity (CNIs and steroids are toxic to islet cells).
- Recurrent transplantation is often necessary.

Hypertension

Hypertension facts and figures

Epidemiology

The WHO identifies hypertension as the *single most important* preventable cause of premature death in developed countries. It is the most common indication for prescription drug therapy (in 2001 the NHS in the UK funded 90 million prescriptions for antihypertensive drugs at a cost of £840 million).

- The 1998 Health Survey for England (sample size 12,000) found a prevalence of hypertension (≥140/90 or on antihypertensive medication) of 40.8% for ♂ and 32.9% for ♀.
- ~$\frac{1}{3}$ of those in middle age and $\frac{2}{3}$ in old age are hypertensive.
- It occurs in association with other CV risk factors rather than isolation
- Significant under-diagnosis and treatment remains common. The 'rule of halves':
  - ½ those with ↑BP have not been diagnosed.
  - ½ of those who have been diagnosed are not on treatment.
  - ½ of those receiving treatment do not have adequate control.

Classifying hypertension

Essential hypertension is a heterogeneous genetic and environmental condition.
Secondary hypertension implies ↑BP is 2° to an underlying disorder. It accounts for ~5–10% cases (📖 p.306).

Hypertension facts and figures

- Systolic BP (SBP) ↑ with age until the 8th decade.
- Diastolic BP (DBP) ↑ up to age 50, after which it ↔ or ↓slightly.
- DBP is the best indicator of CV risk <50 years. With ↑age there is a shift to SBP (then pulse pressure) as the principal predictor.
- Reduction in SBP of 20mmHg systolic or DBP of 10mmHg is associated with reductions in death from stroke and IHD of ~50% (slightly more in younger patients, slightly less in older). This is consistent down to 115/75—there is no clear threshold below which further reduction in BP is no longer beneficial.
- Non-pharmacological strategies (i.e. lifestyle measures) have been shown to ↓BP.
- Antihypertensive drug treatment not only ↓BP, but also ↓complications.
- Patient education is paramount: ↑BP is an asymptomatic condition and benefits of treatment may not be immediately apparent to the patient.

Major cardiovascular risk factors

- Hypertension*
- Smoking
- Obesity (BMI ≥ 30)*
- Physical inactivity
- Dyslipidaemia*
- Diabetes mellitus*
- Albuminuria or GFR <60mL/min
- Age (♂ >55 years, ♀ >65 years)
- Family history of premature CV disease (♂ <55 years, ♀ <65 years).

* components of the metabolic syndrome

Target organ damage (TOD)

- Heart: LVH, IHD, LV dysfunction, and CCF
- Brain: stroke, TIA, and vascular dementia
- Chronic kidney disease
- Peripheral arterial disease
- Retinopathy.

SBP, pulse pressure, and CV risk

SBP

- Historically DBP was thought the best predictor of CV disease.
- Now clear that SBP has a continuous independent relationship with stroke and IHD risk.
- It can be difficult to get SBP to target, particularly in the elderly.

Pulse pressure (PP) and risk

- A wide PP (SBP minus DBP) more accurately predicts adverse CV outcome than SBP or DBP.
- PP appears to be a marker of arterial stiffness.
- PP may identify those with SBP at particular risk.
- The majority of trial data is for SBP and DBP so the major guidelines are based on these rather than PP.

What is hypertension?

BP variation in a population follows a normal distribution, so an arbitrary cut-off point defines abnormal. Normal BP varies between races, the sexes, with age, and even throughout the day. Even if an arbitrary definition of ↑BP could be agreed, it would differ depending on the population studied.

Important prognostic differences in systolic vs. diastolic hypertension have only recently been recognized, with systolic pressure (and PP), now thought to be more important in predicting risk.

> Perhaps the most useful definition, then, is:
> *'hypertension is a level of blood pressure which places an individual at increased risk of cardiovascular events'.*
> ▶ An individual whose BP is just below that cut-off has a virtually identical CV risk to one just above it.

The great apes do not get hypertension, nor do present-day hunter-gatherer populations (with a similar diet and lifestyle to that of our ancestors). There is something about our *environment* and *diet* which predisposes to hypertension. Genes and genetics are relevant, but insufficient in isolation.

Important principles in pathophysiology

BP = cardiac output (CO) x systemic vascular resistance (SVR)

The final common pathway in chronic hypertension is increased systemic vascular resistance. The earliest event in the development of hypertension is usually a rise in cardiac output. Increased cardiac output causes an increase in wall: lumen ratio in resistance vessels, (to normalize wall stress). This leads to a sustained rise in SVR, and causes chronic hypertension. Cardiac output is usually *normal* in those with *established* hypertension.

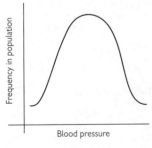

Fig. 5.1 Distribution of BP in any population: the cut-off for defining 'high' BP is arbitrary.

Central role of the kidney

- Sodium excretion depends on renal perfusion pressure (the Guyton hypothesis). So ↑renal perfusion → pressure natriuresis. In hypertension this curve is pushed to the right (see Fig. 5.2).
- Monogenic (rare!) forms of ↑BP suggest tubular ion transport mechanisms are important mediators of blood pressure control.
- There is much redundancy in control of BP. Many neuro-endocrine systems contribute to it in overlapping and interlocking ways. And any or all of these may lead to abnormal blood pressure.

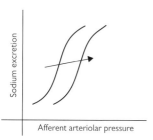

Afferent arteriolar pressure

Fig. 5.2 In the normotensive individual, salt balance is maintained at a normal BP. The slope of the curve is very steep, such that dietary salt loading does not significantly alter BP. In hypertensive individuals the curve is shifted to the right, though it remains parallel. Thus on a normal sodium diet, salt balance is maintained, but at a higher BP. In salt sensitive individuals the rightward shift is accompanied by a depression of the slope (not shown). Thus not only is the BP set point on a normal diet elevated, but the BP also increases in response to dietary salt loading.

Salt intake and blood pressure

A high dietary salt intake is an important but not absolute condition for the development of hypertension. The Intersalt trial showed that populations with a low intake of dietary sodium have a low prevalence of hypertension—essential hypertension is seen mainly in societies with a salt intake >6g per day. Modest reduction in salt intake for people on a typical Western diet results in a BP drop of 5.3/3.7mmHg in hypertensive patients and 1.9/1.1mmHg in normotensives. Were salt intake to be reduced over many years, the population benefits may be substantial.

'Salt sensitive hypertension' is said to occur when BP varies with salt intake. In most people the renal pressure natriuresis curve is steep (a small ↑ in BP → to a large ↑ in salt excretion). If this curve is shallower, then BP will vary with salt intake. This occurs in patients with CKD, but also in others with more subtle disruption of renal tubulo-glomerular feedback (📖 p.620). It is more common in black and obese patients.

In societies in which salt is consumed in vast excess of physiological requirements, to have a blood pressure which is sensitive to salt intake may predispose to hypertension.

Pathogenesis

Genetics

Inheritance is not Mendelian. No one gene is responsible.

Blood pressure levels are similar amongst close relatives (even those with 'normal' range BP), suggesting alleles on several different genes may have an effect on BP.

Rare monogenic causes of hypertension (see box below) have been identified using linkage analysis in afflicted families. Defects in these genes may also be important in *essential* hypertension (gene defects coding the β and γ subunits of the epithelial Na^+ channel (linked to Liddle's syndrome) are associated with BP variations in the general population. Research focus has been on likely culprit genes (esp. the angiotensinogen gene). Our understanding remains far from complete.

Genes which have been associated with essential hypertension include:

- ACE polymorphisms (I/I and I/D phenotypes associate with salt-sensitive hypertension).
- α-adducin polymorphisms—a cytoskeletal protein which regulates ion transport in the renal tubule. Polymorphisms may relate to salt sensitivity, diuretic sensitivity, and essential hypertension.
- 11 β-hydroxysteroid dehydrogenase (GG phenotype correlates with salt sensitivity).
- AT-1 receptor gene—in experimental studies AT-1a +/+ mice have higher blood pressures than –/– mice. Clinical relevance unknown.

Rare single gene causes of hypertension

Liddle's syndrome: mutations affect the epithelial sodium channel (ENaC). Autosomal dominant, with ↑BP characterized by ↓renin, ↓aldosterone, and ↓K^+ (📖 p.536).

Glucocorticoid-remediable aldosteronism (📖 p.310)

Syndrome of apparent mineralocorticoid excess (📖 p.312)

Pregnancy associated hypertension: a gene defect → partial activation of the mineralcorticoid receptor by progesterone (rare).

Phaeochromocytoma: may occur with one of the following:
- Multiple endocrine neoplasia type 2A: mutations in the RET proto-oncogene. Autosomal dominant, phaeochromocytoma, medullary thyroid carcinoma, and hyperparathyroidism
- Von Hippel–Lindau disease: mutations in the VHL tumour suppressor gene, autosomal dominant. Presents with adrenal phaeochromo-cytomas, renal cell carcinomas, cerebellar and retinal haemangio-blastomas
- Neurofibromatosis type 1: mutations in the NF1 tumour suppressor gene, autosomal dominant. Presents with phaeochromocytomas, multiple neurofibromas, café au lait spots, Lisch nodules of the iris.

The renin–angiotensin system (RAS)

Plays a central role in salt and water homeostasis, and BP control. Abnormalities in the RAS affect blood pressure and the system is a therapeutic target (ACE inhibitors, AII receptor blockers, 📖 pp.342 and 344). In the juxtaglomerular apparatus, granular cells synthesize and release renin. Renin converts inactive angiotensinogen into angiotensin I, which in turn is converted by ACE in the lungs to active angiotensin II (AII). AII binds two receptors, AT-1 and -2 (see below).

Renin release is mediated by

- ↓ afferent arteriolar (ie renal perfusion) pressure of any cause.
- Sympathetic nervous system activation (granular cell β1-receptors).
- ↓ Na^+ delivery to the distal tubule (sensed by the macula densa).
- Prostacyclin, ACTH.

Increased renin

Renal artery stenosis, renal cell carcinoma, benign reninoma (very rare), other renin secreting malignancies (also very rare).
▶ Many patients with essential hypertension have ↑plasma renin levels *not* related to any of the above, nor of any therapeutic use.

Angiotensin

Circulating AII binds vascular receptors, but *locally released* AII works at tissue level in a paracrine fashion. Levels in tissue have no correlation with systemic levels, but may correlate better with disease pathogenesis.

Actions of angiotensin II

- Arteriolar vasoconstriction (and venules to a lesser extent)
- Efferent renal arteriolar vasoconstriction
- Aldosterone secretion
- Epinephrine (adrenalin) release
- Smooth muscle hypertrophy
- Increased reabsorption of sodium in PCT
- Inhibits renin release (negative feedback loop)
- Renal mesangial cell growth and matrix expansion
- Myocardial growth and matrix expansion
- Stimulates thirst and ADH release.

Most effects are mediated by the angiotensin type 1 (AT-1) receptor. The role of AT-2 receptors remains unclear, but angiotensin binding may regulate vasodilatory, proliferative and apoptotic effects of AII.

Aldosterone

Aldosterone synthesis occurs mainly in the zona glomerulosa of the adrenal cortex, and is tightly regulated by the RAS, or by electrolyte imbalance: ↑K^+ or ↓salt intake → aldosterone synthesis. Aldosterone acts at the collecting duct to promote Na^+ retention and K^+ excretion (📖 p.628). Cortisol *also* activates the mineralocorticoid receptor—so aldosterone-sensitive tissues contain high levels of 11-β hydroxysteroid dehydrogenase 2 (this converts cortisol to cortisone, which is incapable of activating the receptor) and this protects the mineralocorticoid receptor from states of high circulating cortisol.

Extra-renal actions of aldosterone

- Paracrine action in non-epithelial tissues (brain, heart, epithelium).
- Associated with vascular inflammation and cardiac fibrosis. The same may be true of other non-vascular tissues.
- Activates pro-fibrotic and growth factors in other tissues (including the kidney).

Arterial stiffness

Arterial pressure depends in part on the compliance of conduit arteries. Stiff arteries are less able to dampen a surge in pressure in systole, so systolic pressure is higher. A stiffer artery will also conduct a pulse wave more rapidly. Normally, the pulse wave is reflected back from the small vessels, arriving back at the heart during diastole. If conducted more rapidly, the reflected pulse wave may reach the heart during systole, further ↑systolic pressure, and ↓diastolic pressure. Coronary artery perfusion, which occurs predominantly during diastole, may be affected. Commoner causes of reduced compliance (or ↑stiffness) include:

- Ageing: loss of elastin, calcification of arterial walls, lipid deposition, and defective endothelial function all contribute.
- Diabetes: ↑arterial stiffness is accelerated (even if ↑BP is absent), as non-enzymatic glycosylation of connective tissue, high insulin levels ± activation of the sympathetic nervous system alter compliance.
- Chronic kidney disease, and esp. ESRD: oxidant stress, impaired endothelial function, abnormal lipid profile, calcification of the arterial wall (exacerbated by disordered calcium, phosphate and PTH), and a variety of putative uraemic toxins are thought important (📖 p.158).

⚠ Increased arterial stiffness and pulse wave velocity are *independent predictors* of all cause mortality and cardiovascular morbidity and mortality in patients with hypertension.

Endothelial dysfunction and nitric oxide

↑BP is associated with impaired endothelium-dependent relaxation of the vessel wall. A number of factors influence endothelial function:

- Nitric oxide (NO)
  - → relaxation of vascular smooth muscle. Released by endothelium in response to shear stress (i.e. blood flow)
  - Endogenous NO synthase (eNOS) → continuous normal basal release. Inducible iNOS → high concentrations of NO in response to inflammatory cytokines.
  - ↓NO has been reported in hypertensive patients (+ their offspring).
- Oxidative stress: free radicals scavenge NO, forming potentially toxic by-products. Radicals themselves (such as superoxide, O_2^-) are potent vasoconstrictors.
- Prostaglandins: prostacyclin (PGI_2) is released by endothelial cells in response to shear stress and has a synergistic effect on tone with NO.
- Angiotensin II: a vasoconstrictor, also contributes to free radical generation, and to endothelin release.
- Endothelin: a potent vasoconstrictor, opposing the actions of NO. Also cause renal Na^+ retention, ↑aldosterone, vascular smooth muscle cell proliferation, cardiac hypertrophy, and fibrosis. Their causal role in hypertension is unclear.

Sympathetic nervous system (SNS)

Activation of the SNS is clearly linked with acute hypertension—chronic activation may have a role in the genesis of long-term hypertension in those with a genetic predisposition. SNS activation causes:

- ↑ in stroke volume (via α-1 and -2 receptors).
- ↑ in heart rate (via β-1 receptors).
- ↑ in systemic vascular resistance (via α-1 receptors).
- Activation of the RAS (via β-1 receptor mediated renin release).

Other factors

- Insulin resistance has a clear relationship with hypertension:
  - Fasting insulin levels correlate with BP in insulin resistant patients.
  - Relatives of those with ↑BP are more likely to have insulin resistance.
  - Insulin resistance predicts the subsequent development of ↑BP
  - Mechanisms may include SNS activation and Na$^+$ retention.
- Natriuretic peptides, including:
  - ANP (atrial natriuretic peptide). Released by atrial tissue in response to stretch i.e. volume overload.
  - BNP (brain natriuretic peptide), first discovered in the brain but synthesized and secreted by ventricular myocardium.
  - CNP (C-type) and DNP (Dendroaspis): more recently discovered. Relevance not yet clear.
  - Urodilatin. Similar structure to ANP but confined to the kidney. Synthesized in distal tubular cells, causing natriuresis.

The natriuretic peptides are secreted in response to volume overload, leading to a compensatory natriuretic effect. Other effects include vasodilation, modulation of vascular smooth muscle function, and control of the RAS system. Their role in the pathogenesis of hypertension is less clear. In experimental studies defects in natriuretic peptide production cause salt sensitive hypertension.

BP measurement

Clinic

The mercury sphygmanometer remains the gold standard, though semi-automated devices are increasingly popular. Validation and maintenance are vital: for a list of approved apparatus, see www.bhs.org.

Procedure

- No coffee, strenuous exercise, or smoking just before measurement.
- Sit the patient in a quiet room for a few minutes.
- Measure with the patient sitting and support the arm at heart level.
- The cuff bladder should encircle ≥80% of the upper arm. The standard adult bladder is 12x26cm (some consider 12x35cm standard).
  - Cuff too large → underestimation.
  - Cuff too small → overestimation.
- In elderly or diabetic patients, check for orthostatic hypotension by repeating after 2 minutes standing.
- Use Korotkoff phase I (appearance) for SBP and phase V (disappearance) for DBP. If phase V goes to zero, use phase IV (muffling).
- Take 2 measurements 1–2min apart and read to the nearest 2mmHg.
- Measure in both arms. If there is a significant difference, use the arm giving the higher value for subsequent readings.
- Don't round up or down to preconceived values (observer prejudice).
- Document the time of measurement in relation to tablets.

Home

Wrist monitors are not as accurate as upper arm devices and not recommended. Explain the device to patients, and ensure it is used properly.
- Pros include involving patients in their own management (? better compliance), allows multiple readings on different days, reduces the 'white coat' effect (📖 p.291). ► Home readings predict target organ damage.
- Cons include many monitors being inaccurate and poorly maintained, and that measurements are not taken under standardized conditions.

Clinic readings demonstrably correlate with CV risk. Home readings are generally lower, so what constitutes normal? The British Hypertension Society (BHS) recommends a downward correction of 12/7mmHg for clinic values when comparing with home values (normal is probably <130/85).

Ambulatory BP monitoring (ABPM)

Provides a measure of BP during 'normal life'—may correlate better with CV risk and TOD (◆). Measurements are usually lower than clinic. Presently complements rather than replaces standard measurements. Fitting takes 15–30min. Tell the patient to refrain from strenuous exercise, straighten their arm during measurement (tricky if driving) and to keep a concurrent diary e.g. sleep times. BP is measured at repeated intervals (commonly every 30min), throughout the day and night. SBP and DBP can be plotted over time, with most devices providing average day, night, and 24 hour pressures.

ABPM readings and interpretation

	Normal	**Abnormal**
Daytime	<135/85	>140/90
Night-time	<120/70	>125/75
24 hours	<130/80	>135/85

A relatively high nocturnal BP (blunted nocturnal hypotension or 'dipping') without a fall of <10/5mmHg, may indicate an adverse prognosis.

Potential indications for ABPM

- Unusual clinic BP variability, or other discrepancies in readings.
- Hypertensive clinic values but hypotensive symptoms.
- Possible 'white-coat hypertension' (first and last hours ignored).
- Evaluation of real or apparent drug resistance.
- Investigation of autonomic dysfunction.

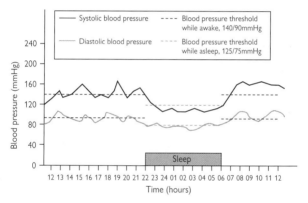

Fig. 5.3 Example of variation in daytime and night-time BP

'White coat' hypertension (isolated clinic hypertension)

- Clinic BP is consistently elevated, though ABPM readings are normal.
- Consider when BP appears elevated, but there is no TOD.
- The anticipation of BP measurement → alerting reaction → ↑BP.
- Can result in normotensive patients being diagnosed with hypertension. Also occurs in treated hypertensive patients.
- Prevalence ↑ with age and is higher for milder forms of hypertension (10–30% for grade 1 and <10% for grade 2 and 3 📖 p.294).
- May be a precursor of sustained hypertension.
- May in itself confer ↑CV risk (✦ not in all studies).

Clinical assessment

History and examination
- Duration of elevated BP. Previous monitoring, treatment, and control.
- Other CVD risk factors.
- Anything to suggest secondary hypertension (□ p.306)?
  - Young age (<30 years, esp. if non-obese and Caucasian)
  - Sudden-onset hypertension
  - Presents as malignant hypertension (□ p.350)
  - Sudden deterioration in BP control
  - Severe or 'resistant' (≥3 drugs) hypertension
  - Other diagnostic clues? (□ p.307)
- Other contributory factors?
  - Drugs
  - Overweight (especially abdominal obesity)
  - Excess C_2H_5OH
  - Excess salt intake
  - Lack of exercise
  - Environmental stress
  - Smoking.
- Evidence of hypertensive complications?
  - Stroke, TIA, cognitive decline, carotid bruits
  - IHD, cardiomegaly, CCF
  - Peripheral vascular disease
  - Fundi: hemorrhages, exudates or papilloedema (retinopathy grades I and II have little prognostic value)
  - Renal impairment or proteinuria
  - Sexual dysfunction.
- Previous drug treatment and side effects.
- Contraindications to specific drugs; e.g. bronchospasm.
- Family history: ↑BP, stroke, diabetes, ↑lipids, renal disease, premature IHD.

Investigations

Routine
- Urinalysis (?protein ± blood).
- U+E (& eGFR).
- Blood glucose—preferably fasting.
- Lipid profile—preferably fasting.
- ECG for LVH (± LV strain—higher risk) and evidence of IHD.

Desirable
- Echocardiogram
- Uric acid (↑ in the metabolic syndrome)
- Hb and Hct
- CRP (may predict CV risk)
- Microalbuminuria
- Vascular US
  - Plaque detection
  - Measurements of intima media thickness
  - Pulse wave velocity to estimate large artery compliance.

Classification of hypertension

Drawing up guidelines is easy. Transferring them into clinical practice isn't.

Grade 1 (SBP: 140–159 and/or DBP: 90–99mmHg)

Encouraged lifestyle measures. Recheck BP within 3 months. Offer drug treatment if:
- Evidence of complications.
- Coexistent diabetes.
- Estimated 10-year CVD risk is >20% (Joint British Societies CVD risk chart 📖 p.298).
- The patient is willing to accept it.

If untreated, annual (minimum) monitoring of BP is mandatory; 10–15% will need treatment within 5 years and overall CV risk ↑ with age.

Grade 2 (SBP 160–179 and/or DBP 100–109mmHg)

Encourage lifestyle measures. Recheck BP within 2 months. Offer drug treatment if:
- Evidence of complications.
- Coexistent diabetes.
- Elevated BP persists after 2 months despite lifestyle measures.

Grade 3 (SBP>180–219 and/or DBP>110–119mmHg)

Encourage lifestyle measures. Recheck BP within 2 weeks. Offer drug treatment if:
- Elevated BP confirmed.

Severe hypertension

- ▶ BP >220/120mmHg: treat immediately.
- ⚠ Malignant hypertension (papilloedema ± hemorrhages and exudates) or acute cardiovascular complications → admit (📖 p.350).

Isolated systolic hypertension (ISH)

- Grade 1
  Treat if sustained SBP 140–159mmHg. If:
  - TOD (📖 p.281)
  - Established CV disease
  - Diabetes
  - 10-year CV risk >20%.
- Grade 2
  - Drug therapy indicated if sustained SBP >160mmHg despite lifestyle measures.

Table 5.1 British Hypertension Society classification of BP

Category	Systolic blood pressure (mmHg)	Diastolic blood pressure (mmHg)
Optimal blood pressure	<120	<80
Normal blood pressure	<130	<85
High-normal blood pressure	130–139	85–89
Grade 1 hypertension (mild)	140–159	90–99
Grade 2 hypertension (moderate)	160–179	100–109
Grade 3 hypertension (severe)	≥180	≥110
Isolated systolic hypertension (Grade 1)	140–159	<90
Isolated systolic hypertension (Grade 2)	≥160	<90

If SBP and DBP fall into different categories, the higher value is taken.

There are several important sources of guidelines for the classification and treatment of hypertension:
• The British Hypertension Society (BHS)
• The European Society of Hypertension-European Society of Cardiology (ESH-ESC)
• The WHO/International Society for Hypertension (WHO/ISH)
• The Joint National Committee (JNC) (USA)
• The National Kidney Foundation—Kidney Disease Outcomes Quality Initiative (NKF/K-DOQI) (hypertension in the context of renal disease).
• National Institute for Clinical Excellence (NICE).

All draw on the results of large randomized controlled trials and meta-analyses to formulate their recommendations. All are available online.

The above BHS classification is very similar to that of the ESH-ESC and the WHO/ISH. The most recent JNC guidelines differ in designating the high-normal group 'pre-hypertensive'.

Treatment thresholds

Aim for a target of
- <140/85mmHg
- <130/80mmHg if DM, CKD (lower if proteinuria 🕮 p.151) or established CV disease.

The minimum acceptable level of control (audit standard) is 150/90, (140/80 for DM, CKD or established CV disease).

There is now little evidence to support the J shaped curve hypothesis; i.e. generally, the lower the BP the better.

Suggested indications for specialist referral

- Urgent treatment needed
  - Accelerated hypertension (severe hypertension with grade III–IV retinopathy)
  - Particularly severe hypertension (220/120mmHg)
- Impending complications
  - e.g. TIAs, LVF
- Renal disease
- Possible 2° hypertension
- Resistance to treatment (≥3 drugs)
- Multiple drug intolerances
- Multiple drug contraindications
- Persistent nonadherence or noncompliance
- Other situations
  - Unusual blood pressure variability
  - Possible white-coat hypertension
  - Hypertension in pregnancy.

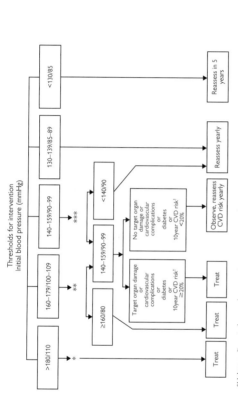

Thresholds for intervention
Initial blood pressure (mmHg)

*Unless malignant phase or hypertensive emergency confirm over 1–2 weeks then treat.
**If CV complications, target organ damage or diabetes present, confirm over 3–4 weeks then treat, if absent remeasure weekly and
treat if BP persists at these levels over 4–12 weeks.
***If CV complications, target organ damage, or diabetes present, confirm over 12 weeks then treat if absent remeasure monthly
and treat if these levels are maintained and if estimated 10 year CVD risk is ≥20%
†Assessed with CV risk chart

Fig 5.4 Thresholds for intervention. Redrawn from BHS guidelines (with permission)

Hypertension and CV risk

⚠ Risk calculators are inappropriate in the presence of pre-existing CV disease.

- The absolute risk of a CV event occurring in a patient with ↑BP varies widely depending according to age, sex, severity of BP, and presence or absence of additional risk factors.
- Intuitive estimates of risk are crude and inaccurate. Complex methods have been developed, many based on Framingham data[*].
- These data have been developed as statistical formulae, tables and charts by various authors. They have been incorporated into many guidelines, including those of the BHS and American College of Cardiology.
- Risk models provide a useful tool for both clinicians and patients. They facilitate informed treatment decisions and allow the need for medication to be reinforced in the context of overall CV risk rather than just BP.
- The BHS endorse the use of the Joint British Societies risk charts (available as a chart and computer programme at www.bhs.org and in the BNF). The latest version gives the risk of a CV event over 10 years (a combined score for CHD and stroke).
- Limitations of risk tables include poor validation in the young and ethnic populations. Framingham studied a white, middle class population on no treatment (including aspirin, statins etc.). It is now several decades old.

[*] The Framingham Heart Study: a cohort of over 5000 men and women aged 30–62, from Framingham, Massachusetts followed up from 1971 to assess the determinants of CV disease.

Notes on cardiovascular disease risk prediction charts
(Figs. 5.5 and 5.6, 📖 pp.302–3)

*Reproduced with permission from The University of Manchester
Department of Medical Illustration, Manchester Infirmary*

These charts are for estimating cardiovascular disease (CVD) risk (non-fatal MI and stroke, coronary and stroke death and new angina) for individuals who have not already developed coronary heart disease (CHD) or other major atherosclerotic disease.

They are an aid to making clinical decisions about how intensively to intervene on lifestyle and whether to use antihypertensive, lipid lowering medication and aspirin.

The use of these charts is not appropriate for the following patients groups. Those with: CHD or other major atherosclerotic disease, familial hypercholesterolaemia or other inherited dyslipidaemias, chronic renal dysfunction, type 1 or 2 diabetes mellitus.

The charts should not be used to decide whether to introduce anti-hypertensive medication when BP is persistently at or above 160/100 or when target organ damage (TOD) due to hypertension is present. In both cases medication is recommended regardless of CVD risk.

Similarly the charts should not be used to decide whether to introduce lipid-lowering medication when the ratio of serum total to HDL cholesterol exceeds 7. Such medication is generally then indicated regardless of estimated CVD risk.

To estimate an individual's absolute 10 year risk of developing CVD choose the table for his or her gender, smoking status (smoker/non-smoker) and age. Within this square define the level of risk according to the point where the coordinates for systolic blood pressure (SBP) and the ratio of total cholesterol to HDL-cholesterol meet. If no HDL cholesterol result is available, then assume this is 1.00mmol/l and the lipid scale can be used for total serum cholesterol alone.

Higher risk individuals are defined as those whose 10 year CVD risk exceeds 20%, which is approximately equivalent to the CHD risk of >15% over the same period.

The chart also assists in the identification of individuals whose 10 year CVD risk moderately increased in the range 10–20% and those in whom risk is <10% over 10 years.

Smoking status should reflect lifetime exposure to tobacco and not simply tobacco use at the time of assessment; e.g. those who have given up smoking within 5 years should be regarded as current smokers for the purposes of the charts.

The initial BP and the first random (non-fasting) total cholesterol and HDL cholesterol can be used to estimate an individual's risk. However, the decision on using drug therapy should generally be based on repeat risk factor measurements over a period of time.

Men and women do not reach the level of risk predicted by the charts for the three age bands until they reach the ages 49, 59, and 69 years respectively. Everyone aged >70 years should be considered at higher risk. The charts will overestimate current risk most in the under forties. Clinical judgement must be exercised in deciding on treatment in younger patients. However, it should be recognised that BP and cholesterol tend to rise most and HDL cholesterol to decline most in younger people already possessing adverse levels. Thus untreated, their risk at the age 49 years is likely to be higher than the projected risk shown on the age-less-than 50 years chart.

These charts (and all other currently available methods of CVD risk prediction) are based on groups of people with untreated levels of BP, total cholesterol and HDL cholesterol. In patients already receiving antihypertensive therapy in whom the decision is to be made about whether to introduce lipid-lowering medication or vice versa the charts can act as a guide, but unless recent pre-treatment risk factor values are available it is generally safest to assume that CVD risk is higher than that predicted by current levels of BP or lipids on treatment.

CVD risk is also higher than indicated in the charts for: those with a FH of premature CVD or stroke (male first degree relatives aged <55 years and female first degree relatives aged <65 years) which increases the risk by a factor of approximately 1.5, those with raised triglyceride levels, women with premature menopause, those who are not yet diabetic, but have impaired fasting glucose (6.1–6.9mmol/L).

In some ethnic minorities the risk charts underestimate CVD risk, because they have not been validated in these populations. For example, in people originating from the Indian subcontinent it is safest to assume that the CVD risk is higher than predicted from the charts (1.5 times).

The charts may be used to illustrate the direction of impact of risk factor intervention on estimated level of CVD risk. However, such estimates are crude and are not based on randomised trial evidence. The charts are primarily to assist in directing intervention to those who typically stand to benefit most.

Non-diabetic men

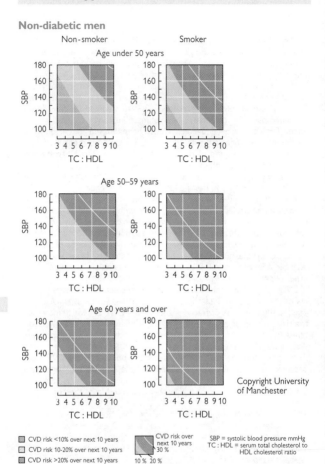

Fig. 5.5 Cardiovascular risk prediction chart for men. Reproduced with permission.

Non-diabetic women

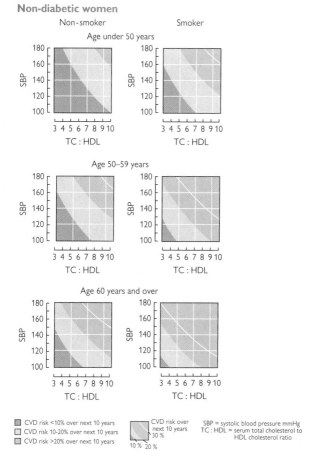

Fig. 5.6 Cardiovascular risk prediction chart for women. Reproduced with permission.

Lifestyle measures

Lifestyle changes can ↓BP, ↓drug requirement, and improve CV risk. They may also ↓ the incidence of hypertensive complications (☛unproven). Clear advice, including culturally appropriate written and audiovisual material, should be provided to all patients, as well as those with a high-normal (pre-hypertensive) BP or +ve family history.

Low sodium diet

↓BP in both normotensive and hypertensive patients, enhancing the latter's response to drug therapy. Usual Na^+ intake is in the range 150–200mmol/day. ↓ to <100mmol/day (~ 2.3g of Na^+ or 6g NaCl) by avoiding salt in cooking, salt on the table, processed foods (including many breads, stock cubes, 'ready meals', numerous breakfast cereals and pre-prepared sauces). Cook using natural ingredients. If necessary, refer to a dietitian. Note: 1g of Na^+ contains 44meq, 1g of NaCl contains 17 meq of Na^+; 5g of NaCl ~ 1 teaspoon.

⚠ Low Na^+ salt substitutes often contain KCl, ∴ avoid in renal patients.

Weight loss

Obesity (BMI ≥30kg/m^2) is fuelling the increasing incidence of ↑BP and T2DM. Weight reduction improves BP, even without dietary Na^+ restriction and has beneficial effects on insulin resistance, lipids, LVH and diabetic control.

Healthy eating

The Dietary Approach to Hypertension Trial (DASH), though short, showed impressive reductions in BP. The diet is rich in fruit and vegetables, provides high amounts of K^+, Mg^{2+}, and Ca^{2+}, limits intake of total and saturated fats and (moderately) restricts Na^+ intake (3g/24h).

The DASH eating plan can be downloaded at:
www.nhlbi.nih.gov/health/public/heart/hbp/dash

Exercise

Brisk walking for 30min ≥5×/week has been shown to ↓ the risk of DM by >50% and reduce BP by up to 10mmHg. Even mild exercise is beneficial. Isometric (weight training etc.) and strenuous exercise tend to ↑BP and are best avoided until BP is under control.

Alcohol

There is a linear relationship between C_2H_5OH consumption and BP, with the incidence of ↑BP increasing ~1.5–2.0× at >2 drinks/day. Patients will no doubt remind you of the apparent paradox that moderate alcohol intake reduces overall CV disease risk, however recommended daily amounts should not be exceeded (♂: <21 units/week; ♀: <14 units/week). Recommend low alcohol alternatives.

Caffeine

Caffeine is an adenosine receptor antagonist (→ vasoconstriction). >5 cups coffee/day is undesirable. Caffeine is also present in tea and cola drinks. Recommend decaffeinated alternatives.

Stress management
E.g. meditation, cognitive therapy, biofeedback, muscle relaxation etc.
A modest, if variable response has been seen in some studies. More are
needed.

Table 5.2 Lifestyle interventions for BP reduction

Intervention	Recommendation	Expected SBP reduction (range)
Weight reduction	Maintain ideal BMI (20–25kg/m^2)	5–10mmHg per 10kg weight loss
DASH eating plan	Consume diet rich in fruit, vegetables, low-fat dairy products with reduced content of saturated and total fat	8–14mmHg
Dietary sodium restriction	↓dietary sodium intake to <100mmol/day (<2.3g sodium or <6g sodium chloride)	2–8mmHg
Physical activity	Undertake regular aerobic activity; e.g. brisk walking for ≥30 min most days	4–9mmHg
Alcohol	♂ <21 units/ week ♀ <14 units/ week	2–4mmHg

Additional lifestyle measures that ↓CV disease risk

- Stop smoking. Does not ↓BP, but will improve overall CV risk. Quitting before middle age returns life expectancy to near that of life long non-smokers.
- Reduce total fat intake.
- Replace dietary saturated fats with mono-unsaturated fats.
- Increase consumption of oily fish.

Secondary hypertension

Probably accounts for ~5–10% of all cases of ↑BP, though true prevalence remains unknown. More common in the subgroup of 'resistant' hypertension 🕮 p.348. History, examination, and routine investigation along with a high index of suspicion should identify those in need of specialist assessment. The diagnoses are important to make as curative treatment is available for many. Diagnostic clues are shown in Table 5.3.

Classification

1. Renal disorders (🕮 p.150 for ↑BP in CKD)
- Renal parenchymal disease: acute or chronic GN, tubulointerstitial disease, APKD, obstructive uropathy.
- Renovascular disease (🕮 p.412).
- Renin producing tumours (🕮 p.310).
- Genetic diseases affecting tubular transport (Liddle's syndrome, 🕮 p.536). Very rare.

2. Endocrine disorders
- Excess mineralocorticoid (🕮 pp.308–13): 1° aldosteronism, apparent mineralocorticoid excess, congenital adrenal hyperplasia, liquorice ingestion, ectopic ACTH secretion, exogenous mineralocorticoids; e.g. fludrocortisone, pseudohyperaldosteronism.
- Others, including phaeochromocytoma, Cushing's syndrome, hypothyroidism, hyperthyroidism (↑SBP), hyperparathyroidism, acromegaly or the carcinoid syndrome.

3. Drugs
Oestrogen-containing contraceptives, sympathomimetics (cold cures), glucocorticoids, NSAIDS (and COX-2 inhibitors), ciclosporin, monoamine oxidase inhibitors, amphetamines, cocaine, sodium bicarbonate.

4. Pregnancy (🕮 p.576)
Pregnancy induced hypertension, pre-eclampsia and eclampsia.

5. Miscellaneous
- Coarctation of the aorta (↓renal perfusion).
- Obstructive sleep apnoea.
- Increased intracranial pressure or spinal cord injury.
- Acute LVF and intravascular volume overload (IV fluids!).
- Hyperdynamic circulation (systolic hypertension):
  - Anaemia
  - Fever
  - Thyrotoxicosis
  - Aortic regurgitation
  - AV fistulae.
- Acute intermittent porphyria.
- Alcohol withdrawal.

Table 5.3 Diagnosis and treatment of secondary hypertension

Condition	Diagnostic clue	Further investigation
Primary renal disease	• ↑C_r • Proteinuria ± haematuria	• Renal USS (?APKD) • Renal biopsy
Renovascular hypertension	• ↑C_r • Acute ↑C_r post ACEI/ARB • Renal asymmetry on imaging • Flash pulmonary oedema • Abdominal bruit (sensitivity: 65%; specificity 90%)	• CT Angiogram • MRA • Duplex USS • ± Formal angiography
Primary aldosteronism	Hypokalaemia (rarely → muscle weakness, polyuria, arrhythmias)	• Plasma aldosterone/renin ratio • Urinary aldosterone excretion (post salt load)
Apparent mineralocorticoid excess	• Mainly children • ↑BP, ↓K^+, ↓renin • Aldosterone not ↑	↑ratio of THF to THE in urine (see text)
Phaeochromocytoma	Paroxysmal symptoms (headache, palpitations sweating)	Urinary catecholamines
Thyroid disease	Both hypo- and hyper- are associated	Thyroid function
Hyperparathyroidism	Serum Ca^{2+} ↑	Serum PTH
Cushing's syndrome	• Corticosteroid therapy • Cushingoid appearance (central obesity, striae bruising etc), muscle weakness, hyperglycaemia, oligomenorrhea	• Urinary cortisol excretion • Dexamethasone suppression tests
Coarctation of the aorta	• Midsystolic murmur (precordium → back) • Weak femoral pulses • Radiofemoral delay • BP in arms ↑, BP in legs ↓	• CT or MRA • ± aortography
Obstructive sleep apnoea	Snoring, daytime somnolence, morning headache, obesity (large collar size)	• Sleep observation with pulse oximetry • Formal polysomnography
Acromegaly	↑sweating, headaches, fatigue, arthralgia, change in shoe or ring size, change in appearance, hyperglycaemia	• ↑IGF-1 • Failure to suppress GH to <2 mU/L post 75g oral glucose load.

Primary hyperaldosteronism

Disorders of autonomous aldosterone hypersecretion with suppressed renin levels. Aldosterone acts on the distal tubule to ↑renal Na^+ retention (with ↑urinary K^+ and H^+ loss), increasing total body Na^+ content and driving hypertension. Thought to account for ~0.1% of the hypertensive population (possibly an underestimate, some say 1–5%) and the most common endocrine disorder leading to 2° hypertension.

Clinical and biochemical findings vary widely. Often asymptomatic, but may present with ↓K^+, metabolic alkalosis and mild ↑Na^+ (helps distinguish from essential BP treated with diuretics, where Na^+ usually low-normal). If severe, ↓K^+ → tetany, myopathy and nephrogenic diabetes insipidus (polyuria and nocturia).

Causes include

- Conn's syndrome (aldosterone-producing adrenal adenoma) ~70%
- Bilateral adrenal hyperplasia ~30%
- Glucocorticoid remediable aldosteronism
- Aldosterone-producing adrenal carcinoma (↑↑aldosterone and ↓↓K^+—may also produce cortisol and sex steroids).

Diagnosis

- Measurement of K^+ has been considered a screening test, but only 50–80% have ↓K^+ early on (∴ underdiagnosis).
- Document renal K^+ wasting (urinary K^+ > 30mmol/d).
- Aldosterone–renin ratio (ARR).
  - Commonly used diagnostic test. Unregulated aldosterone secretion → suppressed renin production and ↑ARR.
  - See box opposite.
- Oral salt loading.
  - High Na^+ diet for 3 days (120 mmol/day—ask your dietician) then measure 24h urinary aldosterone secretion. Adequate salt loading can be confirmed by urinary Na^+ >250 mmol/24h. IV N saline (2L/day) is an alternative salt load. The normal response will be suppressed aldosterone secretion, ∴ lack of suppression can be used to confirm the diagnosis.
  - ⚠ May precipitate ↓K^+ in normokalaemic patients who were previously on a low salt diet.
- Fludrocortisone suppression test: 4 day administration of fludrocortisone further suppresses plasma renin activity without suppressing plasma aldosterone below a threshold value.
- Adrenal CT and MRI are used to localize tumours (>1.5cm).
- Adrenal venous sampling is occasionally necessary—the distinction between an adenoma and hyperplasia is important because of the role of surgery in the former.

General principles of treatment

Spironolactone (a competitive antagonist of the mineralocorticoid receptor 📖 p.335) initially 50–100mg (SE: gynaecomastia, impotence, menstrual irregularities, GI upset). Eplerenone an alternative. Add amiloride 5–20mg if ↓K⁺ persists. Other antihypertensive agents may also be required. Surgical resection if adenoma: 70% normotensive at 1 year (● poorer results in some series—esp. if BP longstanding). Some argue for a trial of spironolactone in all cases of resistant hypertension (📖 p.348).

Doing an ARR: the nuts and bolts

- Tubes: liaise with your biochemistry lab—they will probably require an EDTA or heparinized sample (or both) for aldosterone and give you a special tube for renin. They will definitely want to know that the samples are coming. Transport to the lab on ice.
- Time: 0700–0900.
- Posture: upright (for at least 2 hours).
- Potassium: normalize first using supplements as ↓K⁺ suppresses aldosterone.
- ⚠ Discontinue all drugs influencing RAS (β-blockers, ACEI, ARB, diuretics) for a washout period of 2 weeks (6 for spironolactone). The 'cleanest' drugs are α blockers; e.g. doxazosin.
- Result: aldosterone (pmol/L)/plasma renin activity (ng/mL/h) >750 or aldosterone (ng/dL)/plasma renin activity (ng/mL/h) >30–50. The ↑ the ratio the more likely the diagnosis. Refer equivocal cases to a specialist centre.

Specific causes of hyperaldosteronism

1° hyperaldosteronism

Glucocorticoid remediable aldosteronism (GRA)

Very rare. Autosomal dominant. A chimeric aldosterone synthase/11β-hydroxylase is ectopically expressed in the adrenal fasciculata. ACTH → stimulates enzyme activity → normal cortisol production + aldosterone excess (→ volume expansion and ↑BP). Presents with ↑BP at a young age with a family history (early haemorrhagic stroke in some pedigrees). Diagnosis now confirmed with genetic testing. Dexamethasone → suppress ACTH secretion → ↓enzyme activity → ↓aldosterone production.

Congenital adrenal hyperplasia (CAH)

Inherited enzymatic defects (autosomal recessive) in cortisol production. Clinical features depend on the enzyme affected, but result from (i) ↓cortisol synthesis (ii) ↑ACTH driven steroid production. Two forms (of six) are associated with mineralocorticoid excess and ∴ ↑BP.

- 11β hydroxylase (CYP11B1) deficiency, presenting in childhood; ♀ are virilized and ♂ are sexually precocious.
- 17α hydroxylase (CYP17) deficiency. Extremely rare. Presents with ↑BP, ↓K^+ and hypogonadism—often at puberty.

2° hyperaldosteronism

Occurs when aldosterone hypersecretion occurs secondary to ↑ circulating renin levels—often in response to renal hypoperfusion. ↑Renin → ↑ circulating AII, ↑peripheral resistance and ↑BP (often severe). Associated 2° hyperaldosteronism →↑tubular Na^+ reabsorption (∴ ↓K^+). Causes include:

- Renal artery stenosis
- Renal infarction; e.g. atheroemboli.
- Cirrhosis (vasodilatation → ↓ effective circulating volume)
- CCF (falling CO → ↓ effective circulating volume)
- Nephrotic syndrome
- Renal trauma (so-called 'Page kidney')
- Renin secreting tumours (see box below).

Renin secreting tumours

Very rare. Renin secreting tumour of the juxtaglomerular cells → angiotensin induced ↑BP. Presents with severe ↑BP, ↓K^+ (↑urinary K^+ excretion), ↑renin, ↑angiotensin II, and ↑aldosterone.

Diagnosis: MRA, angiography (tumour blush)

Rx: ACEI and ARBs effectively ↓BP. Surgery may be curative.

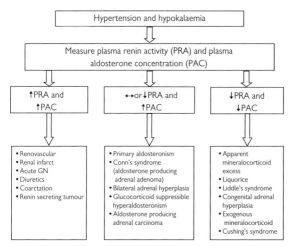

Fig. 5.7 Diagnostic algorithm for hyperaldosteronsim

Other 'hyperaldosteronism' syndromes

Other mineralocorticoids may occasionally be the cause of a clinical syndrome very similar to that seen with ↑aldosterone, namely ↑BP, ↓K⁺ with alkalosis. Crucially, both renin and aldosterone are suppressed. Causes include:
- Apparent mineralocorticoid excess
- Congenital adrenal hyperplasia
- Liquorice ingestion
- Ectopic ACTH secretion
- Exogenous mineralocorticoids; e.g. fludrocortisone.

Apparent mineralocorticoid excess

<1% hypertensives. Autosomal recessive, presenting in childhood. Inactivating mutation in 11β hydroxysteroid dehydrogenase 2 (11βHSD2). The mineralocorticoid receptor (which has an equal affinity for cortisol and aldosterone) is protected from ongoing cortisol stimulation by 11βHSD2, which metabolizes cortisol → cortisone (relatively inactive). As cortisol is present at 100-fold concentrations compared to aldosterone, absence/inhibition of this enzyme allows cortisol to flood the receptor, → chronic activation.

Diagnosis: ↑ratio of urinary tetrahydrocortisol (THF + 5αTHF) (metabolite of cortisol) to tetrahydrocortisone (THE) (metabolite of cortisone).
Rx: block the mineralocorticoid receptor (spironolactone) or suppress ACTH secretion (dexamethasone, suppresses endogenous cortisol synthesis, but does not activate the mineralocorticoid receptor).

Glycyrrhizinic acid in liquorice can bind the 11βHSD2 enzyme creating a state of apparent mineralocorticoid excess. Look out for it in herbal preparations.

'Pseudoaldosteronism'

Caused by abnormalities of renal tubular transport rather than elevated renin or aldosterone. The electrolyte abnormalities mimic those seen with ↑ aldosterone, hence the name. See 📖 p.536. Causes include:
- Liddle's syndrome
- Bartter's syndrome (normotensive)
- Gitelman's syndrome (normotensive).

Other causes of secondary hypertension

Cushing's syndrome

↑BP is very common, affecting ~ 80%. 24h urinary cortisol excretion is a reliable diagnostic rest (>110nmol/day is highly suggestive). Diagnosis confirmed by a 2-day low dose dexamethasone suppression test (0.5mg every 6h for eight doses) or an overnight suppression test (1mg at 2300h). In the 2 day test urinary cortisol excretion >27 nmol (10μg) per day on day 2 indicates Cushing's syndrome, as does plasma cortisol > 140 nmol/L (5μg/dL) at 0800h in the overnight test. Serum ACTH concentrations, a long dexamethasone suppression test ± corticotrophin releasing hormone (CRH) stimulation test and adrenal/pituitary imaging will help distinguish different forms of the syndrome (Cushing's disease most common: overproduction of ACTH by pituitary).

Phaeochromocytoma

Very rare (<0.1% hypertensives). Adenoma (rarely carcinoma) of adrenal medulla → oversecretion of catecholamines (adrenaline → ↑HR and contractility, noradrenaline → ↑SVR). Can arise in extra-adrenal chromaffin tissue (e.g. para-aortic ganglia). Most patients have ↑BP the majority of the time, though symptoms (including pallor, palpitations, anxiety, angina, headache, sweating and nausea) may be paroxysmal. Postural ↓BP also seen. Occasional fulminant presentation. The sensitivity and specificity of various screening tests are shown below. Many centres use 24h urine catecholamines x 3 (acidified container). MIBG scanning may localize the tumour and metastases (~10% malignant). Often large and peri-adrenal ∴ visible on USS or CT. Rx: α and β blockade prior to surgery.

Table 5.4 Sensitivity and specificity of screening tests for phaeochromocytoma.

	Sensitivity (%)	Specificity (%)
Plasma metanephrines	99	89
Plasma catecholamines	85	80
Urinary catecholamines	83	88
Urinary metanephrines	76	94
Urinary vanillymandelic acid	63	94

Reproduced with permission from Pacak K (2001). Recent advances in genetics, diagnosis, localisation and treatment of phaeochromocytoma. *Ann Internal Medicine*, **134**, 315–29.

Coarctation of the aorta

A rare cause of 2° ↑BP in children and young adults. ♂ >♀. Represents <1% of congenital heart disease. A ridge extends into the aortic lumen just distal to the left subclavian artery. Often asymptomatic, may be diagnosed after CV examination (mid-systolic murmur, radiofemoral delay, ↑BP (arms>legs)), or CXR (aortic '3-sign' from pre- and post-stenotic dilatation and posterior rib notching). If undetected in childhood, presents with cardiac failure in middle age and prognosis is then poor.
Diagnosis: CT, MRA or aortography.
Treatment: surgical. BP correction is age-dependent (>90% in childhood).

Drug induced hypertension

📖 p.306.

Obstructive sleep apnoea (OSA)

The number of diagnosed and treated patients with OSA is rising rapidly. ↑BP, which may be difficult to treat, is commonly associated and may be related to disease severity (though obesity and other comorbid factors may contribute more). Treatment of the OSA improves BP.
Rx: weight reduction, alcohol avoidance, correction of airway obstruction, oral prosthetic devices, CPAP, uvulopalatopharngoplasty.

Thyroid disease

Hypothyroidism may influence RAS and is associated with ↑DBP. Hyperthyroidism is associated with an ↑BMR, ↑SBP, and a wide PP.

Drug management of hypertension

Introduction

- The 1° goal of treatment is to achieve a ↓ in long term CV morbidity and mortality risk.
- Patients will be accruing benefit even if they do not achieve target BP.
- The benefits of BP lowering therapy are primarily determined by the level of BP control rather than class of drug used to achieve it ☛. This is an important issue—the difference in cost between older (β blockers and thiazides) and newer (CCBs, ACEI/ARBs) drugs is considerable.
- In general, the lower the BP the better.
- Most patients will require ≥2 drugs to attain target.
- Combination tablets have a role (currently UK physicians prescribe less combination pills than anywhere else in Europe).
- Compliance is improved with once a day formulations.
- Explain the benefits of drug treatment as well as possible side-effects.
- Marked interindividual variation in drug responses reflects heterogeneity in the pathogenesis of ↑BP. Profiling patients according to their hypertensive phenotype with a view to individualizing drug therapy has proved difficult (exceptions: the elderly and ethnic groups).
- Drug withdrawal might be possible if other lifestyle interventions are undertaken and prove successful.
- The patient may benefit from joining local or national forums.
- Once BP is adequately controlled, provide at least an annual review for monitoring.
- The 4 major groups are equally well-tolerated. They are prescribed in ~ equal amounts in primary care, though costs vary considerably.
  - Thiazide diuretics (📖 p.332)
  - β-blockers (📖 p.336)
  - ACEI and ARBs (📖 p.342–5)
  - Calcium channel blockers (CCBs)
  - (α blockers are not recommended first line (📖 p.338)
- ☛ The benefits are probably the same regardless of the initial agent you use. It depends which guideline you follow. In the UK β blockers have recently been 'downgraded' and are not recommended as first line therapy.
- When considering which agent for which patient, it is useful to consider *compelling indications* and *compelling contraindications* (Table 5.5). There are other less definite pros and cons which will assigned different importance by different prescribers.

Aspirin and statins

Consider prescribing other drugs that modify CV risk
- Aspirin 75mg od for all those needing 2° prevention of CV disease and 1° prevention in hypertensives >age 50 with 10 year CV risk >20%. Wait until BP is controlled first.
- Statin therapy in all with overt CV disease, irrespective of baseline total cholesterol or LDL. Also 1° prevention in hypertensives with 10 year CV risk >20%. Targets: ↓total cholesterol by 25%, or LDL cholesterol by 30%, or achieve a total cholesterol of <4.0mmol/L, or LDL cholesterol of <2.0mmol/L (whichever is the greatest reduction).

Table 5.5 Compelling and possible indications, contraindications and cautions for the major classes of antihypertensive drugs (from BHS guidelines. Used with permission)

Class of drug	Compelling indications	Possible indications	Caution	Compelling contraindications
Alpha-blockers	Benign prostatic hypertrophy		Postural hypotension, heart failure[a]	Urinary incontinence
ACE inhibitors	Heart failure, LV dysfunction Post MI or established CHD, type I diabetic nephropathy, 2° stroke prevention[c]	Chronic renal disease[b], type II diabetic nephropathy, proteinuric renal disease	Renal impairment[b] PVD[c]	Pregnancy, renovascular disease[d]
ARBs	ACE inhibitor intolerance, type II diabetic nephropathy, hypertension with LVH, heart failure in ACE-intolerant patients, post MI	LV dysfunction post MI, intolerance of other antihypertensive drugs, proteinuric renal disease, chronic renal disease, heart failure[e]	Renal impairment[b] PVD[c]	Pregnancy, renovascular disease[d]
Beta-blockers	MI, angina	Heart failure	Heart failure[e], PVD, diabetes (except with CHD)	Asthma/COPD, heart block

CCBs (dihydropyridine)	Elderly, ISH	Elderly, angina	—	—
CCBs (rate limiting)	Angina	MI	Combination with beta-blockade	Heart block, heart failure
Thiazide/thiazide-like diuretics	Elderly, ISH, heart failure, 2° stroke prevention			Gout[f]

COPD = chronic obstructive pulmonary disease; ISH = isolated systolic hypertension; PVD = peripheral vascular disease;

[a] HF when used as monotherapy.

[b] ACE inhibitors or ARBs may be beneficial in chronic renal failure but should only be used with caution, close supervision and specialist advice when there is established and significant renal impairment.

[c] Caution with ACE inhibitors and ARBs in peripheral vascular disease because of association with renovascular disease.

[d] ACE inhibitors and ARBs are sometimes used in patients with renovascular disease under specialist supervision.

[e] Beta-blockers are increasingly used to treat stable heart failure. However, beta-blockers may worsen heart failure.

[f] Thiazide/thiazide-like diuretics may sometimes be necessary to control BP in people with a history of gout, ideally used in combination with allopurinol.

Drug treatment of hypertension

Algorithms

Guidelines have become increasingly didactic as previous, less specific, recommendations generally proved ineffective.

The British Hypertensive Society and NICE

Two key UK advisory bodies recently joined forces to produce a new guideline for drug treatment (Fig. 5.8). The major (and fairly bold) change was a downgrading of β-blockers, in response to growing evidence that suggests they may be less effective at ↓ major CV events (particularly stroke) than other drug classes. They may also carry a higher diabetes risk than ACEI or CCBs (particularly in patients also taking a thiazide diuretic (📖 p.336)). However, β-blockers are still recommended as possible first line therapy in ♀ of childbearing potential and patients with evidence of ↑ sympathetic drive.

Renin profiling demonstrates that younger people (<55 years) and Caucasians tend to have higher renin levels relative to elderly and black patients. Since ACEI (and ARBs) act through RAS suppression, they are recommended as initial therapy in younger caucasian patients.

Recommendations

- People age <55: initial therapy with an ACEI (ARB if ACEI intolerant).
- People age >55: initial therapy with a CCB or thiazide diuretic.
- Black patients (any age): CCB or thiazide diuretic (does not include mixed race, Asian, or Chinese patients).
- Second line: add ACEI (or ARB) to CCB/thiazide (or vice versa).
- Compelling indications/contraindications should always be taken into account (📖 p.318).

Joint National Committee (JNC VII)

US guidelines, acknowledging data from several studies (particularly ALLHAT (📖 p.326), also recommend a 'stepped care' approach—though generally starting with a thiazide diuretic.

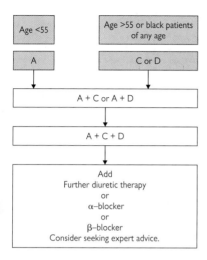

A = ACEI (ARB if ACEI intolerant)
B = β blocker
C = Calcium channel blocker
D = Thiazide diuretic

Fig. 5.8 2006 BHS/NICE recommendations for the drug treatment of hypertension. Reproduced with permission.

Special situations

Hypertension in blacks

The prevalence of ↑BP and complications such as CHD, stroke and renal disease is higher in African-Americans than other ethnic groups. This holds true in the UK, with mortality data for England and Wales showing mortality 3.5x the national average. British Asians have a mortality rate 1.5x the national average.

There is evidence of differential BP lowering efficacy of particular drugs within ethnic groups. Black people, in general suffer with low renin hypertension, so agents (ACEI, ARB and β-blockers) that suppress renin production may not be effective, especially when used as monotherapy. However, they may be effective in combination with other agents, especially diuretics and CCBs.

Hypertension in the elderly

CHD and stroke remain the major killers >age 65, with BP the commonest treatable risk factor.

SBP ↑ with age. DBP ↑ to age 60, plateaus, and then falls. This leads to an age-related increase in PP and isolated SBP. BP variability also increases ∴ more measurements are desirable prior to treatment. Using a relatively conservative definition of ↑BP (≥160/95mmHg), it is estimated that >15% of the 12 million people >60 in the UK are hypertensive (>70% ≥age 80). ↑BP in the elderly is ∴ a major public health issue.

Clinical trials have shown that older people benefit just as much, if not more, from intervention as younger patients.

The elderly are more prone to orthostatic hypertension (→ falls → fractures), so treatment may need to be titrated to the standing value. Other lifestyle interventions still apply. Low renin hypertension is the norm, so begin treatment with a thiazide or CCB. 2nd line, ARBs are demonstrably more effective than β-blockers.

Hypertension in diabetes mellitus (see 📖 p.443)

Hypertension in CKD (see 📖 p.150)

Hypertension in pregnancy (see 📖 p.576)

Oral contraceptives, HRT, and BP

Oral contraceptives

- The combined oral contraceptive (COC) modestly ↑BP in a minority of women (~1%) Occasionally elevations may be severe. The rise in BP may not become apparent for several months or even years after COC introduction. The mechanism(s) of ↑BP remain uncertain and it has not been possible to identify women at particular risk. COC use is also associated with ↑ stroke and MI risk.
- BP should be measured prior to COC use and at least every 6 months thereafter.
- Progestogen-only pills have not been associated with ↑BP and are recommended for women with both COC induced ↑BP and pre-existing ↑BP. In those women wishing to remain on the COC, antihypertensive medication should be given early consideration.
- For older women (age >35), with higher CV risk (e.g. smokers), non-hormonal forms of contraception are preferable.

Hormone replacement therapy (HRT)

- HRT use is not associated with ↑BP and its use is not contraindicated in pre-existing hypertensives.
- Several large randomized trials have established that the CV protection afforded by HRT has previously been overplayed and should not be used as the motivation for their prescription.

Clinical trials in hypertension

The benefits of lowering BP is supported by one of the most authoritative evidence bases in clinical medicine. The foundation of this evidence base is the prospective randomized clinical trial.

Trial designs

- Duration rarely >5 years.
- End-points:
  - All cause mortality.
  - Cause specific morbidity and mortality (usually CHD ± stroke; more recently CCF).
  - The 'composite 1° end point' has emerged (i.e. a combination of events), because trials seldom have sufficient power to examine specific outcomes.
- Early trials compared active therapy with placebo, often among patients with severe ↑BP. Consequently, they had ↑power and could be conducted on a relatively small scale. Such trials became unethical as the benefits of BP lowering became apparent.
- Modern 'head to head' trials tend to assess whether drug classes offer advantages over others (drug companies are desperate to demonstrate benefits 'beyond BP lowering').
- BP differences between treatment arms now tend to be minimal, ∴ ↓ study power and requiring ↑patient numbers.
- Contemporary treatment objectives also influence trial design—most patients now require multiple drugs to achieve target.
- The majority of patients at high CV risk will be receiving concomitant treatment with aspirin ± a statin, further diminishing trial power.
- Trials are hugely expensive.
- The data from clinical trials is often pooled for meta-analysis. This provides increased power to examine drug specific effects.

Controversies ♦

- Do specific classes of drugs offer benefits for CV disease prevention beyond the expected benefits of BP lowering?
  - There are marked drug specific differences in their effect on CV structure and function as well as metabolic end points. The relevance of these effects on longer term outcomes remains unknown.
  - Could certain classes of drugs be potentially harmful with regard to specific outcomes.
- With regard to study design: can treatment be solely measured in terms of CV events, or is the real aim to prevent the evolution of a destructive disease process?
- Clinical trials rarely run for more than 5 years, while life expectancy in middle aged hypertensives is 20–30 years.

Meta-analysis of BP lowering trials: the BPLTTC

The Blood Pressure Lowering Treatment Trialists Collaborative (BPLTTC) is an international alliance of the principal investigators of the largest trials of antihypertensive regimes. The project is based at the George Institute for International Health, a department of the University of Sydney.

Its objective is to address questions concerning safety and outcome with specific drug classes. To achieve this, data from recent trials is pooled and subjected to meta-analysis ($\therefore$ providing the necessary statistical power to examine drug specific effects).

Their most recent analysis, published in 2003*, incorporated data from 29 randomized controlled trials involving ~160,000 patients, with a mean duration of follow-up of 2.0 to 8.0 years (>70,000 patient years). The mean age was 65 years (52% ♂, 48% ♀).

Conclusions
- Treatment with any of the commonly used regimens ↓ the total risk of major CV events.
- Larger reductions in BP produce larger reductions in risk.
- ACEI and diuretics ± β-blockers are more effective at preventing heart failure than regimes based on CCBs . Other differences in regimes 'beyond BP lowering' are less certain (including for stroke).

*Turubull F et al. (2003) Lancet **362**: 1527–1535
www.thegeorgeinstitute.org/bplttc

Table 5.5 Recent major trials in hypertension

Study acronym	Full name	Purpose
AASK	African American Study of Kidney Disease and Hypertension *JAMA* (2002); **288:** 2421–31	To determine whether lowering BP below recommended CV goals or particular agents slowed the progression of hypertensive renal disease (GFR 20–65mL/min). Patients received ramipril or amlodipine, with both compared to metoprolol.
ALLHAT	The Antihypertensive and Lipid Lowering Treatment to Prevent Heart Attack Trial *JAMA* (2002); **288:** 2981–97	The largest double blind, randomized trial of hypertensive patients (n=42,418). Hypothesis: fatal CHD and non-fatal MI would be lower in patients randomized to 'new' drugs (ACEI and CCBs) as compared to those taking a thiazide.
ANBP-2	The Second Australian National Blood Pressure Study *NEJM* (2003); **348:** 583–92	To compare outcomes with an ACEI (mainly enalapril) and a diuretic (mainly hydrochlorothiazide) among elderly patients with ↑ BP (open label).
ASCOT	The Anglo-Scandinavian Outcomes Trial. *Lancet* (2005); **366:** 895–906	To compare the effects on CHD of a β-blocker ± diuretic ('old-fashioned') vs a CCB ± ACEI ('modern') in patients with ↑ BP.
		A second arm (*Lancet* 2003; **361**: 1149–58) compared atorvastatin with placebo for ↑ lipids in hypertensive patients.
HOPE	Heart Outcomes Prevention Evaluation Study *NEJM* (2000); **342:** 145–53	To compare ramipril to placebo for the prevention of CV events in patients with evidence of atherosclerotic CV disease taking standard therapy (~50% non-hypertensive).

Result	Comment
Ramipril was superior in ↓rate of decline. The amlodipine arm was stopped early because of worse outcomes.	Showed (surprisingly) that the level of BP attained did not affect the rate of decline of renal function.
A Doxazosin arm was stopped early (median 3.3 years follow up) after interim data suggested an ↑risk of combined CHD events. Main finding was that thiazides, CCBs and ACEI all provide similar protection from CHD. Thiazides appeared superior to CCBs and ACEIs in preventing some adverse CV outcomes. CCBs not associated with excess CV deaths—a concern in previous studies.	General conclusion: thiazide diuretics are unsurpassed in preventing the major complications of ↑ BP. They are also well tolerated and inexpensive. They became the initial drug of choice in many guidelines. Criticisms: (i) designed in an era of monotherapy, (ii) many conclusions drawn on the basis of 2° end points, (iii) randomization deprived some patients with CCF of their diuretic (iv) old fashioned treatments were used for step up (e.g. clonidine, reserpine).
Similar BP control observed in both arms. The ACEI group had a ↓ incidence of nonfatal CV events (benefits restricted to ♂).	Apparently at odds with the findings of ALLHAT, though the study designs were very different.
Stopped early (median follow-up 5.4 years), because of superior results in the CCB/ACEI arm for several 2° end-points, including all cause mortality and new onset DM (1° endpoints were non-fatal MI and fatal CHD). Atorvastatin treatment resulted in a significant ↓ in the incidence of stroke.	Unique in its focus on combination therapy. Good press for CCBs after a lot of (unjustified) bad press. Likely to reignite concerns regarding new onset DM with diuretics + β-blocker Has been the catalyst for an early review of current guidelines.
Ramipril decreased the combined relative risk of MI, stroke, or CV death by 22%	Provided considerable impetus to the 'beyond BP lowering' hypothesis. There were important BP differences between the groups that probably accounted for the results (and led cynics to dub it the 'HYPE' trial).

Table 5.5 (Contd.)

Study acronym	Full name	Purpose
HOT	Hypertension Optimal Treatment Study *Lancet* (1988); **351**: 1755–62	To assess the relationship of major CV events with 3 target DBPs (≤90, ≤85, or ≤80 mmHg). Also whether low dose aspirin, in addition to ↓ BP therapy, ↓ CV events.
INSIGHT	Intervention as a Goal in Hypertension Treatment. *Lancet* (2000); **356**: 366–72	To compare CV events in high risk hypertensive patients treated with nifedipine or amiloride + hydrochlorothiazide
LIFE	Losartan Intervention for Endpoint Reduction in Hypertension *Lancet* (2002); **359**: 995–1003	To compare the long-term effects of losartan with atenolol on CV mortality and morbidity in hypertensive patients with LVH.
NORDIL	The Nordic Diltiazem Study *Lancet* (2000); **356**: 359–65	To evaluate the potential preventative effects of diltiazem on CV morbidity and mortality compared to a β-blocker ± diuretic
PROGRESS	Perindopril Protection against Recurrent Stroke Study *Lancet* (2001); **358**: 1033–40	To investigate whether perindopril, alone, or in combination with indapamide, influenced stroke recurrence (~50% patients non-hypertensive)
STOP-2	The Swedish Trial in Old Patients with Hypertension-2 *Lancet* (1999); **354**: 1751–6	Patients aged 70–84 were assigned to either an ACEI, a dihydropyridine CCB, or a 'conventional' therapy (β-blocker ± diuretic)
SYST-EUR	Systolic Hypertension—Europe *Lancet* (1997); **354**: 757–64	To investigate whether antihypertensive treatment in elderly patients with isolated SBP could ↓CV events (primarily stroke). Participants received placebo or nitrendipine (with enalapril and hydrochlorothiazide added if needed).
VALUE	Valsartan Antihypertensive Long-term Use Evaluation *Lancet* (2004); **363**: 2022–31	To investigate whether, for the same level of BP control, valsartan is more effective than amlodipine in ↓CV events.

Result	Comment
Achieved BPs were 144/85, 141/83 and 140/81. The lowest incidence of CV events occurred at DBP 83mmHg. The benefit of progressive BP reduction was most marked in patients with DM. Aspirin caused a further significant ↓ in CV events (due entirely to a ↓ in MIs).	Defined a new optimal BP target (DBP 83 mmHg), Further reductions did not ↑ CV events (i.e. did not support the 'J-curve' hypothesis).
Both regimens resulted in equivalent BP control and outcomes.	The diuretic group needed significantly more add on antihypertensive medications. Less new onset DM was seen in the CCB group.
BP control was identical between the two groups. 1° events were fewer, the incidence of new-onset DM lower and LVH regression greater for losartan than for the β-blocker.	One interpretation: the benefits of losartan extend beyond its BP lowering effects. Another: apparent benefits of losartan actually due to negative effects of atenolol.
There were no differences in the incidence of the 1° endpoint (a composite of all stroke, MI and other CV events). 2° analysis indicated a ↓ in the incidence of stroke in the CCB group.	One of the few studies to evaluate a non-dihydropyridine CCB. The protection against stroke probably reflected better BP control in the CCB group.
Those on perindopril had a significant ↓ in recurrent stroke,	Often cited as evidence for the 'beyond BP lowering' hypothesis' for ACEI, but the improved stroke outcome was probably driven by the more pronounced ↓ in BP in the combined perindopril + diuretic arm.
No difference in 1° end-points among the 3 arms. ACEI were associated with a lower risk of MI and CCF than those treated with a CCB.	Suggested newer and older drugs are generally equivalent.
Stopped early because of a 42% ↓ in stroke in the active arm. Cardiac events were also reduced, but not significantly.	Also suggested CCBs may have a protective role in vascular dementia.
There were no differences between treatment groups in CV morbidity or mortality.	Good BP control in groups underscored the importance of achieving target BP, whatever the agent(s) used

The ASCOT study

A large multi-centre study[1], likely to change the drug management of hypertension. For many years the consensus had been that reductions in mortality or morbidity were due to BP lowering rather than any specific drug class. This was reflected in national and international guidelines. Drug effects 'beyond blood pressure lowering', particularly affording cardiovascular protection, had been claimed in many studies over the last 10–20 years, but flawed study designs had called into question the validity of the results.

ASCOT appears to have changed this—robustly designed, the trial has already led to a redraft of the UK BHS/NICE Guidelines (published June 2006). The BP lowering arm is discussed here (a lipid lowering arm showed significantly fewer cardiovascular events in those patients treated with a statin and was also stopped early).

Study design
- 19,257 patients from the UK and Scandinavia.
- Age 40–79.
- Patients all had hypertension + at least 3 other cardiovascular risk factors.

Treatment regimens
- Treatment arm 1: calcium channel blocker (amlodipine) ± ACE inhibitor (perindopril)
- Treatment arm 2: β-blocker (atenolol) ± thiazide diuretic (bendroflumethiazide)
- α-blocker (extended release doxazosin) added if BP did not reach target.

Target BP
140/90 (130/80 for patients with diabetes). Most patients achieved this (mean 2.2 agents).

Median follow-up
5.5 years (< 2% patients lost to follow up).

Results
The primary end-point was fatal coronary heart disease or non-fatal MI. The trial was stopped early when the data monitoring group reported significantly more events in the atenolol-based group.

10% reduction in the primary endpoint was seen in the amlodipine ± perindopril group (p=0.1, so not statistically significant). However this group also had:
- ↓ all cause mortality (11%)
- ↓ cardiovascular mortality (24%)

1 Dahlof B, Sever PS, Poulter NR et al. (2005) Prevention of cardiovascular events with an antihypertensive regimen of amlodipine adding perindopril as required versus atenolol adding bendroflumethiazide as required in the Anglo-Scandinavian Cardiac Outcomes Trial-Blood pressure Lowering Arm (ASCOT-BPLA): a multicentre randomized controlled trail. *Lancet* **366**: 895–906.

- ↓ all coronary events (13%)
- ↓ fatal and non-fatal strokes (23%)
- ↓ new-onset diabetes (30%).

When the primary end-point was adjusted to include coronary revascularization (in line with changing clinical practice during the period of data collection), a significant reduction was observed (of 14%) in the amlodipine ± perindopril group.

BP lowering was better in this group (by 2.7/1.9mmHg). However further analysis, matching patients with similar BP, suggested continued benefit in the amlodipine / perindopril group[2] ∴ BP control unlikely to be the whole reason for the benefit.

Significance of ASCOT

ASCOT is set to shape future guidelines and clinical practice. The likelihood is that:

- ACE inhibitors (or ARB) ± calcium channel blockers will be recommended for first line use except in specific situations.
- Thiazide diuretics may be an alternative first line in the elderly, but second line in younger age groups.
- Beta blockers can no longer be recommended as first line. This has proved to be the case in the recently revised BHS/NICE Guidelines in the UK—others may follow.

2 Poulter NR, Wedel H, Dahlof B et al. (2005). Role of blood pressure and other variables in the differential cardiovascular event rates noted in the Anglo-Scandinavian Cardiac Outcomes Trial-Blood Pressure Lowering Arm (ASCOT-BPLA). Lancet **366**: 907–13.

Diuretics

See also 📖 p.530

Diuretics work by directly inhibiting the Na^+ transporters/channels mediating renal Na^+ reabsorption.

Efficacy depends on active secretion of the diuretic into the proximal nephron, such that high concentrations are achieved at sites of action along the tubule. Renal insufficiency impairs proximal secretion → relative diuretic resistance. Higher doses may still be effective, but risk ↑toxicity.

The Na^+ and volume loss associated with diuretics is initially accompanied by the activation of vasoconstrictor mechanisms (including RAS). This ↑SVR and attenuates their antihypertensive effect. Over a period of days, SVR falls through poorly understood mechanisms, and antihypertensive effects become sustained. This is one of the reasons that diuretics and ACEI/ARBs are a good combination.

Thiazide and thiazide-like diuretics

Examples
- Thiazides: bendroflumethiazide (bendrofluazide), hydrochlorothiazide.
- Thiazide-like: chlorthalidone, indapamide

Mechanism
- Compete with both Na^+ and Cl^- to block the Na^+–Cl^- co-transporter in the DCT (normally responsible for 5–7% of filtered Na^+ reabsorption).
- ↑Na^+ delivery to distal nephron → ↑Na^+/K^+ exchange and, indirectly, ↑H^+ excretion: hypokalaemic metabolic alkalosis often results.
- Blocking the Na^+–Cl^- co-transporter ↑Ca^{2+} reabsorption (mechanism unknown). Thiazides ∴ have a role in renal stone disease and exert a protective effect in osteoporosis.
- Thiazide-like agents differ in several of their actions including duration of action, channel-blocking activity, and inhibitory influence on carbonic anhydrase. The implications for clinical practice are uncertain.

Role
- Effective, good evidence base, and inexpensive.
- Introduced in 1957 and still the first line antihypertensive in several guidelines.
- ↑plasma ½ life and sustained renal actions make them preferable to loop diuretics as antihypertensives (except in special situations 📖 p.334).

Problems
- Hypokalaemia (dose dependent).
- Impaired glucose tolerance (especially when used with a β-blocker).
- Small ↑ in LDL cholesterol and triglycerides.
- Small ↑serum urate.
- Erectile dysfunction.
- Efficacy ↓ in those taking NSAIDS.
- Avoid if history of gout
- Avoid if taking lithium (↑risk of lithium toxicity).

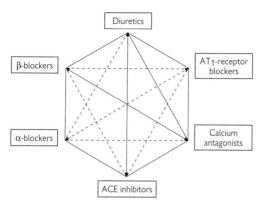

Fig. 5.11 Possible combinations of different classes of antihypertensive agents. The most rational combinations are represented as thick lines. From 2003 ESH/ESC Guidelines for the management of anterial hypertension (*Journal of Hypertension* (2003); **21**: 1011–13). Used with permission.

Loop diuretics

Examples

Furosemide (frusemide), bumetanide.

Mechanism

- Block the type 2 $Na^+K^+2Cl^-$ (NKCC2) co-transporter in thick ascending limb of loop of Henle (usually responsible for 15–20% of filtered Na^+ reabsorption).
- Tubuloglomerular feedback would normally act to compensate by a ↓ in GFR, but this is dependent on an identical (∴ inhibited) co-transporter in the macula densa.
- As for loop diuretics, hypokalaemic metabolic alkalosis may result.
- Initial Na^+ and volume loss may be compensated for by Na^+ retention during the latter part of the dosing interval, with amelioration of BP-lowering efficacy. Twice daily dosing (at least) is ∴ required.

Role

More potent natriuretics than thiazides, but less effective BP lowering agents. Have little place in the routine management of ↑BP, except in patients with CCF (with volume overload), renal impairment (with volume overload) or other oedematous state (e.g. cirrhosis).

Potassium sparing diuretics

Examples

Amiloride, triamterene

Mechanism

- Block the epithelial Na^+ channel (ENaC) expressed in the late DCT and collecting duct.
    - ENaC plays a central role in the control of urinary Na^+ reabsorption, ECF volume homeostasis, and BP regulation.
    - Several hormones, including aldosterone, vasopressin, angiotensin II, insulin, and endothelin, regulate ENaC activity.
    - Liddle's syndrome (📖 p.536) is caused by activating (gain of function) mutation(s) in ENaC.
- K^+ absorption is tightly coupled with ENaC Na^+ absorption. Drugs blocking ENaC ∴ cause K^+ retention. Also has Mg^{2+} sparing effects.

Role

Not first-line. Useful adjuncts to limit ↓K^+ and ↓Mg^{2+} with other diuretics. ↓K^+ may actually ↑BP and is associated with insulin resistance, DM, arrhythmias and sudden death.

Amiloride may be used to prevent ↓K^+ and ↑BP associated with excess glucocorticoids or mineralocorticoids (📖 p.309) and in patients with Liddle's syndrome.

Problems

Hyperkalaemia! Cautions: renal impairment (especially in DM), combination with β-blockers, ACEI/ARB or spironolactone. The incidence of ↓K^+ when amiloride is co-prescribed with a thiazide or loop diuretic is very low.

Mineralocorticoid antagonists

- RAS activation is associated with worse outcomes in patients with CCF and ↑BP.
- Plasma aldosterone levels correlate with mortality in CCF and with LVH in hypertensive patients.
- Patients with 1° hyperaldosteronism appear to have worse CV outcomes.
- Aldosterone activates mineralocorticoid receptors in the heart, vasculature, and brain. Adverse consequences of activation include, endothelial dysfunction, myocardial fibrosis, myocyte hypertrophy, vascular injury, and centrally mediated elevations in BP.
- Pharmacological blockade of mineralocorticoid receptors ↓ LVH and microalbuminuria in hypertensive patients.
- Administration in severe CCF has been associated with a ↓ in mortality (RALES study).
- Although ACEI and ARBs ↓ aldosterone production, with chronic use levels return toward normal.
- Spironolactone and eplerenone are mineralocorticoid receptor antagonists.
  - Spironolactone has long been used in the treatment of conditions associated with 2° hyperaldosteronism and volume expansion such as cirrhotic ascites.
  - Eplerenone is more selective for the mineralocorticoid receptor than spironolactone and may be better tolerated.
- These agents may also have an antihypertensive role in patients with 'resistant' hypertension in whom undiagnosed 1° hyperaldosteronism may be more common than currently appreciated ●.

Adverse effects: gynaecomastia (common), GI upset, impotence, ↑K⁺ (⚠ caution with ACEI and ARB, especially if renal impairment).

β-blockers

Competitive inhibitors of catecholamines at β-adrenergic receptors. Many are available, with marked inter-drug differences in pharmacodynamic and pharmacokinetic properties. In general, these characteristics influence clearance and side effect profile rather than efficacy.

Examples

See opposite.

Mechanism

Remains a matter of debate. See box below.

Putative BP lowering mechanisms of β-blockers

- ↓Cardiac output
- ↓Renin release
- ↓Plasma volume
- ↓Vasomotor tone
- ↓Peripheral vascular resistance
- Improved vascular compliance
- Resetting of baroreceptor levels
- Effects on prejunctional β receptors: ↓ noradrenaline release
- ↓Pressor response to catecholamines with exercise and stress.
- Direct CNS effect.

Role

Downgraded in recent BHS/NICE guidelines in the UK. Still useful if concomitant angina, post-MI (↓mortality risk), arrhythmias or hyperdynamic circulation. Carvedilol, metoprolol, and bisoprolol have been shown to reduce morbidity and mortality in patients with stable CCF. Labetolol is useful in pregnancy (📖 p.576) and when parenteral treatment of hypertension is necessary (📖 p.355). Probably less effective in black patients and in the elderly

Problems

- Avoid in obstructive airways disease, marked bradycardia, AV node disease.
- Can cause lethargy, impaired concentration and memory, vivid dreams, hallucinations, depression (CNS effects may be more prominent with lipid soluble agents), deterioration in peripheral vascular disease, and Raynaud's symptoms.
- Metabolic effects:
  - ↓HDL-cholesterol and ↑triglycerides.
  - ↑Likelihood of new-onset DM, particularly when combined with a thiazide. Avoid this combination if high risk: strong family history of T2DM, impaired glucose tolerance (FPG ≥6.5 mmol/L), clinically obese (BMI >30), or of South Asian or Afro-Caribbean origin. (Combination leads to approximately 1 new case of DM for every 250 patients treated per year.)
  - Worsen glycaemic control and hypoglycaemic awareness in T1DM (worse with non-selective agents).
- Combined with diltiazem or verapamil may cause slowing of SA node ± negative inotropic effect.

Table 5.6 Examples of β-blockers

	β$_1$-selectivity[a]	Intrinsic sympath-omimetic activity[b]	Membrane stabiliz-ing activity[c]	α-blocking activity[d]	Major route of elimination[e]
Acebutolol[1]	+	+	+		Renal
Atenolol[1]	++				Renal
Bisoprolol	++				Both
Carvedilol			++	+	Hepatic
Celiprolol		+		+	Both
Labetolol				++	Hepatic
Metoprolol[1]	++				Hepatic
Nadolol[1]					Renal
Nebivolol	+			+	Renal
Oxprenolol[1]					Hepatic
Pindolol[1]		++	+		Both
Propanolol			++		Hepatic
Sotalol[2△]			†	+	Renal
Timolol[1]					Hepatic

[1]Combination tablet with a thiazide diuretic available. Atenolol also available combined with a CCB.
[2]△Sotalol is not licensed for use in hypertension. †Sotalol has class III antiarrhythmic properties and can prolong the QT interval.

β blockers differ in terms of their β$_1$ selectivity, intrinsic sympathomimetics activity (ISA), membrane stabilizing activity (MSA), α adrenergic blocking ability and pharmacokinetic properties.

[a] β$_1$ selectivity: these agents have less effect on β$_2$ receptors and are therefore relatively cardioselective. Applies at lower doses only. Theoretically an advantage in patients with obstructive airways disease, but should still be regarded as a contraindication. May not block arteriolar β$_2$ receptors, which be an advantage in T1DM with hypoglycaemia.

[b]Intrinsic sympathomimetic activity (ISA): partial agonist activity at β$_1$ receptors, β$_2$ receptors, or both. Identified as slight cardiac stimulation, inhibited by propanolol. Cause less bradycardia and AV node slowing, possibly less negatively inotropic, less effect on peripheral vascular resistance. Appear to have a better lipid profile. Remains unclear if these represent an overall advantage (or disadvantage).

[c]MSA: These agents have a quinidine or local anaesthetic like effect on the cardiac action potential. Usually seen above therapeutic levels and ∴ apparent in overdose.

[d]α-blocking activity: antagonistic properties at both α and β adrenergic receptors. Causes a reduction in peripheral and coronary vascular resistance. The benefit of carvedilol in heart failure is not dependent on this property.

[e]Water soluble agents are predominantly excreted via the kidney and have a longer ½ life. △ Dose reduction is often necessary in renal impairment. Lipid soluble agents mainly undergo hepatic excretion. They are usually shorter acting (requiring bd or tds dosing) and responsible for more CNS side effects (cross the blood–brain barrier).

α-blockers

α adrenoceptors participate in the regulation of vascular tone by the sympathetic nervous system (SNS) and play a role in the genesis of ↑BP and other CV disorders.

Examples

- Selective α_1 antagonists: doxazosin, prazosin, terazosin, indoramin.
- Unselective α_1 and α_2 antagonists: phentolamine, phenoxybenzamine.

Mechanism

- α_1 receptors are post-synaptic. Norepinephrine → ↑intracellular Ca^{2+} flux → ↑smooth muscle contraction → vasoconstriction. Selective α_1 blockade causes ↓SVR and BP with little or no effect on heart rate or cardiac output. α-blockers are essentially vasodilators.
- α_2 receptors are presynaptic. Stimulation → ↓norepinephrine release.
- Non-selective and α_1 and α_2 antagonists were developed first.
- In normotensive patients with normal sympathetic tone and vascular resistance, α-blockers have minimal BP lowering effect.

Role

- Antihypertensive effect only modest when used as single agents. Effects are additive with other antihypertensive classes.
- ALLHAT study (box below and 📖 p.326) provided bad press for α blockers.
- In light of the above, not considered first (or even second) line.
- Favourable lipid effects (↓total cholesterol, LDL, triglycerides; ↑HDL).
- Safe and effective in renal insufficiency.
- BP lowering effect independent of age race and gender.
- Non-selective α blockers useful in the management of phaeochromocytoma (📖 p.314).

Problems

Prazosin has a short ½ life, causing first dose (and postural) ↓BP—generally less of a problem with longer acting agents. Dizziness can persist (even without demonstrable postural ↓BP). Caution with sildenafil (Viagra®), tadalafil, and vardenafil (→ rapid ↓BP). Stress incontinence aggravated in ♀. Can cause fluid retention (∴ good combined with a diuretic).

α-blockers and ALLHAT (📖 p.326)

The doxazosin limb was stopped early (3.3 years follow-up, ~9000 patients) because of a 25% ↑incidence of CV disease (mainly CCF; no difference in 1° end-points—fatal and non-fatal MI) compared to the thiazide group, As a result, α-blockers have fallen in popularity with guideline authors and prescribers alike. However, (i) SBP was higher in the doxazosin arm; (ii) randomization deprived many patients with CCF of diuretics, β-blockers, or ACEI, disadvantaging the α blocker group.

α-blockers remain a good component of multiple drug regimens for moderate-to-severe ↑BP and are particularly useful in ♂ with concomitant prostatic disease. Avoid if coexisting CCF.

α-blockers and bladder outflow symptoms (see 📖 p.515)

- Lower urinary tract symptoms (LUTS) associated with BPH and obstruction are common in ♂ >age 60.
- Bladder emptying involves relaxation of α_1 receptor mediated smooth muscle contraction in the bladder neck and prostate.
- α_1 receptors are integral to the bulbospinal pathways from brainstem → lumbosacral cord which inhibit reflex urination.
- α-blockers relieve the symptoms of outflow obstruction and decrease the need for surgery.
- Newer α-blockers, e.g. tamsulosin (Flomax®), are 'uroselective', acting on the α receptor subtypes α_{1a} and α_{1b}, within the bladder neck and prostate, with limited effect on systemic BP.
- α blockers are effective, with >60% reporting improvement. Medical therapy is now common and TURP rates are in decline.
- α blockers are the best monotherapy for symptom relief of LUTS.
- In those with moderate to severe symptoms and demonstrable prostatic enlargement, combination therapy of an α-blocker and 5α-reductase inhibitor (blocks conversion of testosterone → dihydrotestosterone), e.g. finasteride, provides effective symptom relief and retards disease progression.

Calcium channel blockers

Examples

- Dihydropyridine (vasodilating) CCBs: nifedipine, amlodipine, felodipine, isradipine, lacidipine, lercanidipine, nicardipine, nisoldipine.
- Non-dihydropyridine (cardiac active) CCBs: diltiazem, verapamil.

Mechanism

- Block voltage dependent L-type Ca^{2+} channels → ↓calcium entry into smooth muscle cells → ↓smooth muscle contraction → ↓vascular resistance → arterial vasodilatation.
  - Dihydropyridines: more selective at Ca^{2+} channels in vascular smooth muscle cells ∴ more powerful vasodilators.
  - Non-dihydropyridines: block Ca^{2+} channels in cardiac myocytes and ↓cardiac output. Antiarrhythmic properties via AV node (verapamil > negative inotrope and chronotrope than diltiazem).
- Other CCB effects: ↓aldosterone release, ↓growth and proliferation of vascular smooth muscle cells, anti-atherogenic in animal models.
- Moderately ↑Na^+ excretion via natriuresis. ↓BP effect is not augmented by dietary Na^+ restriction (unlike other classes).
- Undergo first pass metabolizm to some degree. Most are short acting ∴ require multiple dosing regimens or a slow release delivery system.

Role

- BP lowering effect equivalent to most other drug classes. Among CCBs, antihypertensive properties are ~ equivalent.
- Can be combined with all other classes (⚠ avoid diltiazem or verapamil with β-blockers—cardiac effects are additive).
- Good choice in patients with concomitant angina.
- Effective in low renin ↑BP (i.e. black or elderly patients)
- Don't worsen dyslipidaemias.
- ↓BP effect not blunted by NSAIDs.
- ASCOT trial (📖 p.330) has elevated their status.
- Nimodipine is used for the prevention of ischaemic deficits following subarachnoid haemorrhage—not licensed for hypertension.

Problems

- Flushing, tachycardia, or headache; especially short acting agents.
- Dose-dependent peripheral oedema with dihydropyridine CCBs. This is not due to fluid retention (∴ diuretic unresponsive) but 2° to mismatched arteriolar and venous vasodilatation.
- Gum hypertrophy occurs with dihydropyridine CCBs.
- Avoid in systolic LV impairment (esp. non-dihydropyridine)
- CCBs have many drug interactions—worth checking before prescribing. Grapefruit juice inhibits cytochrome P450 CYP3A and ↑ the bioavailability of several dihydropyridine CCBs.
- Several trials have suggested that CCBs are not as effective protection against hypertensive or diabetic renal disease as ACEI or ARBs ∴ not first line in this situation.
- Verapamil use is often accompanied by constipation.

⚠ Early formulations of some dihydropyridines (e.g. capsular or sublingual nifedipine) had a rapid onset of action, unpredictable BP lowering effect accompanied by reflex sympathetic stimulation, tachycardia and RAS activation. These agents have no place in the management of hypertension.

ACE inhibitors (ACEI)

Examples

Captopril, cilazepril, enalapril, fosinopril, imidapril, lisinopril, moexipril, perindopril, quinapril, ramipril, trandolapril.

Mechanism

- Block conversion of angiotensin I → angiotensin II (AII) by angiotensin converting enzyme (ACE). The resulting ↓ in AII → vasodilatation and ↓BP.
- AII has many actions potentially detrimental to the CV system (📖 p.286)
- Alternative pathways of AII production, e.g. chymases and other tissue proteases, are unaffected.
- In the short term, ACEI reduce AII levels, but with chronic treatment they return to normal ('AII escape'). Other mechanisms of BP lowering are ∴ thought to be active. Possibilities: -
  - ↑bradykinin → ↑nitric oxide ± ↑PGI_2 (→ vasodilatation).
  - ↑angiotensin-(1–7), a peptide that is antagonistic to AII.
  - ↓sympathetic nervous system activity.
  - Direct effect on endothelial function and vascular remodelling
- ACEI can be subdivided according to their affinity for tissue ACE. It is possible that lipophilic compounds with high tissue affinity (e.g. ramipril, quinapril, perindopril) exert greater influence on endothelial function and provide CV benefits independent of BP lowering ◆.
- Increasing the dose of an ACEI does not generally alter peak effect, but extends duration of response. Many patients benefit from a second daily dose.

Role

- Comparable BP lowering to other classes (but no better).
- Cardioprotective and renoprotective ∴ good choice if: CCF, post-MI, DM, chronic renal failure (especially proteinuric) or LVH.
- Patients at high risk of CV disease may have improved survival when treated with ACEI (independent of BP reduction ◆).
- Synergistic effects when used in combination with diuretics (diuretics → Na^+ depletion → RAS activation → AII dependent (and ∴ ACEI responsive) ↑BP. Also ameliorate diuretic induced ↓K^+ (↓AII induced aldosterone release).
- Also suitable for combination with β-blockers, α-blockers and CCBs (ASCOT study likely to promote the latter 📖 p.330). Insufficient evidence at present to recommend routine combination with ARB.
- Relatively ineffective monotherapy in certain groups with low renin ↑BP; e.g. blacks, though response highly variable (↓Na^+ diet increases efficacy). Generally effective in the elderly.
- Documenting plasma renin activity or ACE gene polymorphisms to 'individualize' therapy is not useful—neither predict response.
- Lack adverse metabolic effects.

Problems

- *Renal insufficiency*: much feared by clinicians. If glomerular filtration pressure is dependent on AII driven efferent arteriolar tone (e.g. volume depletion, renal artery stenosis, CCF) then ACE inhibition may cause a precipitous decline in GFR.
- ⚠ *Precautions*: ensure patient is volume replete, ask those on diuretic therapy to take first dose before retiring to bed, seek expert help if high index of suspicion of renovascular disease (📖 p.412). Check U&E before commencing treatment and 5–7 days after. Expect (and allow) a rise in Cr of ≤20% or ↓ in eGFR of 15%.
- *Hypotension*: acute falls in BP with ACEI occur when RAS is activated; e.g. over-diuresis, CCF, accelerated hypertension. Rare when therapy initiated in uncomplicated hypertensive patients (admission to hospital for ACEI introduction was commonplace in the 1980s). Postural hypotension is actually comparatively uncommon.
- *Hyperkalaemia*: unusual unless renal impairment ± other drugs causing ↑K^+ (e.g. amiloride, spironolactone, β-blockers).
- *Cough*: common (5–40%, ♀>♂) and generally resistant to all measures except drug withdrawal. (↑bradykinin ± other vasoactive peptides; e.g. substance P → cough reflex activation).
- *Angioneurotic oedema*: rare. Blacks >Caucasians, also bradykinin mediated and potentially fatal. Stop the ACEI and avoid for life.
- ↓*Erythropoietin secretion*: may cause or worsen anaemia.
- *Pregnancy*: contraindicated.
- *Rash and altered taste*: mainly captopril.

AII receptor blockers (ARB)

Examples

Candesartan, eprosartan, irbesartan, losartan, olmesartan, telmisartan, valsartan.

Mechanism

- Developed more recently than ACE inhibitors, ARB essentially block the vasoconstrictive action of AII on smooth muscle.
- There are two AII receptor subtypes:
  - AT_1 mediates (i) vasoconstrictor effects of AII and (ii) AII induced growth in the myocardium and arterial wall.
  - AT_2 function is less well understood. Expressed at high levels in fetal tissues, with ↓expression after birth. Probably responsible for many of the proliferative effects of AII.
- Two major differences between ACEI and ARB:
  - ACEI ↓activity of AII at both AT_1 and AT_2 receptors. ARB only ↓AT_1 activity, with no effect on AT_2.
  - ACE is a kininase, so ACEI lead to ↑kinins. Kinins are responsible for some ACEI side-effects (esp. cough), but may also mediate some of their beneficial effects, including BP lowering and ↑insulin sensitivity.
- AII blockade leads to ↑renin, ↑angiotensin I, and ↑AII, though this accumulation does not appear to overwhelm receptor blockade.

Roles

- Similar BP lowering effect to ACEI and other main classes.
- As with ACEI, synergistic with diuretics.
- Evidence is growing that ARB have similar benefits to ACEI in conditions other than ↑BP, such as CCF (Val-HeFT and CHARM studies) and post-MI (VALIANT).
- Several major trials (IDNT, IRMA-2, RENAAL,) have demonstrated renoprotection with ARB in nephropathy associated withT2DM.

Problems

- Generally well-tolerated, similar side-effect profile to ACEI.
- Less cough than ACEI (as kinin mediated), though angioedema has been reported.
- Altered taste.
- Contraindicated in pregnancy.

Combined ACEI and ARBs

- Good theoretical rationale for using in combination:
  - ACE inhibitors do not completely block the formation of AII (other tissue proteases are involved)
  - ARB are selective for the AT_1 receptor, leaving AT_2 receptor exposed to ↑AII.
  - With ACEI, ↓AII → ↑renin release, eventually returning AII towards baseline ('AII escape').
- Combination therapy is effective in LV dysfunction (Val-HeFT and CHARM studies).
- Growing evidence to support their combined use in proteinuric renal disease (e.g. COOPERATE).
- ON-TARGET is a large study aiming to comparing the effects of telmisartan, ramipril and their combination on CV mortality in high risk patients. Should complete in 2007.
- Insufficient evidence at present to recommend combination therapy for hypertension treatment.

Other antihypertensives

With the exception of methyldopa and moxonidine, these drugs are rarely seen in the routine treatment of ↑BP in the UK. They are still widely used around he world, as generic formulations mean lower costs in many instances.

Centrally acting agents

Methyldopa

Metabolized to a methyl-norepinephrine, a false neurotransmitter that (i) displaces norepinephrine from α adrenergic receptors preventing smooth muscle contraction and (ii) stimulates adrenergic receptors in the central vasomotor centres, inhibiting sympathetic outflow. Large dose range (250mg–3g daily) and remains widely used to treat hypertension in pregnancy (📖 p.572). In non-pregnant, best given with a diuretic.

Problems: positive Coombs' test in 20% (though overt haemolytic anaemia rare), dry mouth, oedema, drowsiness, febrile illness and depression. Avoid in liver disease.

Clonidine

Stimulates adrenergic receptors in the central vasomotor centres, inhibiting sympathetic outflow. Very rarely used in the UK. Clonidine suppression test occasionally used in the diagnosis of phaeochromocytoma (📖 p.314).

Problems: dry mouth, sedation, depression. Associated with severe rebound ↑BP (may require treatment with parenteral α blockers)

Moxonidine

A selective imidazole agonist that acts on central receptors to decrease sympathetic outflow. A useful add on therapy when other classes are insufficient or poorly tolerated. Can be used with caution in renal insufficiency.

Problems: dry mouth, headache, fatigue, dizziness, sleepiness. Avoid abrupt withdrawal (if also on β-blockers, stop them first). Avoid if AV block, severe CCF (worse outcomes) and pregnancy.

Direct acting vascular smooth muscle relaxants

Hydralazine and minoxidil

↓arteriolar resistance. The consequent ↓peripheral resistance and BP causes reflex sympathetic activation with tachycardia and palpitations. This can be offset with a β-blocker.

Problems: flushing, headache, palpitations. Avoid in ischaemic heart disease. Cause Na^+ and water retention (especially minoxidil) ∴ give with a diuretic. Hydralazine can cause a lupus like syndrome, particularly in slow acetylators. Minoxidil causes hirsutism. Hydralazine's metabolites accumulate in renal failure ∴ avoid, minoxidil is OK.

Antihypertensives on the horizon

Endothelin antagonists

The endothelins are a group of potent vasoconstrictor peptides produced in many different tissues. ET-1 is the predominant endothelin secreted by the endothelium, where it acts in a paracrine fashion. Several antagonists are under investigation and it is hoped they will prove reno- and cardio-protective as well as antihypertensive. Bosentan is already licensed for use in 1° pulmonary hypertension.

Vasopeptidase inhibitors

Inhibit both ACE and neutral endopeptidase, a membrane bound metalloprotease involved in the enzymatic degradation of natriuretic (📖 p.288) and various other peptides (including angiotensin II). Several in development (e.g. omapatrilat). Achilles heal appears to be the frequency of angioedema.

Renin inhibitors

Another means of antagonizing RAS. Effects may prove additive to ACEI and ARBs.

Resistant hypertension

Relatively common—up to 20–30% of study populations in clinical trials, usually as a consequence of poorly-controlled SBP. Compliance is often a central issue in apparent resistance, underlying the importance of a good physician-patient relationship.

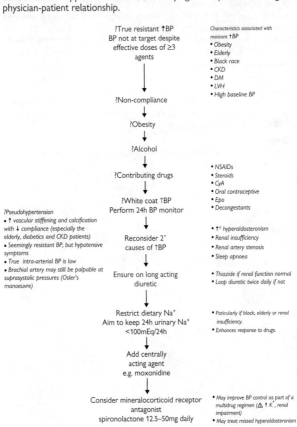

?True resistant ↑BP
BP not at target despite
effective doses of ≥3
agents

Characteristics associated with resistant ↑BP
- *Obesity*
- *Elderly*
- *Black race*
- *CKD*
- *DM*
- *LVH*
- *High baseline BP*

↓

?Non-compliance

↓

?Obesity

↓

?Alcohol

↓

?Contributing drugs

- *NSAIDs*
- *Steroids*
- *CyA*
- *Oral contraceptive*
- *Epo*
- *Decongestants*

↓

?White coat ↑BP
Perform 24h BP monitor

?Pseudohypertension
- *↑ vascular stiffening and calcification with ↓ compliance (especially the elderly, diabetics and CKD patients)*
- *Seemingly resistant BP, but hypotensive symptoms*
- *True intra-arterial BP is low*
- *Brachial artery may still be palpable at suprasystolic pressures (Osler's manoeuvre)*

↓

Reconsider 2°
causes of ↑BP

- *↑° hyperaldosteronism*
- *Renal insufficiency*
- *Renal artery stenosis*
- *Sleep apnoea*

↓

Ensure on long acting
diuretic

- *Thiazide if renal function normal*
- *Loop diuretic twice daily if not*

↓

Restrict dietary Na⁺
Aim to keep 24h urinary Na⁺
<100mEq/24h

- *Paticularly if black, elderly or renal insufficiency.*
- *Enhances response to drugs.*

↓

Add centrally
acting agent
e.g. moxonidine

↓

Consider mineralocorticoid receptor
antagonist
spironolactone 12.5–50mg daily

- *May improve BP control as part of a multidrug regimen (△ ↑ K⁺, renal impairment)*
- *May treat missed hyperaldosteronism*

Fig. 5.12

Hypertensive urgencies and emergencies

Definitions

- ▶ Hypertensive crises are classified as *emergencies* or *urgencies* based on the presence or absence of progressive target organ dysfunction.
  - *Emergencies:* severe ↑BP complicated by evidence of acute or progressive organ dysfunction such as cardiac ischaemia, encephalopathy, stroke, pulmonary oedema or renal failure.
  - *Urgencies:* severe ↑BP *without* evidence of acute or progressive target organ dysfunction.
- The term *malignant hypertension* was coined before antihypertensive therapy improved an appalling prognosis (1 year mortality ~90%). It is a syndrome of ↑BP with progressive target organ damage and papilloedema. Pathologically, arteriolar fibrinoid necrosis is characteristic.
- *Accelerated hypertension* was applied to the scenario of retinal haemorrhages and exudates without papilloedema. The distinction from malignant hypertension is unhelpful, as both carry an identical prognosis.
- There is no threshold of BP above which malignant hypertension develops. DBP ranges from 100–180mmHg, SBP 150–290mmHg.
- ▶ Severity is not determined by the BP alone—it is the clinical context and degree of target organ dysfunction.
- Affects <1% of the hypertensive population, but the hypertensive population is large. ♂>♀.
- Essential hypertension accounts for ~2–30% of episodes in Caucasians, but ~ 80% in blacks. Therefore usually avoidable
- Renal disease (intrinsic and renovascular) accounts for the majority of the rest. Other previously unrecognized forms of 2° BP may also be responsible.
- The duration of hypertension prior to the development of malignant phase may range from days to years.

Pathophysiology

Vascular autoregulation

Auto-regulation describes the ability of organs to maintain their perfusion regardless of BP. ↑BP causes distal arteriolar vasoconstriction, protecting end-organs from hypertensive mechanical stress. Hypertensive emergencies are associated with a failure of this process, resulting in transmission of ↑BP to the microvasculature, where mechanical trauma → endothelial injury → ↑vascular permeability → leakage → platelet and fibrin deposition → fibrinoid necrosis. Release of catecholamines and vasopressin also contributes.

Endocrine and paracrine mediators, including the renin-angiotensin system, are activated with ↑AII leading to further vasoconstriction and ischaemia. Volume depletion due to pressure natriuresis stimulates further renin release and worsens ↑BP. A vicious cycle of vasoconstriction and worsening ↑BP ensues.

Pathological changes

Vascular lesions are due to endothelial injury, and consist of myo-intimal proliferation and fibrinoid necrosis, with sub-endothelial lipid deposition and hyaline thrombi. Vascular smooth muscle hypertrophy and collagen deposition contribute to medial thickening, which, with cellular intimal proliferation, results in the 'onion skin' appearance of small vessels with luminal narrowing. Ischaemia or infarction of end organs may occur. These changes are particularly well seen in the kidney, with proliferative endarteritis of the interlobular arteries, fibrinoid necrosis of the afferent arteriole and glomerular ischaemia (± tubulointerstitial damage).

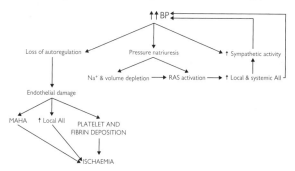

Fig. 5.13 The pathophysiology of malignant hypertension (Redrawn with permission from *Acute Renal Failure in Practice*, Imperial College Press. (MAHA: microangiopathic haemolytic anaemia.)

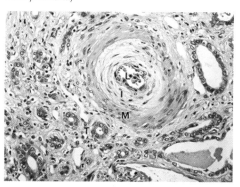

Fig. 5.14 Proliferative endarteritis of an interlobular artery in malignant hypertension. I, arterial intima showing gross proliferative change and 'onion-skin' appearance; L, severely narrowed arterial lumen; M, arterial media; T, tubular atrophy and interstitial fibrosis (reproduced with permission from Davison AMA, Cameron JS, Grunfeld J-P, et al. (eds) (2005) *Oxford Textbook of Clinical Nephrology*, 3rd edn. Oxford: Oxford University Press.).

Assessing urgencies and emergencies

How does the BP compare to previous readings?

- 160/100 may be sufficiently high to cause acute TOD in a previously normotensive patient
- A patient with longstanding hypertension may tolerate a higher BP without any evidence of acute TOD

Clinical assessment

- ▶ Assess degree of target organ involvement.
- **Urgency** is ↑BP without acute or progressive TOD.
- **Emergency** is ↑BP with acute or progressive TOD.

Is there evidence of target organ damage?

Acute TOD:

▶▶*Manage as an inpatient as an emergency*

- Neurological symptoms: at risk for haemorrhagic or thrombotic stroke, encephalopathy (altered consciousness, fits, focal signs).
- LVF.
- Acute renal failure (send U+E, dipstick urine).
- Chest pain ⚠ Acute coronary syndrome → MI or **aortic dissection**. Perform ECG, and check pulses. If in doubt CT aorta.
- Visual symptoms ± *either* grade III *or* IV hypertensive retinopathy
- Pancreatitis due to haemorrhagic infarction (rare).

What medication has the patient been on until now?

- Continue current medication, adding in further treatment as necessary.
- Check adherence to medication (recent non-compliance is very common in this situation). ⚠ Beware precipitating hypotension by restarting multiple anti-hypertensives in the previously non-adherent patient.
- ⚠ Remember recreational drug use (cocaine, amphetamines)

Symptoms and signs

- *BP:* **no pathognomic values**. Usually>220/140 (range: DBP 100–180 mmHg, SBP 150–290mmHg). Check the BP in both arms, look for missing pulses, bruits or an abdominal aortic aneurysm.
- *Eyes:* visual disturbances (35–60%): often present to ophthalmology.
- *Neurological:* headache (60%), dizziness (30%), neurological deficit; e.g. hemiparesis, cortical blindness (<10%). Encephalopathy (from cerebral oedema) is uncommon—confusion, seizures and coma.
- *Renal:* ARF (30%).
- *Cardiovascular:* dyspnoea 2° to LVF (~10%), chest pain (~4%).

Hypertensive retinopathy

Grade 1: arterial narrowing (tortuosity, 'silver wiring' are subjective)
Grade 2: AV nipping
Grade 3: haemorrhages and exudates
Grade 4: papilloedema.

Investigations

- *Urinalysis:* proteinuria (can be nephrotic range—send PCR ± 24h collection), haematuria, cellular casts (red cell casts may indicate parenchymal renal disease).
- *U+E*
  - *Serum creatinine:* ↑2° to acute (or acute on chronic) renal failure.
  - *Potassium:* ↓K^+ (2° hyperaldosteronism → hypokalaemic alkalosis; renin and aldosterone are both raised in malignant hypertension), ↑K^+ (2° to ARF) also possible.
- *FBC:* microangiopathic haemolytic anaemia: ↓Hb, ↓platelets, red cell fragments, ↓haptoglobins. ↑ESR.
- *ECG (± echocardiogram):* LVH, ischaemia, MI.
- *CT brain:* if ↓GCS or neurological signs.
- *Renal biopsy:* a prognostic (rarely diagnostic) renal biopsy may be necessary.

Secondary hypertension?

Some conditions require specific management. Consider the list below.

Causes of hypertensive emergencies

- Essential hypertension
- Renal parenchymal disease
  - Glomerulonephritis
  - Tubulointerstitial disease
- Systemic diseases
  - Systemic sclerosis
  - HUS/TTP
  - SLE
  - Antiphospholipid syndrome
  - Vasculitis
- Renovascular disease
  - Atheromatous
  - Fibromuscular hyperplasia
- Pre-eclampsia/eclampsia
- Coarctation

- Endocrine
  - Conn's syndrome
  - Phaeochromocytoma
  - Cushing's syndrome
- Drugs
  - Cocaine
  - Amphetamines
  - Ecstasy
  - MAOI interactions
  - Erythropoietin
  - Ciclosporin
  - Tacrolimus
- Tumour related
  - Renal cell Ca
  - Lymphoma

Management of urgencies and emergencies

Hypertensive urgency

▶ *Severe uncontrolled hypertension (>130 diastolic BP) with no evidence of acute TOD*

- If no acute TOD, does not require admission.
- Repeat BP after 1–2 hours to confirm. If DBP still >130, → treat.
- Start with a single agent (e.g. amlodipine 5mg daily). Aim for diastolic BP 100–110 mmHg at first. Recheck BP after 24–48h.
- If still uncontrolled, double dose of amlodipine to 10mg daily.

Recheck after every 2–3 days until BP at desired level. Further suggested batting order (titrate doses up, then add in another agent).

- Atenolol 25–100mg daily.
- Ramipril 2.5–10mg daily (⚠ watch U+E carefully to exclude RAS).
- Furosemide 40–120mg 12–24h (esp. if renal failure) or bendroflumethiazide 2.5mg daily.
- Doxazosin (use long acting preparation) 4–8mg daily.

Hypertensive emergency

▶ *Severe uncontrolled hypertension (>130 diastolic BP) with acute TOD.*

- Treat in a high dependency environment.
- Volume depletion may be present—resuscitate with 0.9% NaCl.
- Oral agents usually provide a gradual and controlled ↓ in BP.
- *Use the same order as for hypertensive urgencies*
- Too rapid ↓BP may → cerebral infarction or worsening renal failure.
- Aim for a diastolic BP of 100–110mmHg over 24–36h.

When to use IVI anti-hypertensives

- Hypertensive encephalopathy (especially if fitting).
- Aortic dissection.
- Acute LVF or cardiac ischaemia.
- ▶ Need intensive monitoring, ideally with arterial line.

Aim for 160/100mmHg during first 24 hours, or 20–25% drop in MAP[1] over 4h. Will need to lower faster (to lower target) if aortic dissection.

- Labetalol 20 mg IV stat (can be repeated × 2 within 10–15min), then infusion of 0.5–2mg/min.
- GTN at 2–10mg/hour.
- Sodium nitroprusside 0.25–1.5µg/kg/min, with dose increase of 0.5 µg/kg/min every 5min until response.

Once BP within target range, transfer to oral agent and wean IV infusion down over 4–8h.

Prognosis

Without effective treatment, 1 year mortality ~90%, with it <10%. Many patients who develop renal insufficiency will recover renal function, even if initially dialysis dependent, though this may take several months.

---

1 MAP estimated as DBP + [SBP—DBP]/3

Table 5.8 Drugs used in hypertensive emergencies

Drug	Route and dose	Comment
Calcium channel blockers	• Oral • Start with amlodipine 5–10 mg or nifedipine MR 10mg 12h; max 40mg 12h	• NEVER use rapid release formulations. • Nimodipine used post subarachnoid haemorrhage
β-blockers	• Oral • Useful 2nd line (e.g. atenolol 50mg daily)	• SE: bronchospasm
ACE-inhibitors	• Oral • Start with low dose (e.g. ramipril 2.5mg or captopril 6.25mg) and titrate up	• May cause rapid fall in BP. • Treatment of choice in scleroderma crisis
Diuretics	• Oral/IV • Frusemide 40–120mg 12h	• Beware volume depleted patients
α-blockers	• Oral • Doxazosin MR 4mg 12h (up to 8mg 12h)	• Useful 2nd or 3rd line because of titration range
Labetolol	• IV • Up to 2mg/min as infusion or 20–80mg bolus every 10min	• Safe in pregnancy. Used in eclampsia • SE: bronchospasm, LVF, heart block
Esmolol	• IV • 25–200µg/kg/min • Initial bolus of 0.5–1.0mg/kg	• Very short ½ life. • SE: bronchospasm, LVF, heart block
Sodium nitroprusside	• IV • Start 0.25–1.5µg/kg/min. (↑ 0.5µg/kg/min every 5min until response). Range 0.25–10 µg/kg/min	• Potent, rapid acting, vasodilator. • Requires close monitoring (?arterial line) and light resistant delivery equipment • SE: nausea, vomiting, thiocyanate accumulation (esp if renal impairment)
Nitrates (GTN)	• IV • 10–200µg/min	• Familiar • SE: headache, tachycardia, vomiting
Hydralazine	• IV • 5–10mg bolus, repeated after 1h. Infusion: start 200–300µg/min, maintenance 50–150µg/min	• Arterial vasodilator used in eclampsia • SE: Na^+ and water retention, headache tachycardia, vomiting
Phentolamine	• IV • 1–5mg repeated as necessary	• Phaeochromocytoma • SE: tachycardia, dizziness, flushing, nausea
Fenoldopam	• IV • 0.1–0.3µg/kg/min	• Newer agent—a dopamine-1 agonist and peripheral arterial vasodilator. Also ↑urine flow and both Na^+ and K^+ excretion ∴ attractive if renal impairment • SE: headache, tachycardia, flushing.

Orthostatic hypotension

A frequent clinical problem, particularly in the elderly. Generally defined as a 20/10mmHg (symptomatic) fall in BP within 5min of assuming an upright posture. Symptoms include weakness, dizziness, visual disturbance, pre-syncope, blackouts and falls.

Normal response

Standing → splanchnic and lower limb blood pooling → ↓venous return → ↓cardiac output → ↓BP → reflex sympathetic and parasympathetic activation → ↑peripheral vascular resistance → ↑venous return → cardiac output → ↑BP.

Causes of orthostatic hypotension

- Hypovolaemia
- Drugs
- Autonomic dysfunction
  - ↓ Baroreceptor sensitivity (elderly)
  - Pure autonomic failure
  - Multiple system atrophy (Shy-Drager syndrome)
  - Parkinson's disease
  - Diabetes mellitus
  - Amyloidosis
  - Postural tachycardia syndrome (POTS)
  - Paraneoplastic autonomic dysfunction
- Endocrine disorders
  - Addison's syndrome
  - Hypoaldosteronism
  - Phaeochromocytoma
- Miscellaneous
  - Paroxysmal syndromes
    —Micturition syncope
    —Cough syncope
  - Varicose veins
  - Carcinoid syndrome
  - Mastocytosis

Volume depletion

Requires exclusion in all cases

Antihypertensive drugs

A frequent culprit. Other drugs include nitrates, opiates, tricyclic antidepressants and alcohol

Pure autonomic failure

Characterized by orthostatic ↓BP with a static heart rate, ↓sweating, impotence, nocturia, constipation, anaemia, and supine ↑BP. Symptoms are slowly progressive and often worse early morning and postprandially. Associated with ↓levels of plasma noradrenaline and degeneration of post-ganglionic neurons (with Lewy body inclusions).

Multiple system atrophy

Progressive neurodegenerative condition of unknown aetiology. ♂ > ♀, >age 50. Autonomic dysfunction (often first symptom) is accompanied by combinations of extrapyramidal, pyramidal and cerebellar dysfunction.

Postural tachycardia syndrome (POTS)

Relatively common; age <40, ♀ >♂. Aetiology uncertain, but abnormalities of autonomic regulation implicated. The presence of tachycardia distinguishes it from autonomic failure. Often little or no fall in BP. Tilt-table testing diagnostic.

Decreased baroreceptor sensitivity in the elderly
Mild postural ↓BP in the elderly associated with abnormal responses to baroreceptor reflexes such as tilting. May be associated with ↑ mortality.

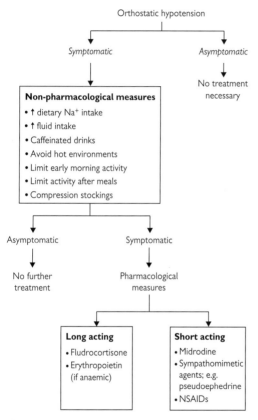

Fig. 5.15 Treatment of orthostatic hypotension (reproduced with permission from Jordan et al (1998). *Am J Med* **105**; 116–24).

Diseases of the kidney

Approaching glomerular disease

Glomerulonephritis (GN) is classified by clinical presentation, histological appearances, or by aetiology (e.g. lupus or post-streptococcal GN).

By clinical syndrome
- Asymptomatic urinary abnormalities (📖 p.12)
- Acute nephritis (📖 p.364)
- Nephrotic syndrome (📖 p.386).

These may all be accompanied by ↑BP ± renal impairment.

Asymptomatic urinary abnormalities
Common, and usually detected on routine urinalysis for unrelated problems. A positive dipstick for haematuria or proteinuria should always be repeated (e.g. after 72 hours). Trace to +ve on dipstick may be spurious.

Microscopic haematuria
Dipstick analysis is very sensitive, but non-specific. If persistent, arrange urine microscopy to confirm haematuria (defined as >2rbc/hpf), and to examine red cell morphology. Dysmorphic red cells, acanthocytes, or red cell casts imply glomerular bleeding (📖 p.50).

Dipstick positive proteinuria
Always repeat dipstick analysis. Transient proteinuria is not uncommon, esp. in concentrated urine.

'Benign proteinuria' may be caused by
- Orthostatic (postural)
- Vigorous exercise
- Febrile illnesses and infectious diseases
- Congestive heart failure.

Arrange for urine microscopy to exclude pyuria or casts, and culture to exclude infection. Proteinuria can be quantified on spot samples (protein:creatinine ratio, PCR, 📖 p.19), or by 24 hour urine collection.

Haematuria and proteinuria
Usually requires referral and further investigation to exclude an early glomerular lesion. Repeat dipstick to confirm findings.

Helpful investigations (📖 p.12)
- Urine microscopy for red cell morphology
- Quantify proteinuria
- U+E, albumin
- USS kidneys.

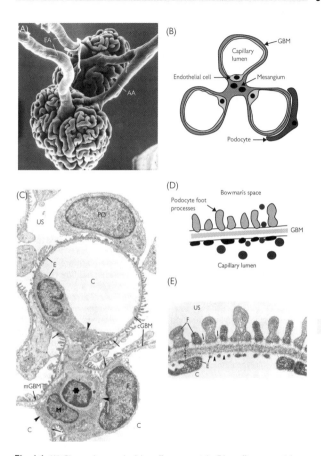

Fig. 6.1 (A) Glomerular vessels: AA = afferent arteriole; EA = efferent arteriole. (B) Cartoon of the glomerular capillaries: GBM = glomerular basement membrane. (C) EM of glomerular capillaries: C = capillary; E = endothelial cell; cGBM = capillary GBM; mGBM = mesangial GBM; PO = prodocyte; US = ultrafiltration space. (A–C) Reproduced with permission from Davison AMA, Cameron JS, Grunfeld J-P, et al (2005) *Oxford Textbook of Clinical Nephrology*. Oxford University Press, Oxford. (D) Cartoon of glomerular filter. (E) EM of glomerular filter: (F) = prodocyte foot process.

Histology of glomerulonephritis

Renal tissue is sampled at renal biopsy (📖 p.636), and prepared for:
- Light microscopy: various histochemical stains (eg, H+E, periodic acid–Schiff [PAS], Jones [silver] stains). Useful for morphology, chronicity and diagnosis.
- Immunohistochemistry: usually by immunofluorescence but also immunoperoxidase staining. Localizes immune reactants (particularly immunoglobulins or complement fractions) within glomeruli using fluorescein-labelled antibodies. Their nature and pattern of staining are characteristic for certain GN.
- Electron microscopy: useful for examining glomerular deposits and cell and membrane structure.

When examining a preparation of renal cortex, many glomeruli (10–30 on average) are sampled. The following descriptive terms are then used:
- Focal or diffuse? *Focal* lesions affect some (<50%) of the sampled glomeruli, but not all. *Diffuse* lesions involve most (>50%) if not all of the glomeruli.
- Segmental or global? *Segmental* lesions affect *part* of an affected glomerulus, whilst global lesions involve most of any tuft.
- Proliferative or not? *Proliferative* lesions describe an increase in local cell number. For instance, an increase in mesangial cells ('mesangial proliferative') is a feature of IgA nephropathy.
- Crescentic or not? Glomerular parietal epithelial cells (lining Bowman's capsule) proliferate in response to local inflammatory and pro-coagulant signals, with fibrin deposition and adhesions filling some or all of Bowman's space.
- Matrix or membrane? *Expansion* of matrix produced by mesangial cells as found in IgA nephropathy, or increase in GBM width (and thus capillary wall thickness) as found with immune deposits.
- Necrosis or sclerosis? *Necrosis* refers to fresh cell death as a result of ongoing injury, while *sclerosis* reflects a scarred glomerulus or glomerular segment.

As an example:
Focal and segmental glomerulosclerosis affects some glomeruli, but not all, and only part of any affected tuft. The disease leads to scarring within glomeruli.
Diffuse proliferative crescentic glomerulonephritis affects most glomeruli, with hypercellularity (increased cell number) and the formation of crescents in Bowman's space.

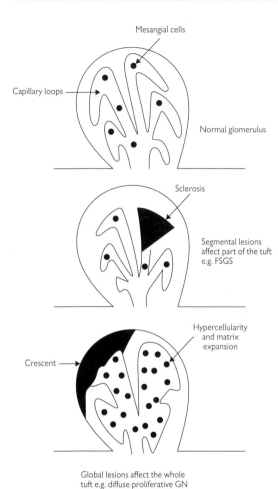

Fig. 6.2 Defining terminology used in describing glomerulonephritis

Acute nephritic syndrome

The underlying pathology is glomerulonephritis. Presents (rapidly) as:
- Impaired renal function
- Haematuria and proteinuria
- Oliguria with signs of salt and water retention.

It is a spectrum of disease with a variety of aetiologies marked by a common site of primary injury: the glomerulus. Onset may be insidious, with urinary abnormalities alone, or fulminant, with a rapidly progressive crescentic GN and acute renal and other organ failure.

Mechanisms of glomerular injury

The injury leading to most GN is immunologically mediated, with loss of tolerance to auto-antigens provoking both arms of the immune system (cellular and humoral). These antigens may be native to the glomerulus itself (occurring normally within the tuft, e.g. the GBM in anti-GBM disease), or circulating antigens or antigen-antibody complexes that become fixed in glomerular structures.

Antigen–antibody binding may then fix and activate complement (forming immune complexes, ICs) or recruit inflammatory cells causing injury that differs depending on the site of the IC (e.g. IgA containing complexes in the mesangium activate these cells to cause IgA nephropathy). Local complement activation and recruited cells (neutrophils, macrophages) generate oxidant species and proteases, inflammatory cytokines, growth factors, vasoactive factors, and procoagulants.

Damage to and activation of surrounding cells and matrix then leads to the changes seen on histology: haematuria, proteinuria and impairment of glomerular filtration. This damage is determined by the number of ICs formed, and host responses to such ICs. Cellular immunity may add to or cause further structural changes in the glomerulus (esp. true of pauci-immune GN, where ICs play no role).

Resolution from inflammation may return an inflamed glomerulus to normal, or, if the healing phase is poorly regulated, may lead to cellular drop-out, scarring and CRF.

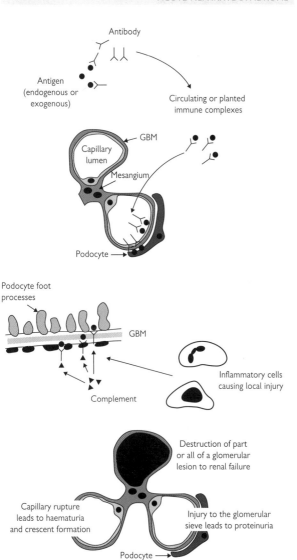

Fig. 6.3 An example of an immune-complex mediated GN

Approaching acute nephritis

Causes of an acute nephritic syndrome

- IgA nephropathy and Henoch–Schönlein purpura
- Lupus nephritis
- Post-infectious GN
- Anti-GBM disease
- ANCA positive small vessel vasculitis and idiopathic pauci-immune GN
- Idiopathic crescentic GN
- Mesangiocapillary GN

Investigations

- Dipstick urine for haematuria, proteinuria.
- Urine microscopy for red morphology ± casts. Red cells originating from the lower urinary tract are usually normal in appearance. Bleeding from glomerular capillaries means red cells traverse the tubules, exposed to osmotic stress. Dysmorphic red cells ± acanthocytes (thorn-like spicules on the rbc membrane) may be seen. Red cell casts present.
- 24 hour proteinuria variable (often <1g/day, but may be nephrotic range), and urinary light chains.
- U+E, bone profile, LFT.
- Acute phase markers (ESR, C-reactive protein).
- Full nephritic screen.
- USS kidneys.
- Renal biopsy.

General principles of management of nephritis

Salt and water restriction

▶ It is vital to correctly assess volume status.

- Fluid overload ± pulmonary oedema often complicate oliguric GN
  —limit salt intake <80mmol/day (<5g/day).
- Set oral intake at 500–1000mL/day (adjusted according to volume status and UO).
- Diuretics may promote a natriuresis and provide symptom control: use loop diuretic, e.g. furosemide 40–160mg/day po or IVI titrated against response and renal function.
- Less commonly, dehydration may be present, in which case increased oral intake or rehydration with IVI 0.9% NaCl may be needed.

Review volume status and monitor weight daily, and chart input and output to plan following day's fluid balance. Indwelling catheter only required in unwell patients.

Control BP

↑BP may be significant, and is usually volume-related. Aim for target BP of ≤130/80. ACE inhibitors or ARB offer theoretical advantages in the control of ↑BP secondary to renal disease, due to their anti-fibrotic and anti-proteinuric effects, but their use may precipitate further decline in renal function:

- Diuretic as above.
- Step-wise add-on therapy using β-blockers ± calcium channel blockers.
- ACEI (e.g. ramipril) or ARB—titrate up from low-dose with daily increments.

Dialysis if required according to standard indications
(📖 p.118)

Likely to be needed early in cases of ARF secondary to GN: plan ahead for insertion of dialysis access.

Other supportive measures

General measures involving prompt treatment of infection, adequate nutrition and management of the other organ complications often associated with systemic diseases causing GN.

Specific therapies: immunosuppression

Almost always tailored to a histological diagnosis, so renal biopsy usually indicated as soon as feasible.

See under particular diagnosis, and 'Starting immunosuppression', 📖 p.370.

Management of glomerulonephritis

Starting immunosuppression

❶ Treatment of glomerulonephritis often involves toxic therapies in the short-term to improve long-term renal and patient survival. The initial goal is to achieve *remission* prior to altering therapy to *maintain* remission. When starting a drug, the dictum of 'first do no harm' always applies. These are dangerous drugs: does risk:benefit really justify their use?

Monitor toxicity

⚠ FBC, U+E and LFT weekly to fortnightly at induction of therapy.

Preventing drug toxicity

- Issue patients with a steroid card, and counsel as to the risks of abrupt steroid withdrawal and the need to increase dose with stressors (such as intercurrent illness or anaesthesia).
- Prophylaxis against gastric irritation: proton pump inhibitor or H_2 receptor antagonist by convention (evidence poor).
- Offer prophylaxis against PCP with cotrimoxazole for duration of cyclophosphamide therapy (480mg bd po).
- Warn diabetics and those with impaired glucose tolerance to monitor blood sugars closely, and inform their diabetic team.
- In those at high risk for tuberculosis (e.g. previous TB, recent exposure, patients from endemic areas), consider primary prophylaxis with isoniazid + pyridoxine (evidence poor).
- Steroid-induced bone demineralization is an early event (within first months of treatment). Ensure bisphosphonate use (e.g. risedronate SR 35mg weekly or alendronate SR 70mg weekly) in those at risk (if >5mg prednisolone/day for >3 months). Intended to prevent osteoporosis. Calcium (1500mg/day) and vitamin D_3 (800 IU/day) containing preparations (eg Calcichew D3 Forte®) are a less effective alternative. Many bisphosphonates require 50% dose-reduction with renal impairment.
- Treat steroid-exacerbated hyperlipidaemia with HMG-CoA reductase inhibitors (statins). If proteinuric, should be considered as higher risk for cardiac events.

Commonly used drugs

(I)nduction brings about disease remission. (M)aintenance obviously maintains remission.

Prednisolone (I, M)

- To induce remission, either as high dose po (1 mg/kg/day) or by IV pulse (0.5–1 g/day for 3 days).
- Steroids are also used to maintain remission at lower doses. Acts as a potent anti-inflammatory agent, modulating both B and T cell mediated immunity, as well as inhibiting the effector function of both monocytes and neutrophils through regulation of cytokine-driven responses.
  ▶ Ensure bone and gastric prophylaxis in those at risk, and monitor for impaired glucose tolerance or worsening glycaemic control in diabetics.

Cyclophoshamide (I)

Either orally, or as periodic (monthly) IV pulses. An alkylating cytotoxic agent that impairs cellular DNA replication, leading to reduced cell turnover and cell death. Restricts lymphocyte proliferation, influencing auto-immune inflammatory states.

Using IVI cyclophosphamide

- Body surface area is calculated as $\sqrt{}$ (height (m) x Wt (kg)/3600).
- Advise re: risks (📖 p.372).
- Check WCC at d10–14
- Ensure prophylaxis v PCP with cotrimoxazole 480mg bd for duration
- Protect the bladder: vigorous oral fluids, with 1L 0.9% NaCL over 4 hours after therapy. Oral mesna at −2, +2 and +6 hours as (0.2 x cyclophosphamide dose in mg) per dose.
- Anti-emetics as granisetron 1mg (can repeat at +12 hours) + dexamethasone 10mg po at −2 hours.

Ciclosporin (I, M) orally in two divided doses (can be IVI). A calcineurin inhibitor that limits IL-2-driven nuclear transduction, and thus T-cell activation. *Tacrolimus* is increasingly used for similar indications.
▶ Monitor GFR over longer term for signs of ciclosporin nephrotoxicity.

Azathioprine (M) orally in a single daily dose. Anti-proliferative pro-drug metabolized to 6-mercaptopurine, restricting lymphocyte proliferation through inhibition of folate-dependent DNA synthesis.
⚠ Avoid or stop allopurinol as may precipitate profound leucopenia.

Mycophenolate mofetil (I, M) orally in two divided doses (can be IVI). A newer anti-proliferative inhibiting lymphocyte expansion and antibody production. Promotes T-cell programmed cell death, and affects cell:cell interactions.

Rituximab (I) a novel anti-CD20 monoclonal antibody directed against against a B cell surface marker, resulting in widespread B cell and anti-body depletion over time. Shows promise in lupus nephritis and other GN, but best used in centres with specialist expertise.

Important side-effects

❶ All immunosuppressants predispose to infection by nature

Prednisolone
Insomnia, weight gain, ↑BP, impaired glucose tolerance, dyslipidaemia, poor wound healing, osteoporosis.

Cyclophosphamide
- Leucopenia, and ↑risk of infection, esp. herpes zoster.
- Gonadal toxicity (discuss loss of fertility prior to starting treatment—in ♀, measure LH/FSH before therapy, and limit total exposure).
- Haemorrhagic cystitis → longer term bladder cancer (⚠ use mesna if giving IVI, and have low threshold for investigating new haematuria in those previously exposed).
- ⚠ Oral cyclophosphamide is more toxic to *ovaries* and *bladder* than IVI, particularly if >10g cumulative dose used.
- Nausea and vomiting if given IVI.
- Teratogenic.
- Can cause SIADH.

Azathioprine
Myelosuppression, hepatotoxicity (check WCC, LFT by day 14–21 after starting drug). Long term risk of skin cancers.

MMF
Myelosuppression, gut toxicity. Diarrhoea in particular is not uncommon—divide dose qds rather than bd, or reduce drug. Is teratogenic.

Ciclosporin (C) and tacrolimus (T)
↑BP (C), tremor, hirsutism (C), gum hypertrophy, dyslipidaemia, IGT (T>C), gout (C), nephrotoxicity, microangiopathy, amongst others.

Tapering steroids

Prednisolone is the most widely used oral corticosteroid. Its use in renal disease is usually for >3 weeks, and thus often requires slow tapering to allow recovery of a suppressed hypothalamic-pituitary axis.
▶ May not need to taper steroids if used for <6–8 weeks.
A potential regimen from 20mg/daily prednisolone might be:
- Reduce by 5mg every fortnight until on 5mg/day.
- Reduce to 5mg alternating with 2.5mg daily for 2 weeks.
- Reduce to 2.5mg daily for 2 weeks.
- Reduce to 2.5mg alternate days for 2 weeks.
- Stop drug.

Advise re: Addisonian symptoms, and warn to seek medical help if unwell.

IgA nephropathy

Is the most common primary glomerulonephritis in the world, often presenting with haematuria in the 2nd and 3rd decades. Although usually idiopathic, IgA nephropathy (IgAN) is often found in association with Henoch–Schönlein purpura, gut disorders (alcoholic cirrhosis, coeliac disease, inflammatory bowel disease) and skin and joint disorders (spondyloarthropathies, dermatitis herpetiformis, psoriasis). Generally, IgAN is an indolent glomerulopathy, but long-term renal damage is common—renal survival is 50–80% at 20 years.

Pathogenesis

Abnormally galactosylated IgA1 is deposited in the mesangium of the glomerulus. IgA binding of mesangial Fc receptors activates mesangial cells to produce platelet-derived and other growth factors and cytokines, resulting in mesangial cell proliferation and matrix synthesis, with inflammatory cell recruitment and subsequent local injury.

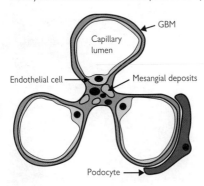

Fig. 6.4 Cartoon of mesangial IgA deposits

Symptoms and signs

Often presents as asymptomatic urinary abnormalities, particularly microscopic haematuria. Haematuria may be macroscopic, classically timed with upper respiratory illnesses (so-called 'synpharyngetic haematuria'). Associated proteinuria is common, although nephrotic range proteinuria (> 3g/day) is unusual (<15%). IgAN may present as a rapidly progressive GN with acute renal failure (🕮 p.58). Hypertension is common and often difficult to control.

Investigations

U+E, alb, bone profile, lipid profile. Elevated serum IgA in ± 50%. Urine microscopy for dysmorphic red blood cells and red cell casts. PCR or 24 hour urinary protein collection. If associated skin rash, skin biopsy may show IgA deposition on immunofluorescence. In adults, *renal biopsy*.

Histology

Mesangial cell proliferation and increased mesangial matrix that may be focal or diffuse seen on LM. IF confirms mesangial IgA deposits with C3. May be co-deposited IgG. EM shows mesangial deposits near the paramesangial GBM.

Henoch-Schönlein purpura

HSP is a systemic vasculitis affecting predominantly children, presenting with as a tetrad of abdominal pain, arthralgia, a skin rash, and renal involvement. It is most prevalent in winter, often precipitated by an upper respiratory tract infection, with a 2:1 ♂:♀ ratio.
- Purpuric rash affecting legs, buttocks, and arms with leucocytoclastic vasculitis with vascular IgA deposition on IF.
- Abdominal colic and often GI bleeding related to bowel vasculitis.
- Symmetrical polyarthralgia.
- GN presenting as haematuria, proteinuria ± renal impairment and hypertension secondary to IgAN.

In children the illness is usually self-limiting (<2 month duration), with skin manifestations predominating. In adults, HSP more commonly affects the kidneys. Complete resolution is the norm, but persistent urinary abnormalities (esp. proteinuria) impart a worse outlook, and long-term follow up is required. Crescentic IgAN in the context of HSP should be treated as 📖 p.377.

Management of IgA nephropathy

Unsatisfactory because of heterogeneity of patients and the disease itself. Few adequate trials have been performed, adding to the therapeutic dilemma faced. Prevention of progressive renal impairment is the key goal.

Poor prognostic features at presentation include:

- Impaired renal function.
- Heavy proteinuria (>3g/day).
- (Difficult to control) hypertension.
- Tubulo-interstitial fibrosis and glomerulosclerosis on biopsy.
- Rapidly progressive crescentic IgAN.

Low risk patients (no poor prognostic features) and,
- Normal renal function
- Episodic macroscopic haematuria
- <1g/day proteinuria
- No hypertension.

No treatment necessary, but regular surveillance (measure BP and Cr, dipstix urine for worsening proteinturia), initially yearly.

Medium risk (no poor prognostic features), and
- Older age
- Proteinuria >1g/day
- Hypertension.

▶ *Treat BP and reduce proteinuria.*

Aim for target BP of ≤125/75mmHg, ideally with ACEI as first agent. If normotensive but proteinuric, treat with ACEI for proteinuria reduction. Dual blockade of AII using combined ACEI + ARB may offer additional benefit (unproven). Aim to increase ACEI/ARB dose for proteinuria <1g/day.

✒ *Fish oils* (ω-3 fatty acids) have been given to limit progression. Presumed to act through modulating eicosanoid production and action. Given as fish oil (Maxepa®) 3g qds–often limited by tolerability (GI upset). It is safe, and is given for 6 months. Definitive evidence supporting its use is still awaited, but it remains a reasonable adjunct to ACEI alone.

High risk
▶ High risk patients are often difficult to treat with frequent progression to ESRD despite therapy.

If treatment with ACEI ± ARB, ± fish oil does not stabilize renal function, and reduce proteinuria to < 1 g/day: consider trial of prednisolone 0.5 mg/kg alt. days for 6 months (♦).

If nephrotic range proteinuria, prednisolone 0.5–1mg/kg/day for 8 weeks (♦).

If crescentic IgAN, treat aggressively to spare renal function: prednisolone 0.5–1mg/kg/day + cyclophosphamide 2mg/kg/day for 8 weeks, followed by tapering prednisolone and conversion to maintenance azathioprine 2mg/kg/day.

There is no robust evidence to support treatment of IgAN by removing the nephritogenic IgA1 through diet, tonsillectomy or drug therapy. Whether antiplatelet agents and anticoagulants (as warfarin + dipyridamole) or HMG CoA reductase inhibitors add benefit is also uncertain.

Recurrence after transplantation

Mesangial IgA deposition occurs in ±50% of patients receiving a renal transplant for the treatment of ESRD secondary to primary IgAN, but does not usually cause accelerated graft loss. It is no contra-indication to transplantation. The same is true for HSP.

Post-infectious glomerulonephritis

Classically post-streptococcal GN, but infection of almost any cause may be associated with an acute GN and similar findings on kidney biopsy (a diffuse proliferative GN). These include:

- Staphylococcal or pneumococcal sepsis
- Syphilis
- Influenza B, mumps, coxsackie, hepatitis B and Epstein–Barr virus
- Malaria, toxoplasmosis, or schistosomiasis.

▶ Infection on heart valves (endocarditis, 📖 p.486), on foreign bodies (shunt nephritis, opposite page) or abscess formation (deep-seated sepsis) often provides the source of chronic infection.

Acute post-streptococcal GN

An immune-complex mediated GN usually occuring in childhood (<7 years old), and is now rare in developed countries. Classically, the trigger is a streptococcal sore throat some 10–21 days prior to the nephritis, although streptococcal infection elsewhere (or other organisms) may be implicated. Tonsillitis or pharyngitis (commonly), impetigo, otitis media, or cellulitis are common sites of associated infection.

Infection with nephritogenic Lancefield group A [β]-haemolytic streptococcus (esp. types 12 and 49) is followed by a latent interval in which immune complex formation and glomerular deposition occurs, before symptoms manifest.

Symptoms and signs

Often gross haematuria (red-brown discolouration), oliguria, oedema (peri-orbital and ankle), ↑BP, and pulmonary oedema. Bilateral loin pain or renal angle tenderness 2° renal engorgement.

Investigations

Urine microscopy for red cell casts ± pyuria. U+E, Ca^{2+}, LFT. PCR or 24h proteinuria. Anti-streptolysin-O titre (ASOT) or anti-DNase B (for Gr A streptococci) may be positive. ↓C3 with normal C4. Rheumatoid factor may be positive.

Histology

Diffuse and proliferative changes with hypercellularity. Cellular crescents and frank necroses are unusual. Extensive neutrophilic infiltration and red cell casts. Sub-epithelial IgG and complement deposition on immunofluorescence. EM: electron-dense deposits in the sub-epithelial aspects of the capillary walls, with endothelial cell swelling. 📖 p.380 for graphic of the biopsy changes seen with PIGN—they are very similar to that of MCGN.

Clinical course

Generally, PIGN is self-limiting if the underlying infection resolves, and is associated with a full renal recovery (even after ARF). Diuresis usually begins after 7–10 days, and heralds resolution. Urinary abnormalities may persist for many years after recovery. All patients should be offered long-term follow-up, as hypertension and impaired renal function is more common in this group (probably reflecting post-GN scarring).

Treatment

▶ *Ensure the predisposing infection has resolved, or treat vigorously.*
- Restrict salt (<5g/day) and fluid. Assess volume status and weight daily. Monitor UO to tailor fluid restriction (500–1000 mL/day).
- Treat hypertension: as salt and water overloaded, start with loop diuretics (e.g. furosemide 40–160mg po/IV). Add in ACEI such as ramipril 2.5–10mg od, or CCB such as amlodipine 5–10mg od.
- Haemodialysis for standard indications (📖 p.118).
- Penicillins or other antibiotics only have a role in ONGOING infection.

Shunt nephritis

Originally coined to describe a GN associated with chronically infected ventriculoatrial (but *not* ventriculoperitoneal) shunts sited to treat hydrocephalus. In the contemporary era bacterial biofilms on indwelling central lines or pacing wires are more likely to →low-grade infection, immune complex formation and deposition in the glomerulus. Clinical features in patients with implanted foreign bodies include:
- Fever
- Haematuria, proteinuria and ↑ Cr
- Splenomegaly.

Characteristic findings include ↑ESR, CRP, ↓Hb, and ↓C3. Histology is that of a PIGN. Removing the foreign body is essential for resolution.

Mesangiocapillary glomerulonephritis

Also called *membranoproliferative glomerulonephritis*. It is a descriptive histological term rather than a distinct GN with a single cause. MCGN is more commonly found at biopsy in the developing world: it has been suggested that chronic or repeated infection predisposes to the disease. As such, MCGN is frequently described in association with a variety of conditions (see opposite). Tends to affect ♂=♀ aged 8–30, and is thought of as carrying a poor renal prognosis: 50% ESRD at 10 years.

Glomerular deposition of immune complexes localizing in mesangium and subendothelial space reflects a common mechanism of injury.

- *Type I MCGN* is described either in the *presence* of cryoglobulinaemia (and usually hepatitis C), or less commonly in their *absence* as a true primary, or idiopathic MCGN.
- *Dense deposit disease* or type II MCGN is related to deficiency in complement factor H (often with partial lipodystrophy and retinal abnormalities).
- *Type III MCGN* is similar to type I, but with added membranous change (there are 3 distinct varieties if type III!).

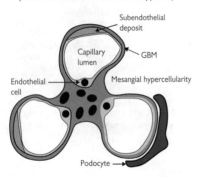

Fig. 6.5 Cartoon of subendothelial deposits in MCGN

Symptoms and signs

↑BP common. All may present as asymptomatic urinary abnormalities, acute nephritis, nephrotic syndrome or rapidly progressive renal failure.

Investigations

▶ Consider underlying cause!

U+E (↑Cr), ↓Alb, ↑Chol, LFTs, immunoglobulins and protein electrophoresis, PCR or 24h proteinuria, microscopy for red cell casts, hepatitis B+C, C3 nephritic factor, cryoglobulins, rheumatoid factor.

📖 p.484 *for hepatitis C and MCGN*

Complement in MCGN

Type I MCGN: the classical pathway is activated by immune complexes, leading to (↑C4 and normal/↑C3).

In DDD (type II), the alternate pathway is activated: (↑C3, normal C4).

▶ A stabilizing IgG binding a C3 convertase (C3Bb) occurs in DDD → persistent cleavage of C3 (the so-called C3 nephritic factor)
Findings are similar to DDD in type III, but without the C3NF

Histology

All subtypes have a characteristic 'double contour' or 'basement-membrane splitting' appearance of GBM caused by mesangial cell cytoplasm intervening between endothelium and GBM.

- *Type I:* diffuse mesangial hypercellularity ± mesangial immune complex deposition. Lobular pattern to tufts (monocyte infiltration). May show crescentic change. IF shows granular IgG and C3 in capillaries and mesangium.
- *DDD (type II):* widespread ribbon-like intramembranous electron dense deposits containing C3 but no Ig.
- *Type III:* is similar to type I, but with prominent subepithelial deposits (membranous change).

Associations with MCGN

With cryoglobulins:

- Hepatitis C or B
- Mixed cryoglobulinaemia unrelated to HCV (malignancies)
- SLE, Sjogren's.

Without cryoglobulins:

- Shunt nephritis and other chronic infections (☐ p.378)
- Visceral abscesses, schistosomiasis, malaria, leprosy
- Complement deficiencies.

Treatment

❶ *Always exclude causes of 2° MCGN prior to planning treatment.*
For treatment of hepatitis C-related MCGN, ☐ p.484.
▶ Evidence-based treatment strategies are lacking for primary MCGN.
General measures:

- Stop smoking (as in all progressive nephropathies).
- Restrict salt intake ± diuretic (☐ p.368).
- Control BP.
- Control proteinuria: ACE inhibitor or ARB (aim for full dose).
- Treat dyslipidaemia: HMG-CoA reductase inhibitor.

In the context of progressive renal failure, or persistent heavy nephrotic syndrome (limited evidence):

- Trial of aspirin 500mg + dipyramidole 75mg daily x 1 year.

❧ The following strategies may offer benefit in non-responders, although no good evidence *in adults* exists supporting use:

- Corticosteroids (tapering prednisolone started at 1mg/kg/day) ± cyclophosphamide 2mg/kg/day for 10 months (significant toxicity! ☐ p.370).
- MMF ± corticosteroids.

Hereditary nephropathies

Include Alport's syndrome and thin membrane disease (or benign familial haematuria).

Alport's syndrome

Classically presents as a triad of:
- Hereditary progressive nephropathy
- Sensori-neural deafness
- Ocular abnormalities.

Defective basement membrane formation in the glomerulus, cochlea and eye accounts for these findings. Although inheritance is varied, an X-linked-inherited mutation in the gene encoding α5 type IV collagen accounts for 80% of cases. This leads to afflicted ♂, with ♀ carriers having thin GBMs and microscopic haematuria (but rarely renal impairment).

Thin membrane disease (TMD)

An AD-inherited familial condition presenting with urinary abnormalities (esp haematuria) almost always with normal renal function. The normal GBM is ± 350nm thick—in TMD it is often less than 200 nm.

A thin GBM may occur in 5% of people, but urinary abnormalities are less common. The underlying defect probably affects type IV collagen integration into the GBM, but results in a partial failure of basement membrane function.

Symptoms and signs

Both hereditary nephropathies present with asymptomatic haematuria early in life (in childhood with Alport's).

Alport's: proteinuria (often nephrotic range) and ↑BP usually present by adolescence. Progressive renal impairment → ESRD by the 4th decade. High-tone sensori-neural deafness and lenticonus (conical rather than spherical lens leading to distorted vision) are typical.

TMD is often a diagnosis of exclusion: proteinuria, ↑BP or renal impairment RARE, though stone formation and gross haematuria does occur.

Investigations

- Inheritance may differentiate TMD from Alport's in early cases.
- U+E, LFT, bone profile, lipid profile. Urine for microscopy (📖 p.12), PCR or 24 hour urinary protein collection.
- Audiometry and ophthalmic assessment. Skin biopsy using monoclonal antibody against α5 type IV collagen may assist in earlier accurate diagnosis. Proceed to *renal biopsy*.

Histology

Alport's: non-specific glomerulosclerosis and tubulo-interstitial scarring on LM (esp. if ↑Cr). A thin GBM on EM with a characteristic 'basket weave' pattern is diagnostic, and negative staining using antibodies directed against type IV collagen in the GBM secures the diagnosis.

TMD: normal light microscopy. EM demonstrates reduction in GBM diameter.

Treatment

- Patients with uncomplicated TMD can be re-assured, but should be followed up at yearly intervals (dipstick, BP and creatinine).
- No specific treatment for Alport's syndrome exists. As with all progressive nephropathies, good control of BP and use of ACEI should be considered early (📖 p.150).
- Family members should be screened for haematuria and ↑BP.

Transplantation and Alport's syndrome

In <5% of cases, transplanted Alport's patients may develop *de novo* anti-GBM antibodies and a rapidly progressive crescentic glomerulonephritis, as donor α5 type IV collagen is recognized as non-self. It is not a contra-indication to transplantation.

TMD or Alport's?

	TMD	Alport's
Haematuria	+ to +++	++
Proteinuria	±	+++ (>3g/day)
↑BP	–	+++
Renal dysfunction	±	+++
Deafness/lenticonus	–	++
History of ESRD	–	+
Father-to-son transmission	+	–

Other glomerulonephritides

Often referred to as 'mesangial proliferative GN', C1q and IgM nephropathies remain ill-characterised and unusual lesions, thought by some to represent a spectrum of minimal change nephropathy. Patients present with proteinuria (often nephrotic range), haematuria ± ↑Cr. Focal or diffuse mesangial proliferation, a relatively non-specific glomerular response to a variety of injuries, is found at biopsy.

The differential diagnosis includes:
- Lupus nephritis
- IgA nephropathy
- Mild post-infectious GN.

C1q nephropathy

Is a mesangial proliferative GN that closely resembles lupus nephritis histologically, but without any serological or clinical criteria for the diagnosis of SLE. Histology shows a characteristic heavy deposition of C1q-containing deposits in the mesangium and elsewhere, with varying degrees of mesangial hypercellularity and 'wire loop' capillary wall thickening. Secondary FSGS-like lesions occur as well.

IgM nephropathy

Is a similar lesion, presenting with the nephrotic syndrome, and characterised by prominent IgM and complement deposition in the mesangium.

Idiopathic mesangial proliferative GN

Is a diagnosis of exclusion, with mesangial proliferation on biopsy, but immune complex deposition on IF.

There is considerable uncertainty over the efficacy of specific treatment. It seems reasonable to treat these GN presenting with nephrotic syndrome with corticosteroids as for MCN, and perhaps those with progressive renal impairment with a cytotoxic agent as well (□ p.370).

The nephrotic syndrome

Is a clinical syndrome defined as >3.5g proteinuria/1.73m^2/day with hypoalbuminaemia, oedema, hyperlipidaemia, and lipiduria. The syndrome arises as a result of a failure of the glomerular filtration barrier to restrict the passage of protein into the urine, and reflects structural abnormalities within the glomerular filter (made up of a charged endothelial cell glycocalyx layer, the endothelium and its fenestrations, the glomerular basement membrane (GBM) and interdigitating podocytes with the slit diaphragm).

The passage through the glomerular filter of albumin in particular, with its net negative charge, is prevented by size-specific factors (such as the slit diaphragm), and charge specific factors (the anionic endothelial glycocalyx and GBM). Albumin escaping into the proximal tubule is efficiently absorbed by receptor—mediated endocytosis, degraded, and returned to the circulation as peptide fragments.

Many primary and secondary causes of the nephrotic syndrome are now thought to be due to abnormalities of or injury to podocytes and the slit diaphragm.

Causes of the nephrotic syndrome

- Diabetic glomerulosclerosis
- Membranous nephropathy
- Minimal change nephropathy
- Focal and segmental glomerulosclerosis
- Mesangiocapillary glomerulonephritis
- Collapsing glomerulopathy (HIVAN)
- Renal amyloidosis
- Light chain deposition disease
- SLE.

Investigation of the nephrotic syndrome

- U+E, TP and Alb, bone profile, LFT.
- Fasting lipid profile.
- MSU for microscopy for casts or lipid bodies.
- 24 hour urinary protein excretion, including a selectivity index (calculated as the transferrin:IgG ratio). Selective proteinuria is the loss of smaller proteins of <100kDa such as albumin or transferrin, whereas non-selective proteinuria includes larger molecular weight proteins such as immunoglobulins appearing in the urine.
- Creatinine clearance or estimated GFR.
- Full nephritic screen (📖 p.84).
- Ultrasound of the kidneys.
- Renal biopsy.

General principles of management

Salt and fluid restriction

$\uparrow Na^+$ retention and $\uparrow$blood volume $\rightarrow$ dependent oedema. A fall in plasma oncotic pressure as a result of hypoalbuminaemia may contribute further to fluid losses into the interstitium.

- Salt restrict to 80mmol/day (<5g/day).
- Diuretics: a loop diuretic such as furosemide, at 40mg/day po increasing to 250mg daily. If grossly oedematous, may require IV diuretics to overcome impaired oral absorption of drugs secondary to gut oedema.
- Furosemide with salt poor albumin (as 50–100mg in 100mL 20% human albumin solution over 1 hour) may enhance diuresis.
- ►Monitor for volume overload.
- Add-on thiazide-type diuretics such as metolazone 2.5–5mg alt. day to daily may promote diuresis with high dose loop diuretics.
- ►*Requires daily measurement of Na^+ and K^+ to prevent profound electrolyte imbalance—use cautiously if out-patient.*

Fluid losses are best measured by regular weighing, aiming for 0.5–1kg loss/day. Intake and output should be charted (indwelling urinary catheters are rarely needed).

Protein restriction and reducing proteinuria

Proteinuria itself leads to tubulo-interstitial inflammation and fibrosis, accelerating declining renal function. Hypoalbuminaemia leaves nephrotic patients susceptible to infection and malnutrition

- Anti-proteinuric drugs (ACEI or ARB) titrated carefully toward full dose (administer nocte if hypotension) may reduce proteinuria by up to 50% by 8 weeks and prevent progression.
- Treat hypertension aiming for 125/75.
- Protein restriction to 0.8g/kg/day with careful nutritional assessment.

Hypercoagulability

Increased hepatic synthesis of pro-coagulant factors, $\uparrow$platelet aggregation, and $\uparrow$urinary losses of anti-coagulant factors occur with nephrotic syndrome. Up to 20% of patients with membranous nephropathy (📖 p.392) as an underlying cause will develop a deep vein thrombosis.

- Breathlessness in a nephrotic patient may imply pulmonary emboli.
- New onset haematuria and flank pain may imply renal vein thrombosis (📖 p.416).
- Anticoagulate all patients with proven DVT with warfarin.
- Prophylactic anticoagulation for high risk patients with heavy nephrotic syndrome.
- Treat for the duration of the nephrotic syndrome for an INR 2–3.

Infection

Infections should be treated promptly, with cover for encapsulated organisms (low IgG levels predispose to infection). Persistingly nephrotic patients should be offered vaccination against pneumococcal disease.

Dyslipidaemia

Increased hepatic synthesis and reduced catabolism of LDL cholesterol occurs, possibly as a response to reduced plasma oncotic pressure. Successful treatment of elevated LDL cholesterol may prevent cardiovascular morbidity and slow decline in renal function.

- Dietary restriction is usually insufficient.
- HMG-CoA-reductase inhibitors (statins).

Minimal change nephropathy

The most common cause of the nephrotic syndrome in children, though less common in adults (± 25% of cases). In adults, ♂:♀. Generally, the prognosis is excellent.

The pathogenesis of minimal change nephropathy (MCN) is unknown, but impaired T-lymphocyte activity and a disorder of podocyte function is suspected. Subsequent albuminuria may be a result of loss of net membrane negative charge leading to failure of the glomerular filter.

Symptoms and signs

Oedema, often massive, with facial and peri-orbital swelling, ascites, pleural and pericardial effusions. Proteinuria and uncommonly microscopic haematuria. Urine may be foamy (protein has a detergent effect) ± lipiduria, visible on microscopy as fat bodies. May present with infections (esp. skin and soft tissue) or hypotension (secondary to hypovolaemia). Abdominal pain may be due to spontaneous peritonitis.

Certain factors have been reported to trigger the nephrotic syndrome: allergens and immunizations, malignancies (esp lymphomas), viral infections and NSAIDs. Clinical course may be complicated by renal or deep vein thrombosis, or oliguric ARF secondary to ATN.

Investigations

U+E, ↓Alb, LFT, bone profile, ↑cholesterol. Urine microscopy (may show hyaline or granular casts). 24 hour urinary protein collection (selective proteinuria, 🕮 p.386). No specific markers of MCN. Adults require *renal biopsy*.

Histology

Normal on light microscopy (hence 'minimal change'), and immunofluorescence is negative. EM reveals diffuse effacement of podocyte foot processes.

Treatment

Symptomatic treatment as outlined on(📖 p.387).

In both adults and children, true MCN remits rapidly to cortico-steroids. 80–90% of adults will be in remission by 12 weeks on therapy.

- Prednisolone 1mg/kg daily (to maximum of 80mg/day) until remission achieved. Taper prednisolone fortnightly, then weekly, until discontinued. Treat for not less than 12 weeks at first presentation.
- Relapse can be expected in 30–70% cases.
- Relapse should be treated as above, but taper steroids immediately on remission aiming for short courses.
- 📖 p.370 initiating immunosuppression.

Certain sub-groups will experience recurrent relapses off steroids after responding to treatment ('frequently relapsing', 2 relapses inside 6 months), or relapse during or within 2 weeks of steroid withdrawal ('steroid-dependent') or not respond to steroids at all (no remission within 12 weeks of treatment, 'steroid-resistant').

▶ *Ensure the histological diagnosis is MCN rather than FSGS (📖 p.396)— may require repeat kidney biopsy to ensure adequate sampling.*

Consider

- Ciclosporin 4–5mg/kg/day in two divided doses for 12 months. Monitor GFR (^{51}Cr-EDTA GFR is an accurate method for monitoring subtle decline in GFR) to exclude ciclosporin nephrotoxicity.
- Cyclophosphamide 2mg/kg/day for 12 weeks then stop.
- If remission not achieved with one regimen, consider the other.
- 📖 p.370 initiating immunosuppression.

Membranous nephropathy (MN)

One of the most common world-wide cause of the nephrotic syndrome, with a peak incidence in the 4th to 6th decades, 2♂:1♀. May be idiopathic (IMN), or secondary (📖 p.394).

It is characterized by IgG-rich immune deposit accumulation on the outer aspect of the GBM, possibly due to antibodies directed against an as yet unknown antigen expressed on the 'sole' of podocyte foot processes. Antibody-mediated complement activation and formation of membrane attack complex leads to free radical generation, podocyte injury, and abnormal GBM synthesis. Trapped circulating immune complexes derived from exogenous antigens may be responsible in secondary forms of the disease.

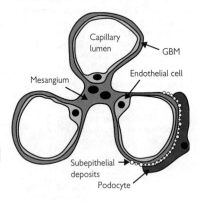

Fig. 6.6 Cartoon of subepithelial deposits in MN

Symptoms and signs

Proteinuria, occasionally asymptomatic, but often with the nephrotic syndrome. Oedema, microscopic haematuria, hypertension. Consider underlying disease.

Investigations

U+E, ↓↓Alb, LFT, bone profile, ↑LDL Chol, ↓immunoglobulins common (IgG > IgA). 24 hour urinary protein collection (non-selective proteinuria, 📖 p.386). Hepatitis B/C. Proceed to *renal biopsy*.

Histology

May be normal to light microscopy, or in more advanced cases show GBM thickening and 'spikes' of GBM extending around subepithelial deposits: often best seen on silver stains. Loss of podocyte foot processes. Variable degree of ATN and tubulo-interstitial fibrosis. Granular IgG ± C3 deposits within capillary wall on IF. Presence of the IgG4 subclass may be a pointer to 2° MN. Subepithelial electron dense deposits with foot process effacement on EM.

Treatment

Symptomatic treatment 📖 p.387
Disease modifying treatment

The natural history of MN is variable, with 20%–30% progressing to ESRD, and about 25%–40% remitting spontaneously. Aim to predict the course of the disease:

Low risk

- Normal renal function.
- Proteinuria <4g/day or spontaneously waning proteinuria.
- Symptomatic treatment.
- Expect remission (up to 4 years after diagnosis), but regularly re-assess risk. Measure U+E, Alb and proteinuria regularly.

High risk

- ♂ >50.
- Impaired renal function.
- Proteinuria >10g/day.
- Persistent proteinuria >4g/day for >1 year.
- Interstitial scarring on renal biopsy.

▶ Disease modifying therapy reduces proteinuria, spares renal function and induces remission.

- Alternating monthly steroids and alkylating agents for six months. Steroids as methylprednisolone as 1g IV daily x 3 days, then prednisolone 0.4mg/kg/day for the remainder of month. Two alkylating agents have been used successfully: either chlorambucil 0.1–0.2mg/kg/day, or cyclophosphamide 1.5–2.5mg/kg/day.
- Can be given as daily po prednisolone 1mg/kg/day + cyclophosphamide 1.5mg/kg/day, tapering steroids against response (easier!).
- Treatment often limited by toxicity (📖 p.370).
- With declining renal function, may need to persist with steroids and alkylating agent for up to one year.
- Alternatively, ciclosporin 3.5mg/kg/day in two divided doses with low dose steroids for 6–12 months. Monitor GFR to exclude ciclosporin nephrotoxicity.
- MMF may also induce remission.
- Rituximab, a monoclonal anti-CD20 antibody, has been used with success.

Secondary MN

Is more common world-wide than IMN. Presentation with nephrotic syndrome may not coincide with presentation of underlying disease. Malignancies in particular may be preceded by MN by many years. Causes include:

Infections
- Hepatitis B and C
- Malaria
- Streptococcal infection
- Syphilis or leprosy
- Schistosomiasis.

Neoplasms
- Solid tumours (lung, colon, breast, kidney, stomach)
- Hodgkin's Disease
- Non-Hodgkin's lymphoma.

Multi-system disease
- SLE
- Autoimmune thyroiditis
- Dermatitis herpetiformis
- Sarcoidosis.

Drugs and toxins
- Captopril
- Gold
- D-penicillamine
- NSAIDs.

Approaching MN

Take a careful history focusing on:
- Medications, particularly NSAIDs.
- Risk factors for hepatitis viruses or other infections (travel, sexual history, transfusions).
- Malignancy. If history and physical examination alone do not suggest an associated neoplasm, extensive investigation is unwarranted and unlikely to reveal any tumour. Some older patients (>50) may need further imaging or endoscopy.

Treatment of secondary MN

Involves treating the underlying condition and leads to remission of the nephrotic syndrome in many cases.

Focal and segmental glomerulosclerosis

FSGS is a histological description rather than a disease. *Secondary FSGS* occurs against a background of glomerular damage and drop-out in an already abnormal kidney, causing haemodynamic stress on remaining nephrons, and a so-called 'hyperfiltration injury'. *Idiopathic* or *primary FSGS* differs from secondary FSGS in being a *de novo* glomerulopathy rather than as a result of an associated disease.

FSGS occurs more often in ♂ (2:1) and $^2/_3$ of the nephrotic syndrome in the black population is due to FSGS.

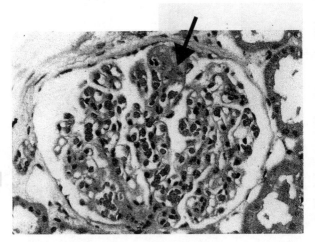

Fig. 6.7 A segmental sclerosis in an affected tuft

Primary FSGS

The cause remains unknown. Because the disease recurs, often immediately after transplantation, a circulating permeability factor has been implicated, but not yet identified. Injury to podocytes, and a subsequent abnormal podocyte response to injury are features of the disease.

Symptoms and signs

Proteinuria, often heavy, microscopic haematuria and ↑BP. Impaired renal function is common. Young black males presenting with heavy proteinuria (>10g/day), profound hypoalbuminaemia (Alb <20g/L) and renal impairment tend to follow a more severe course, often ending in ESRD.

Investigations

U+E, ↓Alb, LFT, bone profile, ↑LDL Chol. 24 hour urinary protein collection (non-selective proteinuria, 📖 p.386). Proceed to renal biopsy.

Histology

A focal (affecting some but not all glomeruli) and segmental (affecting part but not all of a glomerular tuft) process with mesangial matrix expansion, glomerular sclerosis, and hyalinosis. No abnormality may be seen if the sample size is small, reflecting the focal nature of the disease. Some IgM and C3 may be trapped in sclerotic lesions on IF. EM demonstrates foot process effacement and degeneration of podocytes. Tubulo-interstitial fibrosis is not uncommon. Sub-classification into 5 different variants may have prognostic importance: the presence of 'tip lesions' (segmental scleroses affecting the outer 'tip' of the glomerulus alongside the proximal tubule) implies a better, more steroid-responsive course.

Secondary FSGS

May be found with the following conditions:

Reduced nephron number
- Reflux nephropathy
- Renal dysplasia
- Renovascular disease
- Morbid obesity.

Glomerular disease and obsolescence
- Diabetic nephropathy
- HIV-associated nephropathy
- Heroin-associated nephropathy
- Pre-eclampsia
- Sickle cell disease
- Membranous nephropathy
- Alport's syndrome.

Any cause of quiescent glomerulonephritis with scarring
Secondary FSGS tends to present with less proteinuria and hypoalbuminaemia than the primary variant.

Collapsing glomerulopathy describes a FSGS-like lesion with glomerular tuft collapse, GBM wrinkling; and cystic tubular changes with interstitial fibrosis. It is usually due to HIVAN (📖 p.480), but occurs in an idiopathic form that may be related to other viral diseases (parvovirus) and high dose *pamidronate* (possibly other bisphosphonates as well). Presents with torrential nephrotic syndrome and declining renal function, and generally carries a poor renal prognosis.

Treatment of FSGS

In secondary FSGS, treat the underlying cause if possible. The general approach is as for any progressive proteinuric nephropathy (📖 p.150). Even in biopsy-proven primary FSGS, in those with less 2g/day proteinuria, symptomatic treatment and watchful waiting is advised.

Symptomatic treatment for the nephrotic syndrome, 📖 p.387. Particular attention to anti-proteinuric agents should be given.

Disease-modifying treatment

- Prednisolone 1mg/kg/day (max 80mg) for a minimum of 16 weeks, and ideally 24 weeks. FSGS is slow to respond and shorter courses of steroids are of little use. If response (remission of nephrotic syndrome), taper steroids to stopping after a further 12 weeks. Unlike minimal change disease, a degree of proteinuria inevitably persists.

▶ Presence of 'tip lesions' (📖 p.397) improves the likelihood of response.

After a 6 month course of steroids, 30–40% of patients will achieve a meaningful reduction (>50%) in proteinuria. Those that relapse whilst on (tapering) steroids are defined as 'steroid-dependent', and those in whom no reduction in proteinuria is achieved 'steroid resistant'.

In these groups,

- Continue low dose (10–15 mg/day) prednisolone.
- Add ciclosporin 5–6mg/kg/day in two divided doses. Aim for trough levels 125–225ng/mL. Check isotopic GFR prior to starting therapy. Treat for one year, then taper dose and stop if response.
- Alternatively, cytotoxic agents (see below).

In small trials, response rates of 70% have been reported. Many responders will be ciclosporin-dependent, relapsing with drug withdrawal.

▶ Little data exists on how to treat the more aggressive form of the disease, presenting as torrential nephrotic syndrome and progressive renal impairment in younger patients.

An alternative to ciclosporin in such patients is:

- High dose prednisolone as above with,
  - Cyclophosphamide 2 mg/kg/day for a minimum of 12 weeks.
  - Or chlorambucil 0.1–0.2 mg/kg/day for a minimum of 12 weeks.

The toxicity of all such treatment regimes needs to be considered on an individual basis.

Thrombotic microangiopathies

The thrombotic microangiopathies are a disparate group of systemic disorders characterized by a triad of haemolysis, a consumptive thrombocytopenia and tissue ischaemia caused by platelet aggregation and thrombotic occlusion of small vessels.

Causes

- Thrombotic thrombocytopenic purpura (TTP)
- Haemolytic-uraemic syndrome (HUS)
- HELPP syndrome and pre-eclampsia (📖 p.576)
- Disseminated intravascular coagulopathy (DIC)
- Malignant hypertension (📖 p.350)
- Systemic lupus erythematosus (📖 p.468), systemic sclerosis (📖 p.474), rheumatoid arthritis (📖 p.476) and system vasculitis (📖 p.456)
- Antiphospholipid syndrome (primary or as part of SLE, 📖 p.472) or paroxysmal nocturnal haemoglobinuria
- Metastatic malignancies
- HIV.

General points

Take a careful history for diarrhoeal illness. Examine for petechiae, purpura. Dipstick for haematuria, proteinuria and bilirubinuria (haemolysis). Check BP and fundi. ?Skin signs of systemic sclerosis. ?Splenomegaly.

Investigations

- FBC (↓Hb, ↓↓Plt), film for red cell fragments, clotting, D-dimers/FDP, G+S, ↓haptoglobins, Coombs' test (negative).
- β-HCG. ↑↑LDH, U+E, LFT (↑bilirubin), urate. Blood and stool cultures.
- ANF, dsDNA, complement, anti-phospholipid antibodies (📖 p.472).
- Renal biopsy only once (if) platelet count normalizes.

Histology

All TMAs share similar renal histology. Fibrin thrombi are present in the glomerular capillaries with resultant ischaemia. Fluorescence for Ig and complement negative. EM shows capillary thrombi, fibrin deposition, and endothelial injury and swelling.

Thrombotic thrombocytopenic purpura

Von Willebrand factor is released from endothelial cells as a large polymer, and cleaved to form the mature polypeptide that acts as a matrix for haemostasis. The protease responsible for this cleavage is the zinc metalloproteinase ADAMTS13. If the vWF cleaving protein activity is impaired (IgG auto-antibody directed against the protease or inherited mutations encoding ADAMTS13), abnormally large vWF multimers enter the circulation, and under shear stress, bind and activate platelets. This leads to spontaneous platelet aggregation, platelet-rich (though fibrin-poor) thrombus formation and a **systemic** microangiopathy.

Drug-related TTP occurs with ticlopidine and clopidogrel: IgG against ADAMTS13 has been found during this rare complication of treatment.

Symptoms and signs (in addition to general features, 📖 p.400)

Pentad of fever, microangiopathic haemolytic anaemia, thrombocytopenic purpura, renal, and central nervous system involvement (confusion, fits, or any other neurological abnormality). Oliguria, anuria, and advanced renal failure (Cr >300)—↑BP is thus more common with HUS than TTP.

Investigations (📖 p.300)

Monitor disease: ↓↓Plt, red cell fragments on film, ↑↑LDH
↓haptoglobins. Low ADAMTS13 activity (<5% normal) in the correct clinical setting is diagnostic.

Management

Aim to restore ability to cleave vWF.

Plasma exchange (PEX), allows large volume plasma infusion as well as removal of vWF cleaving protein inhibitor, esp. if oligo-anuric.
• Daily PEX until plt count and LDH normalized (usually 7–16 days).
• Exchange one plasma volume/day (📖 p.642).
• May require hydrocortisone 100 mg + chlorpheniramine 10 mg IVI to prevent allergic reactions to large volumes of plasma.

Fresh frozen plasma (ideally platelet poor) or cryosupernatant infusion IF URIC as: 25–30mL/kg/day until improvement. Is inferior to plasma exchange, but *is* efficacious if PEX unavailable. Beware fluid overload.

⚠ Avoid platelet transfusion unless life-threatening bleeding ('fuels the fire'). No role for aspirin or anticoagulants. Resistant disease may be treated by increasing PE to twice daily, or using rituximab (anti-CD20 monoclonal antibody). Alternatives include add-on prednisolone 1mg/kg/day or IV immunoglobulin.

If prompt plasma infusion or exchange instituted, patient survival should be up to 90%. Renal survival is good, with dialysis-requiring ARF unusual. A third may be expected to relapse.

Haemolytic-uraemic syndrome

May be associated with diarrhoea (**D+**), with peak incidence in summer. Usually affects children < 5 years. Occurs after food poisoning (undercooked meat, unpasteurized milk). Pathogenic bacteria produce a Shiga-like exotoxin that translocates across inflamed colonic mucosa, binding intra-renal vasculature and platelets. ↑pro-thrombotic factors, and ultra-large vWF multimers are released from activated endothelial cells.

In the absence of diarrhoea (**D–**), deficiency in factor H (a complement regulatory protein) is responsible for relapsing or familial HUS. Many drugs and other infections may cause a HUS-like syndrome. There is NO reduction of ADAMTS13 in HUS (ie different pathophysiology to TTP). HUS is a renal-limited TMA with widespread complications.

Infections associated with D+ HUS

- *E. coli* O157:H7
- *Shigella dysenteriae* serotype 1
- *Salmonella*, *Campylobacter*, or *Yersinia*.

Associations with D-HUS

- Inherited HUS.
- Drugs: quinine, ciclosporin, tacrolimus, rapamycin, ciprofloxacin, the contraceptive pill, heparin, chemotherapy
- *S. pneumoniae* or Rickettsial infection.

Symptoms and signs (in addition to general features, 📖 p.400)
Triad of microangiopathic haemolytic anaemia, thrombocytopenia + renal involvement. Watery or bloody diarrhoea. Fever, ↑BP, oliguria, and fluid overload. May progress rapidly to multi-organ failure with pancreatitis and a cardiomyopathy.

Investigations (📖 p.400)
- ↑WCC common. Fresh stool for culture.
- Monitor disease: ↓↓Plt, red cell fragments on film, ↑↑LDH

Management
⚠ If in doubt, treat as TTP until diagnosis apparent.

For D+ HUS, management is supportive alone, and dialysis if required. No role for anticoagulation. Antibiotics may paradoxically increase Shiga-toxin release, and should be avoided. PEX does not improve outcome HUS as there is no underlying exchangeable causative factor

Poor prognostic factors: ↑age, high WCC, D- HUS, *S. pneumoniae* or *Shigella* infection, anuria.

Tubulo-interstitial diseases

Acute interstitial nephritis

AIN, or acute tubulo-interstitial nephritis, is a common parenchymal cause of unexplained acute renal failure, usually in response to drugs. $\sigma = Q$, usually in their 50s and 60s, but can occur at all ages. Although the spectrum of causative drugs has changed, drug-induced AIN now accounts for 70–90% of cases.

The provoking agent is associated with an inflammatory cell infiltrate in the renal interstitium, sometimes with delayed-type hypersensitivity reaction phenomena (fever, arthritis, rash) elsewhere. Rechallenging with drugs often leads to recurrent disease, confirming the immune-mediated nature of AIN.

Commoner causes of AIN include
- Drugs
  - NSAIDs (incl COX-2 inhibitors)
  - Penicillins, cephalosporins, rifampicin and sulphonamides
  - Diuretics
  - Allopurinol
  - Proton pump inhibitors
  - Anti-retrovirals
- Infections
- Tuberculosis, legionella and leptospirosis
- Auto-immune disease, esp. TINU (see below)

Symptoms and signs

Classically, a triad of fever, arthralgia and rash presenting with renal impairment—this is rare in the contemporary antibiotic era. Nausea, vomiting, and oliguria may reflect renal failure. Flank pain (renal swelling stretches the capsule). Causative drugs may have been started 3–21 days previously, although AIN may occur up to 18 months after prescription.

Investigations

Urine dipstick may be bland, or have modest haematuria and proteinuria (often <1g/day). Microscopy may reveal eosinophiluria and white cell casts. U+E, bone profile (? $\uparrow Ca^{2+}$), LFT, FBC + diff (?eosinophilia), $\uparrow$ESR.

USS shows normal sized (or slightly enlarged) kidneys. EMU for AFB in high-risk patients. CXR and serum ACE if ?sarcoid. ANF, anti-Ro and La if ?Sjogren's syndrome.

Renal biopsy: if clearly drug-related, and the renal dysfunction mild, withdraw drug and observe. If resolution does not occur <10 days, biopsy. All dialysis-requiring patients should be biopsied to exclude other diagnoses and predict longer term outcome.

Histology

Glomeruli are normal. An intense inflammatory cell infiltrate of lympho-cytes and monocytes (± eosinophils) in the interstitium. Giant cells and granulomata may point to TB or sarcoidosis. The presence of interstitial fibrosis imparts a worse prognosis, as in all renal diseases.

Treatment

Depends on the cause—the treatment of tubulo-interstitial nephritis with uveitis syndrome (TINU) and sarcoidosis is outlined elsewhere. Concentrating on drug-related AIN:

The outcome is generally good, with most of those requiring dialysis regaining independent renal function. Of those with milder disease, a majority will return to their baseline renal function, and almost all will achieve a Cr < 200μmol/L. The mortality rate is reported at < 5%.

▶▶ *Stop* offending drug(s).

✒ Corticosteroids: have been widely used, if only to hasten renal recovery—there is no good evidence to support use. Nevertheless, convention remains to treat those most at risk. A reasonable algorithm is:
- Dialysis-requiring: treat with corticosteroids.
- Dialysis-independent: observe for 10 days.
  - If improving renal function, expectant management.
  - If no improvement, treat with corticosteroids.

Treatment as prednisolone 1mg/kg/day po, tapering against response for a 3–6 month course.

Tubulo-intertsitial nephritis and uveitis syndrome (TINU)

Unlike AIN, affects predominantly young women, presenting as anterior uveitis (often bilateral) and AIN (may be separated in time). Additional features include weight loss, ↓Hb, ↑ESR, deranged LFT. Opthalmology opinion should be requested urgently. Treat with 1mg/kg/day prednisolone tapering against resolution for 3–6 months. Differential diagnosis includes auto-immune disease (SLE, Sjogren's) and sarcoidosis amongst others.

Chronic tubulo-interstitial diseases

Chronic tubulo-interstitial disease includes a wide range of disorders of varying causes linked by a common histological appearance on kidney biopsy. Glomeruli are largely spared (although obsolescent glomeruli may be seen as a result of nephron drop-out), and the tubulo-interstitium is extensively fibrosed, often with a lymphocytic infiltrate in scarred areas. Many tubules are dilated and atrophic.

Although chronic tubulo-interstitial nephritis exists as a distinct diagnosis (AIN of any cause may progress if exposure is not limited, or the underlying condition is not treated), *any* glomerular renal lesion associated with impaired renal function over time will develop the above histological changes (📖 p.144).

Specific causes include:
- Drugs (NSAIDs)
- Reflux nephropathy
- Sarcoidosis
- Tuberculosis
- Auto-immune diseases (Sjogren's syndrome)
- Metabolic causes, e.g. chronic $\downarrow K^+$
- Heavy metals (see overleaf)
- Balkan endemic and Chinese herbal nephropathies.

> **Features include**
>
> - Impaired urinary concentration (nocturia, polyuria)
> - Often normal BP (due to salt-losing state)
> - Low molecular weight tubular proteinuria (β_2-microglobulin)
> - Glycosuria (impaired tubular handling) ± renal tubular acidosis
> - Impaired renal function
> - Small, symmetrical kidneys on USS (exception is reflux nephropathy).

Investigations
MSU for MC+S, EMU for AFB, PCR or 24 hour proteinuria (often <1g/day), U+E, bone profile (?$\uparrow Ca^{2+}$), serum ACE, ANF, anti-Ro/La, rheumatoid factor, USS kidneys.

Lithium-induced nephropathy
Lithium therapy for bipolar disorder is associated with nephrogenic DI (📖 p.527), and may be associated with tubulo-interstitial fibrosis and tubular dilatation. Lithium dosing should aim for the lowest levels that control symptoms, with yearly Cr to monitor for $\uparrow$Cr. Avoid thiazide diuretics, as use leads to $\uparrow$lithium retention. It is usually a mild and non-progressive renal lesion, taking years to evolve, and rarely requires discontinuing drug in well-controlled patients.

Balkan endemic nephropathy (BEN)

Presents in men and women from the lands drained by the Danube >30 years old, with a tubulo-interstitial atrophy and scarring. The cause remains unknown. Patients are usually normotensive with a urinary concentrating defect (polyuria), and may have LMW tubular proteinuria (<1g/day) and glycosuria. USS shows small but symmetrical kidneys. There is an increased tendency to transitional cell carcinoma of the entire urinary tract: new haematuria should be investigated, and urine cytology should performed for atypia regularly.

Chinese herb nephropathy

A histological disorder similar to BEN, with tubulo-interstitial scarring and spared glomeruli the principal features. Although not conclusively proven, it appears to be due to aristolochic acid, an ingredient in many Chinese herbal preparations (notably used as a slimming agent). The clinical presentation and histology is so similar to BEN that some have suggested a similar aetiology: this remains to be proven. The incidence of urothelial malignancies is very high, and surveillance is mandatory. In those considered for transplantation after ESRD, bilateral native nephrectomies has been proposed to reduce the risk of malignant disease with immunosuppression.

Lead nephropathy

Occupational or other exposure to lead may cause chronic lead poisoning, with a chronic and progressive tubulo-interstitial nephritis. Tubular injury results in decreased urate excretion, and hyperuricaemia and gout. In at risk individuals with unexplained CRF associated with high urate concentrations, the total lead burden should be established by bone X-ray fluorescence, or an EDTA lead chelation test. Treatment includes long-term lead-depletion with EDTA or succimer. Lead has also been shown to be an important determinant of progression of CRF of other causes. *Cadmium* exposure causes a similar nephropathy.

Analgesic nephropathy

Analgesic nephropathy (AN) was first described after chronic phenacetin (a pro-drug of paracetamol, with toxicity independent of the latter) use, but is now recognized as a common cause of ESRD, accounting for up to 10% of cases. 2♀:1♂ after the 5th decade.

Combination analgesic preparation use accounts for most AN (e.g. paracetamol + codeine, paracetamol + aspirin). Aspirin alone does not usually cause AN, though paracetamol, if used in sufficient amounts, may (>2kg cumulatively, equivalent to about 8 years of daily full-dose ingestion). Injury begins in the medulla, with ischaemic changes, and progresses to tubulo-interstitial scarring, glomerulosclerosis, and papillary necrosis (PN, see overleaf).

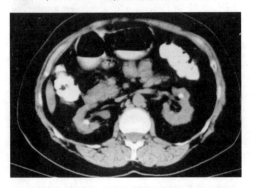

Fig. 6.8 Irregular, ragged renal outline characteristic of AN. Reproduced with permission from Davison AMA, Cameron JS, Grunfeld J-P, *et al.* (2005) *Oxford Textbook of Clinical Nephrology*. Oxford University Press, Oxford.

Symptoms and signs

Hx of analgesic use may be difficult to elicit: direct questioning for chronic headaches or backache. Dyspepsia is common. Nocturia and polyuria (loss of concentrating ability), episodic colicky flank pain and frank haematuria due to papillary necrosis—sloughed papillae may be evident in the urine. ↑BP as CRF develops.

Investigations

Dipstick often bland, or modest proteinuria. Sterile pyuria on microscopy. ↓Hb. ↑Cr. IVU may show small kidneys ± clubbed calyces.

Management

Stop all analgesics. This is often difficult, but reducing the analgesic burden slows disease progression.

▶ Surveillance for urothelial malignancies (transitional cell carcinoma occurs in up to 10% of confirmed AN). May be multiple, in unusual sites, or even bilateral. New haematuria merits investigation (± cystoscopy), and yearly urine cytology provides a useful screening tool.

Analgesic nephropathy is also associated with accelerated atherosclerosis, though the mechanism is unclear.

Papillary necrosis

Is the end result of chronic medullary hypoxia: the vulnerable renal papilla suffers a further (acute) ischaemic injury, undergoes necrosis and is shed into the renal pelvis. This may be associated with:

- Colicky flank pain (as the papilla traverses the ureter)
- Passage of a papilla (or part thereof)
- Frank haematuria
- Unilateral obstruction.

CT kidneys show calcified papillae and an irregular renal contour, and offers a safe and contrast-free investigation to confirm AN. Alternatively, on IVU, contrast tracking into eroded papilla, ring shadows around detached papilla ± calcification may be apparent.

Differential diagnosis of PN on IVU

- Analgesic nephropathy
- Diabetes mellitus
- Post-obstructive uropathy
- Sickle cell nephropathy
- Tuberculosis
- Following severe acute pyelonephritis.

Renovascular disease

Renovascular disease (RVD) remains an imprecise term for diseases of the large, medium-sized and small renal vessels, excluding auto-immune vasculitis. Atherosclerotic renal artery stenosis (ARAS) and fibromuscular dysplasia (FMD) predominantly affect the larger vessels. We use the umbrella term *'ischaemic nephropathy'* to describe the vasculopathy of small intra-renal vessels. The treatment of each differs, so careful diagnosis has real benefits.

ARAS and ischaemic nephropathy

Is common with ↑age (± 7% in people >65), and in those known to have atherosclerosis (± 50% if known PVD). However, anatomically proven ARAS is often haemodynamically unimportant, and associated with ↑BP in only 50% of cases. Generally, stenoses >70% tend to be functionally important, as is bilateral ARAS or disease in the artery to a single functioning kidney. Patients with ARAS or ischaemic nephropathy have a substantial excess risk for cardiovascular death (MI and stroke).

Suspect in older patients with known peripheral, coronary or cerebrovascular atherosclerotic disease, with known risk factors (dyslipidaemia, smoking, diabetes, ↑BP).

Clinically
- Hypertension, often difficult to control (i.e. >140/90 on 3 drugs).
- Renal dysfunction.
- ↑Cr (of > 20% above baseline) with ACEI or ARB.
- Fluid retention, often resistant to diuretics.

Pathophysiology

Atherosclerotic plaque involves the ostium or proximal 2cm of the renal artery, often extending from the aorta. Disease is caused by a fall in renal perfusion, resulting in sympathetic over-activity and renin release. This leads to over-production of the vasoconstrictor angiotensin II, and aldosterone release with salt and water retention. The pro-fibrotic actions of these factors in time cause renal scarring and CRF.

Symptoms and signs

Evidence of central or PVD is perhaps the most important clinical finding. ↑BP, ankle oedema, orthopnoea, and pulmonary congestion, abdominal bruits (low predictive value in isolation), palpable AAA, bland urine on dipstick. Flash pulmonary oedema refers to sudden and episodic pulmonary oedema with hypertension without any precipitating cardiac event, caused by exaggerated activation of renin-angiotensin system and salt and water retention. Loin pain, a sudden decline in renal function and new haematuria may signify renal infarction.

Investigations

U+E (?↓K$^+$ due to ↑aldosterone), cholesterol, urine dipstick (bland or modest proteinuria), ☞ plasma renin (therapeutically unhelpful). Screen for evidence of hypertensive end-organ damage (ECG/echo for LVH, spot urine for PCR or 24 hour urine collection for proteinuria, dilated fundoscopy). Potential imaging includes:

USS kidneys for renal size and symmetry. A difference of >1.5cm in renal length is suspicious

- Duplex USS with Doppler examination for resistive index (RI) as a surrogate for impeded flow. *Only* in experienced hands, a useful dynamic test. May predict responders to angioplasty and stenting.
- Captopril isotope scintigraphy. With captopril, affected kidneys may show a 30 % decline in GFR using DTPA or MAG-3 (📖 p.42).
- Gadolinium-enhanced magnetic resonance angiography (MRA) or multi-slice CT angiography is increasingly good at visualizing ostial lesions.
- Angiography. Secures diagnosis and allows intervention.

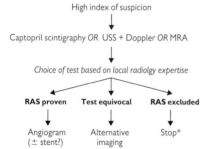

*If captopril scintigraphy is unequivocally negative, but a high index of suspicion remains, consider angiography.

Fig 6.9 A suggested algorithm for the investigation of suspected ARVD.

Management of ARAS

General management

Modify risk factors—stop smoking, HMG-CoA reductase inhibitors, exercise, and low salt diet. Consider aspirin 75 mg od.

Control BP

Aim for <130/85 using non-ACEI/ARB drugs, e.g.
- Loop diuretic (furosemide 40–160mg) titrated vs. response.
- β-blocker
- Vasodilator (calcium channel blocker ± centrally acting agent).

Prevent renal complications

The prime aim is to prevent loss of renal function. Two treatment options exist, conservative or interventional. Selection can be very difficult.

Interventional management

Includes percutaneous transluminal renal angioplasty (PTRA) ± stenting, or surgical revascularization. PTRA alone is associated with a high incidence of re-stenosis—stenting is thus recommended. However, with PTRAS:
- ~ 30 % will see an improvement in Cr
- ~ 50 % will experience no change
- ~ 20 % *will deteriorate.*

Selected candidates do better with PTRAS (or surgery):
- Known recent onset
- Bilateral ARAS or ARAS to a single functioning kidney
- Uncontrolled BP and fluid overload
- Flash pulmonary oedema
- Rapidly declining renal function.

The kidney(s) should be > 7.5cm in length, implying meaningful nephron mass capable of recovering renal function, and the stenosis high grade (> 70 %). The absence of scars on ^{99M}Tc-DMSA isotope scintigraphy may usefully predict recoverable renal function. The presence of heavy proteinuria may imply hyperfiltration injury in a scarred kidney (◻ p.144).

The risk of cholesterol emboli, arterial dissection and contrast nephrotoxicity should be weighed against the potential benefits. Drug-eluting stents may alter the indications for PTRAS.

Surgical revascularization is usually reserved for those undergoing simultaneous aortic surgery.

Conservative management

- As a trial of ACEI/ARB.
- Patients must be well hydrated (check for postural drop). Start with low-dose ACEI (e.g. ramipril 2.5mg od) and measure Cr daily. Continue and increase therapy as long as *efficacious* (BP control) and *no deterioration of > 10%* in Cr. Many physicians would allow 20% deterioration in Cr.
- ACEI/ARB will reduce CV risk, and may prevent progression of CRF, as well as blocking AII-mediated vasoconstriction and fibrosis. *will* drop perfusion pressure, and *may* precipitate ARF.

Other renovascular diseases

Fibromuscular dysplasia

Affects otherwise asymptomatic young women (15–50 years), often with hypertension. Much less common than ARAS. FMD is caused by arterial fibroplasia that may affect many vascular beds (intracranial, carotid, coronary, and limb). May affect both renal arteries, and classically affects the mid-distal renal artery (rather than the ostia as in ARAS).

Angiography shows a 'string of beads' appearance with otherwise normal caliber vessels on either side. ↑BP of FMD may be *cured* (withdrawal of all drugs) or improved by angioplasty, particularly in woman <50 years with hypertension of < 8 years duration, and few stenoses in other arterial beds.

Renal vein thrombosis (RVT)

RVT is usually found in association with the nephrotic syndrome (particularly membranous nephropathy, MN, 📖 p.392), when it may be uni- or bilateral. It is very rare outside of the hypercoagulable state found with hypoalbuminaemia and nephrotic-range proteinuria: it may be seen with tumours (esp. renal cell carcinoma) invading and distorting the renal vein.

May present as:
- Pulmonary emboli
- Renal infarction (loin pain, haematuria, ↑Cr and ↑LDH).

Spiral CT or Doppler of the renal veins should be diagnostic—proven RVT should be treated with anticoagulation until non-nephrotic (Alb > 35). Prophylactic anticoagulation is controversial: no benefit has been proven in routine anticoagulation of either nephrotics in general, or those with MN. Torrentially nephrotic patients (Alb <20), or those immobilized for any reason may be candidates for anticoagulation, initially with IVI heparin, then oral warfarin until albumin normalizes.

Cholesterol emboli

May cause partial occlusion of the renal small vessels, with resultant luminal changes leading to downstream ischaemia. Showers of emboli may present suddenly as ARF, or more commonly as a more gradual decline in renal function. Usually occurs in elderly patients known to have extensive atherosclerosis with recent:
- Instrumentation of or surgery to the aorta (usually angiography).
- Thrombolysis or anticoagulation.

ARF in this setting may suggest the diagnosis. Patients may have embolic infarcts in end-arterial territories (digits, retina), abdominal colic (gut emboli) or livedo reticularis. The urine is usually bland (though heavy proteinuria may be a feature). Eosinophilia, eosinophiluria and ↓C3/C4 are typical. Renal biopsy shows characteristic intravascular clefts. No specific therapy works, though aggressive BP and cholesterol lowering may improve longer term patient survival.

Adult polycystic kidney disease (APKD)

APKD is the most common inherited disease, affecting ± 1:800 live births, and responsible for 5-10% of any ESRD programme.

Inherited in an autosomal dominant manner, mutations in the genes *PKD-1* (located on chromosome 16) and *PKD–2* (chromosome 4) result in defective synthesis of the proteins polycystin –1 and –2 respectively. *PKD-1* mutations are 7 times more common than *PKD-2* mutations, and are associated with more aggressive disease.

Polycystin-1 is a signalling membrane receptor protein that co-localizes with polycystin-2 (a calcium-permeable channel) in the cilia of renal collecting duct epithelial cells. The polycystin complex acts as an extracellular mechanosensor (flow in the lumen disturbs cilia and triggers the complex) regulating cell proliferation, adhesion, differentiation, and maturation to maintain normal tubular calibre.

Failure of normal polycystin complex formation results in dysregulated cell turnover, with uncontrolled cell proliferation in response to normally occurring growth factors. Proliferating tubular cells form disorientated cysts that rapidly close off from the original nephron, and expand in size over time. These changes are accompanied by the release of mitogenic and pro-fibrotic cytokines that exacerbate local ischaemia and scarring, leading to progressive renal failure.

Understanding the pathogenesis of APKD offers the best hope for meaningful therapies aimed at preventing the development of cysts. As cyst formation begins *in utero*, tailored therapy would require early diagnosis and treatment in childhood. In animal models, some experimental therapies seem promising:

- *Vasopressin receptor antagonists* inhibit cyst formation through ↓cAMP
- *Rapamycin or paclitaxel* to block disordered cell proliferation
- Therapies that block the actions of *epidermal growth factor*

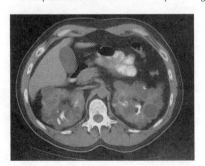

Fig. 6.10 Contrast-enhanced CT scan of a patient demonstrating the number, size, and location of the cysts in the anterior portion of the left kidney and the posterior aspect of the right kidney.

Reproduced with permission from Watson ML, Torres VE (eds) (1996) *Polycystic Kidney Disease*, p214. Oxford: Oxford University Press.

Symptoms and signs

Most patients will present with a family history of APKD—a careful history for familial ↑BP, intracranial bleeds or premature death may point to carriers of the gene mutations. Importantly, 25–40% of new patients will have *no* family history. Inheritance is autosomal dominant, so 50% of offspring should be affected. Patients being investigated for APKD *should* be counselled before and after testing.

Clinical features include:
- Flank or loin pain arising from large cysts.
- Nocturia and polyuria (loss of urinary concentrating ability).
- Dipstick positive haematuria ± episodic frank haematuria.
- Microalbuminuria or less commonly, proteinuria (usually <1g/day).
- ↑BP.
- If presenting late, uraemic symptoms.

Investigations

Ultrasound remains the test of choice. As APKD is an evolving disease, the timing the scan is important. In otherwise asymptomatic at risk individuals, USS should be performed at 20 years old for best negative predictive value. For confirming a diagnosis, use the Ravine criteria:

Age	+ Family history	− Family history
<30 years	2 cysts in either kidney	5 cysts in either kidney
30–60 years	4 cysts in either kidney	5 cysts in either kidney
>60 years	8 cysts in either kidney	8 cysts in either kidney

These criteria are valid for PKD1 mutation alone. As PKD2 mutations present with disease later, the criteria tend to give false negative results.
- Increased renal size is common (often 20cm in length). Cysts in other organs (liver, pancreas, spleen) are suggestive of APKD.
- Genetic testing is available, though not widely used as yet.

Complications of APKD

Hypertension

↑BP is often the first sign of APKD, affecting ± 60% with normal renal function. It is thought to be due to ↑renin generation from ischaemic renal tissue compressed by expanding cysts. Tight BP control (aiming for target BP ≤ 130/80) protects this often young cohort from end-organ damage. Choice of agent:

- ACE inhibitor/ARB as first-line therapy.
- Add in calcium channel blocker, β-blocker or diuretic.

Renal failure

Many patients with APKD will never reach ESRD: however, once renal impairment is established progression, though variable, is relentless. Men diagnosed at a younger age, early hypertension, large kidneys, and black people tend to have a worse renal prognosis: those with PKD2 mutations tend to develop symptoms and CRF later than those with PKD1 mutations.

Once on dialysis, APKD patients have a better survival on dialysis and with transplantation than the general ESRD population

Cyst haemorrhage

Presents as abrupt onset unilateral flank pain ± haematuria (cysts may rupture without communication into the urinary space). Management is conservative with bed rest, hydration and analgesics.

Cyst infection

Suspect if febrile and systemically unwell APKD patient with flank pain. Culture blood and urine, and give a prolonged course of ciprofloxacin or co-trimoxazole (good penetration into cysts). Consider pyelonephritis as a differential diagnosis—may require gentamicin or cephalosporin as well. CT scanning or ^{99M}Tc-ciprofloxacin scanning may demonstrate infected cysts in cases of doubt.

Nephrolithiasis

20% of patients have associated renal stones, usually uric acid or calcium oxalate in origin. Diagnosis is best made with CT scanning, and preventative measures are outlines on 📖 p.434.

Haemorrhage, infection, or stone?

	Haemorrhage	Infection	Stone
Fever	±	++	±
Leucocytosis	±	++	−
Frank haematuria	++	−	+
Renal colic	−	−	+
+ blood cultures	−	+	−

Extra-renal cysts

Particularly hepatic, occur in 10–40% (most commonly multiparous women). They do not interfere with synthetic liver function, and rarely complicate. Those that do may be amenable to surgical de-roofing. Pancreatic and splenic cysts also occur, usually without symptoms.

Intracranial aneurysms (ICAs)

4–10% of patients have ICAs: specific mutations appear to predispose to aneurysm formation, so certain families have a history of intracranial bleeds. These families merit screening with MR angiography.

Symptomatic ICAs or those >10mm diameter need correcting surgically. It is less certain what to do with asymptomatic ICAs <10mm.

Rupture presents as subarachnoid haemorrhage, most commonly in patients <50 years with poor BP control, and results in 50% mortality or severe disability.

Other manifestations

Mitral valve prolapse and aortic regurgitation, diverticular disease and abdominal and inguinal hernias are more common in APKD patients.

Other cystic kidney diseases

Simple cysts

Solitary or multiple renal cysts are common in the elderly: 50% of those aged 50 years or more have one or more such cysts. So-called 'simple' cysts are usually asymptomatic and are found on imaging the urinary tract for other reasons. Simple cysts have no further significance—complex (echoic) cysts need detailed and rapid evaluation by CT scanning to exclude renal malignancies.

Acquired cystic disease

Acquired cysts refer to cysts arising in the context of renal failure with tubulo-interstitial scarring. These can be multiple and bilateral, and may be confused for APKD. Unlike APKD, acquired cysts occur in scarred and thus small kidneys, and are rarely >2–3cm in size (most are ± 5mm).

The age at presentation, a family history, the presence of hypertension, and the site of the cysts on imaging can discriminate the various cystic renal diseases.

Table 6.1 Classification of cystic kidney diseases.

	Age	Family history	↑Cr	↑BP	Site
APKD	Any	++	±	+	Cortex
Juvenile PKD	<10	±	+	+	Cortex
Simple cysts	>65	−	−	±	Cortex
Medullary sponge kidneys	Any	−	−	−	Medulla
Medullary cystic kidneys	20–30	++	++	−	Medulla
Nephronophthisis	<15	+	++	−	Medulla

Autosomal recessive polycystic kidney disease (ARPKD)

Is caused by a rare mutation on *PKHD1* gene (located on chromosome 6) encoding for polyductin. It is a disease of infancy and childhood, presenting with polycystic kidneys progressing to ESRD, congenital hepatic fibrosis and portal hypertension.

Juvenile nephronophthisis

Is a related recessively inherited condition characterized by cystic change and tubulo-interstitial fibrosis presenting in early childhood (>1 year) leading to ESRD in adolescence. Unlike medullary cystic kidney disease, extra-renal manifestations (cerebral degeneration, bone abnormalities and hepatic and portal fibrosis) occur.

Medullary sponge kidney

Is a benign, common condition characterized by diffuse medullary cyst formation. It is a developmental rather than genetic anomaly.

Clinically, there is no family history, and patients are identified incidentally or when investigated for UTI or stones. Impaired calcium handling in the collecting ducts predisposes to formation of calcium-containing stones (often in cysts). Medullary sponge kidney should be considered particularly in young women presenting with calcium stones. Haematuria (microscopic or gross) and recurrent UTI also complicate the disorder.

Diagnosis is made on IVU, with a typical 'calyceal brush' seen with adequate studies. Renal impairment is very rare, and management should be directed to treating infection and preventing stone formation.

Medullary cystic kidney disease

Has autosomal dominant inheritance, presenting in early adulthood with progressive renal impairment. The affected genes, *MCKD-1* and *−2*, encode key signalling proteins located in the renal cilia. This manifests as small cysts (1–10mm) forming at the cortico-medullary junctions with associated tubulo-interstitial inflammation and scarring, with unaffected glomeruli.

Clinically, affected individuals have a positive family history, presenting with nocturia, polydipsia, and polyuria (impaired concentrating ability). Urine dipstick is usually bland, and BP often normal (due to salt losses). Investigation shows small- to normal-sized kidneys on USS. CT kidneys may demonstrate cystic change. Impaired urate excretion and hyperuricaemia (± gout) may occur. Renal function declines to ESRD usually by 60 years of age. Treatment includes correcting salt and water depletion—there is no specific therapy.

Table 6.2 Sponge or cystic kidney disease?

	Medullary sponge kidney	Medullary cystic kidney disease
Age	Any	20–30 years
↑ Creatinine (ESRD)	−	++ (ESRD <60)
Salt-losing state	−	++
Calcium stones	++	−
UTI	+	−
+ Family history	−	+

Urinary tract infections

The incidence of UTI (including bacterial infections of the bladder and kidneys) is roughly 50,000 per million population, making it by far the most common disease of the renal tract. 50% of women will experience UTI in their lifetime, predominantly cystitis, usually occurring in a normal urinary tract.

A second infection is common in women who have had one UTI, but only 3–5% will have recurrent UTIs (📖 p.427). In men and children, UTI is rare, and almost always associated with abnormalities in the urinary tract needing further investigation (📖 p.426). Although serious morbidity from UTI is usually low, Gram negative septicaemia and renal scarring do result from sporadic or recurrent infections. UTI in pregnancy is discussed on 📖 p.568.

Pathogenesis

In women, the pathogens responsible for UTI are found in the colonic flora. Subsequent UTI is usually ascending, ie after perivaginal, perineal and transurethral colonization, often triggered by intercourse. *Lactobacilli* found as commensals in the vagina prevent urinary pathogens colonizing the perineum—changes in the vaginal pH, or antibiotic treatment may lead to failure of this defence mechanism.

Bacteriology

- *Escherichia coli* 70–90%
- *Staphylococcus saprophyticus* 5–20%
- *Klebsiella* sp
- *Enterococcus faecalis*
- *Proteus mirabilis.*

Some women express an inherited and unique receptor on urothelium that aids *E. coli* binding. Also, *E. coli* expressing type P fimbriae (pili), an adhesin that promotes bacterial attachment to urothelium, and particularly likely to cause pyelonephritis.

Host factors predisposing to UTI

- Recent or frequent intercourse.
- Highly concentrated urine (>800mOsm/kg) or failed urinary acidification (pH >5).
- Urinary stasis or incomplete bladder emptying.
- ↑Age (oestrogen vaginal pH)↓.
- Eradication of vaginal commensal organisms (use of spermicides).
- Renal or bladder stones.

Diagnosis of UTI
Symptoms and signs
Cystitis or lower UTI

Dysuria, frequency, urgency, and nocturia. Suprapubic pain or tenderness. Offensive urine or frank haematuria. Ask about sexual intercourse, new partners, and spermicidal or condom use. Recent antibiotic use, or previous episodes of UTI.

▶ In the **elderly**, may present as confusion ± incontinence. Vaginal irritation ± discharge makes UTI less likely (vaginitis more so).

Pyelonephritis or upper UTI

Fever, chills, nightsweats, ± rigors. Nausea ± vomiting. Loin pain, costovertebral (renal) angle tenderness. May be systemically unwell or even incipient septic shock.

▶ In the immunocompromised and children, all the above may be absent—maintain high index of suspicion if unwell.

Investigations
- Dipstick urine: positive leucocyte esterase ± nitrite reductase. May be modest haematuria or proteinuria. *In low risk cases, no further investigation is needed if positive dipstick with characteristic symptoms.*
- Clean catch MSU for microscopy at ×40 magnification (ie high powered field), pyuria (≥10 WBC/hpf) ± organisms (1–10/hpf). WBC casts strongly suggestive of pyelonephritis.
- Culture: sample should be cultured within 2 hours of sampling. If not possible, store at 4° for < 48 hours.

Positive diagnosis of UTI

A pure growth of a urinary pathogen:
- ≥10^5 colony forming units/mL urine remains the standard.

However, at this cut-off, 30–50% of UTI will escape diagnosis. In addition, then:
- ≥10^3cfu/mL in young women with suspected uncomplicated cystitis, or in men.
- ≥10^4cfu/mL if pyelonephritis suspected, or childhood UTI.

If suspected pyelonephritis: ↑WCC, ↑CRP. U+E. Imaging is only required in complicated cases (requiring admission), in those at risk (next page) or after a second episode: USS is the initial investigation of choice.

Persisting or repeated symptoms
Exclude urethritis or vaginitis if persistent symptoms despite treatment. Re-infection is common, often < 1 year after the first episode. Approach as a new infection. Usually due to persistent predisposing factors (colonization).

Who needs closer attention?
- Symptoms >14 days
- Recurrent UTI
- Men
- Children
- Pregnant women
- Diabetics
- The immunocompromised
- *Proteus* UTI—?associated stones
- Known abnormal urinary tract
- Indwelling catheter.

Possible investigations include
- *Plain AXR* for suspected stones (radio-opaque).
- *USS kidneys* with pre- and post-micturition imaging of bladder: will identify parenchymal pathology, hydronephrosis and incomplete bladder emptying (but *not* many pelvic and ureteric abnormalities).
- *IVU* will exclude anatomical abnormalities: should be performed after resolution of acute symptoms. Best examination of pelvi-calyceal system and ureters, and may identify renal stones.
- ^{99M}Tc-DMSA scanning detects scars (reflux nephropathy) and is less invasive than IVU (ideal for children)
- In men, assessment of the prostate (incl PSA) and bladder emptying with *urodynamic flow studies* of lower urinary tract function.
- *Cystoscopy* is indicated in those at risk for bladder or prostate cancer, or those with evidence of impaired bladder emptying that may benefit from urethral dilatation.
- *CT scanning ± contrast* is superceding the above investigations.

Treatment of UTI
Duration of therapy varies widely, as does antibiotic prescribing. The choice of antibiotic should always be informed by local resistance patterns among common causative organisms. Suggested therapies include:

Uncomplicated lower UTI (cystitis)
Either: short course (3 days) therapy:
- Trimethroprim 200mg bd (or co-trimoxazole 960mg bd).
- Fluoroquinolones such as ciprofloxacin 250mg bd or levofloxacin 250mg od. Oral cephalosporins offer a useful alternative.

Or: long course (7–10 days) therapy:
As above, or nitrofurantoin (as monohydrate macrocrystals) 100mg bd (not useful with renal impairment).

▶ If symptoms persist, (re-)culture the urine.

Encourage high fluid intake of > 2L/day. Ampicillin/amoxicillin is less effective at eradicating vaginal and peri-urethral colonization.

Complicated lower UTI

See 'at risk patients' for criteria, p.424. Antibiotic therapy should *always* be tailored against urine culture results. Empirical therapy should be started immediately, and modified once sensitivities known, e.g.
● Fluoroquinolones for 7–10 days

Pregnant women, p.568. In the immunocompromised, consider additional single dose aminoglycoside (e.g. gentamicin 3–5mg/kg IVI or IMI). For renal transplant recipients, p.266.

Acute pyelonephritis

After full assessment, if well, treatment can be as an out-patient. If nausea and vomiting predominate, or if systemically unwell, admit.
▶Antibiotic therapy should *always* be tailored against urine culture results.
● Fluoroquinolones (e.g. ciprofloxacin 250–500mg bd po) or levofloxacin 250mg od for 14 days.
● Alternatives include amoxicillin/clavulinic acid, or a third generation cephalosporin IVI then po for 14 days.
● If unwell, consider IVI therapy ± single dose gentamicin 3–5mg/kg IVI.
● Rehydration with 0.9% NaCl.
● Anti-emetics for nausea and analgesia.

Catheter-related UTI

A common problem in hospitalized patients. Treatment is only effective after removal of the catheter (if possible). Diagnose if cultures positive for > 10^5cfu/mL *and* heavy pyuria (colonization in the absence of pyuria does not merit treatment in most cases). Generally only treat if significant local symptoms or systemically unwell.

Recurrent UTIs

Defined as *>4 culture-proven UTIs in a year*. Establish whether UTI related to intercourse. Investigate and manage for abnormal urinary tract.
● Advise to increase fluid intake >2L/day and frequent voiding.
● Double voiding *may* help bladder emptying.
● Spermicides or spermicide-coated condoms should be discouraged.
● Oestrogen creams per vagina in post-menopausal women.

The following *do not* predispose to UTI: wiping patterns, voiding after intercourse, personal hygiene, showering, hot baths or saunas, pantyhose, tights or synthetic fabrics.

Prophylactic antibiotics should be offered if no underlying cause identified. Ensure any current infection is successfully eradicated.
● If UTI related to sexual activity: trimethroprim 200mg, co-trimoxazole 480mg or nitrofurantoin 50mg after intercourse.
● If no relation, offer nightly low-dose prophylaxis in a monthly rotation in three month cycles as: trimethroprim 100mg then nitrofurantoin 50mg then cephalexin 250mg. Alternatives include co-trimoxazole 480mg or amoxicillin 250mg.

Offer prophylaxis for 1 year.

A *recurrence* is not the same as a *relapse* (defined as return of symptoms with culture of the same organism following UTI). Relapse should be treated with a prolonged (4–6 week) course of antibiotics.

Interstitial cystitis

A difficult to treat sterile inflammatory cystitis, presenting in women >40 years (often with a history of recurrent UTI). Symptoms include frequency, dysuria and disabling suprapubic or pelvic pain. May be sterile pyuria. Patient sensitivity to intravesical potassium solutions may aid diagnosis. Cystoscopy and biopsy may show characteristic inflammation and ulceration. Tricyclic antidepressants treat neuropathic pain. Oral (or intravesical) pentosan polysulfate sodium seems efficacious.

Xanthogranulomatous pyelonephritis

A chronic unilateral pyelonephritis associated with calculi causing widespread parenchymal destruction. Affects women > 40, often with history of recurrent UTI. Presents as fever, nausea, anorexia, weight loss with a palpable kidney. Urinalysis confirms UTI, usually *Proteus sp* or other Gram negative organisms. Diagnosis on CT kidneys—often requires nephrectomy. May be confused with renal cell carcinoma.

Reflux nephropathy

Reflux nephropathy (RN) describes a progressive lesion caused by repeated infections in either or both kidneys, almost always developing in childhood in the setting of an abnormal renal tract. The long term renal scarring and insufficiency resulting from early injury is called RN or *chronic pyelonephritis*. RN causes 5–12% of ESRD in the developed world.

The anatomical abnormality is usually vesico-ureteric reflux, but RN can occur with incomplete bladder emptying or outflow obstruction as well (see opposite). By adulthood, the ureter inserts obliquely through the bladder wall, forming a compressible tunnel that acts as a one-way valve.

Too short a tunnel may allow reflux of urine into the ureters with bladder contraction and micturition. As the bladder is rarely empty, superinfection is the norm. The renal papillae do not restrict refluxing, infected urine, so the tubulo-interstitium becomes chronically infected and inflamed, leading to localised scarring in an affected area.

Symptoms and signs in adults

In children, all UTIs should be referred and evaluated for RN. In adulthood, the presentation usually reflects evolving CKD.

A history of renal colic, haematuria, or the passage of a stone may be offered. ↑BP (± 50% of adults), sterile pyuria, and WBC casts on microscopy. Proteinuria (<1g/day) unless progressive CKD (often secondary FSGS at biopsy), when may be heavy.

Investigations

A single infection with complete recovery and a normal USS of the urinary tract requires no further assessment

^{99M}Tc-DMSA scintigraphy (which is taken up in functioning renal tubules) will demonstrate renal scars as areas of reduced uptake. IVU: renal scarring (as parenchymal loss), and 'clubbed calyces' (Fig 6.11). Localized papillary scars do not take up contrast well, blunting the normal appearance of the renal calyx.

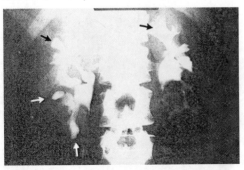

Fig. 6.11 Clubbed calyces (arrows) on IVU. Reproduced with permission from Warrell D, Cox T, Firth J, and Benz EJ (eds) (2004) *Oxford Textbook of Medicine*, 4th edn, p.326. Oxford University Press, Oxford.

Histology

Demonstrates typical features of chronic tubulo-interstitial scarring, with dilated and atrophied tubules, and an infiltrate of inflammatory cells. Secondary hyperfiltration injury develops over time, with compensatory hypertrophy of undiseased segments, vessel changes and glomerular collapse.

Vesico-ureteric reflux

Is genetically heterogeneous but:
- Affects 0.1–1% of newborns.
- Underlies 12–50% of children with a proven UTI.
- Is almost always present in children with proven renal scars.
- Is a leading cause of childhood ↑BP and ESRD.

Scar formation ceases at about 6 years, when the renal papilla no longer allows reflux into the renal parenchyma itself. VUR ceases around puberty, when the bladder base thickens, the ureteric tunnel elongates, and free reflux no longer occurs. Surgical correction of incompetent valves offers no benefit over antibiotic prophylaxis in long term outcome.

Management

Given no new scar formation occurs in adulthood, treatment is aimed at preventing progression of CKD.
- Treat ↑BP and proteinuria.
- ACE inhibitor or ARB as first-line.
- Add-on anti-hypertensives aiming for target BP <130/80.
- Treat new infections vigorously.
- Ureteric re-implantation is no longer widely practised.

Unilateral RN does not cause CRF if BP control is good.

Pregnant women with RN frequently develop UTI, functional deterioration or hypertension ± pre-eclampsia, and should be referred early for specialist care.

Adults with UTI and a NORMAL renal tract will not develop RN.

Salt-losing nephropathy

Refers to inappropriate sodium (and thus) water losses in hypovolaemic patients with chronic tubulo-interstitial disease. Losses rarely exceed 2–3L/day (or 100mmol Na^+) as increased delivery of Na^+ to the macula densa causes a protective afferent arteriolar vasoconstriction and ↓GFR (so-called 'tubulo-glomerular feedback).

Nephrolithiasis

Kidney stones affect 8–15% of people. 2σ:1φ, aged 20–60 years. After a single stone, the likelihood of a second within 7 years is ± 50%. Prophylaxis is highly effective in most cases.

Stones form around a nidus when the solubility of a urinary salt is exceeded: high solute delivery, concentrated urine (low volume) or areas of stasis (anatomically abnormal urinary tract), and an excess of stone promoters over inhibitors predispose to their formation. The key to management is identifying the stone components and any metabolic predisposition to stone formation.

Calcium oxalate/phosphate stones

Occur with an associated metabolic abnormality in most cases, but may be idiopathic. Family history positive. Risk factors (in addition to predisposing factors above) include increased Ca^{2+} or oxalate urinary delivery, or factors that promote solubility:

- *Hypercalciuria*: increased Ca^{2+} absorption from the gut, or renal wasting due to reduced reabsorption. Common.
- *Hyperparathyroidism* and other hypercalcaemic states.
- *Hyperuricosuria*: uric acid forms a nidus for calcium oxalate stone formation.
- *Hyperoxaluria*: increased dietary oxalate, or enhanced oxalate uptake due to ileal inflammation (Crohn's disease) or resection.
- *Hypocitraturia ± chronic acidosis*: citrate forms a soluble complex with calcium.

Uric acid stones

Hyperuricosuria is most commonly associated with the formation of calcium oxalate stones! Pure uric acid stones are less common. ↑urinary urate with ↓urinary pH < 5.5 → insoluble uric acid stones. ↑urinary urate occurs with hyperuricaemia (10–20% will have frank gout) of any cause.

Cystine stones

Cystinuria may be suspected in childhood stone-formers. Mutations in the gene encoding an amino acid transporter leads to wasting of the cationic amino acids cystine, ornithine, lysine and arginine.

Stone composition and incidence

Calcium oxalate/phosphate	60–80%
Struvite	10%
Uric acid	5–10%
Cystine	1%

▶ *Calcium-containing or struvite stones are radio-opaque. All stones will cast acoustic shadows on USS. Cystine stones are seen well on CT.*

Bladder stones

Occur in abnormal bladders, often following surgical reconstruction. Predisposing factors include UTI, bladder diverticulae, neurogenic bladders, ± bladder outflow obstruction.

Staghorn calculi

Struvite or magnesium ammonium phosphate stones. Infection by *Proteus*, *Klebsiella*, or *Serratia*, capable of splitting urea to ammonium and hydroxyl ions (thus ↑ urinary pH), predisposes toward struvite stones. Such stones act as a reservoir for infection, and often expand to fill much of the collecting system. Typically seen on KUB. Treatment depends on size, but often involves nephrolithotomy then lithotripsy. Infection should be treated vigorously.

Investigating recurrent stone-formers

In patients presenting with a first urinary stone, investigation into an underlying cause with a view to prevention is *not* cost-effective. There is no need to fully evaluate patients with ≤1stone/ 3 years.

In patients with +ve family history, or recurrent stones:
- Urinary pH and specific gravity (on random sample)
- Dipstick for haematuria ± proteinuria
- Biochemical analysis of passed stones
- Microscopy for crystals, urine culture
- U+E, urate
- Calcium, phosphate, alkaline phosphatase
- Parathyroid hormone
- Urinary stone screen (see below)
- Imaging (see below).

Urinary values for 24 hour 'stone screen'

Ensure that the collection is adequate. Urine creatinine of ± 0.15mmol creatinine/kg body weight/day implies a complete sample. Normal ranges:
- Calcium <0.1mmol/kg/day (4mg/kg/day)
- Oxalate <0.44mmol/day (45 mg/day)
- Uric acid <4.4mmol/day (>750mg/day)
- Citrate >2.4mmol/day (250mg/day)
- (Phosphate <35mmol/day—*wholly* diet dependent)
- Sodium <200mmol/day
- Cystine negligible.

Collect stones screen in acidified container for all above, except urinary uric acid, which requires a plain container.

Imaging in nephrolithiasis
- Unenhanced CT kidneys offers single best test.
- Plain KUB allows monitoring of radio-opaque stones.
- IVU offers a reasonable alternative to CT.
- USS kidneys if abnormal urinary tract or obstruction suspected.

Management of recurrent nephrolithiasis

General measures:
- Increase fluids for daily UO > 2.5L/day
- Reduce animal protein intake (esp. meat): ↓acid formation, so preserved urinary citrate excretion. Aim <52g/day animal protein. Advise regarding non-animal protein substitutes.
- Reduce salt intake <3g/day NaCl (50mmol/day): salt enhances calciuria.
- *Normal* calcium intake of >1200mg/day (30mmol/day), as low Ca^{2+} intake leads to ↑ oxalate excretion and predisposes women to osteoporosis.
- Reduce dietary oxalate: spinach, tea, nuts, chocolate.
- Increase intake of citrus fruits.
- Monitor urinary stone screen for efficacy of therapy.

Calcium oxalate/phosphate stones

If u-Ca^{2+} *normal*: potassium citrate 450mg bd (↑ to 900mg bd).

If u-Ca^{2+} *raised*: potassium citrate as above + *either* indapamide 2.5–5mg daily or amiloride 2.5–5mg/hydrochlorothiazide 25–50mg daily.
- Potassium citrate: ↑ urinary citrate and pH.
- Amiloride and thiazide diuretics: ↑ tubular Ca^{2+} reabsorption.
- Add-on therapies might include:
  - Allopurinol 100–300mg/day if hyperuricaemia/uria.
  - Pyridoxine 50 mg/daymay reduce oxalate production. Calcium carbonate 500–1500 mg tds before meals may reduce oxalate absorption

Struvite stones require eradication therapy for associated UTI: aim for 3–6 months directed antibiotic therapy against cultures and sensitivities.

Cystine stones are treated with D-penicllamine 250–500mg bd, or α-mercaptopropionylglycine 1000–2000mg/day (considered less toxic than D-penicillamine).

Acute renal colic

Is the syndrome caused by a stone(s) passage down the urinary tract. Patients, usually ♂ in their 4th decade, are often in severe pain.

Symptoms and signs

Colicky abdominal pain, often severe, radiating from loin to groin. Nausea and vomiting. Renal angle tenderness. Haematuria, often macroscopic. Dysuria, strangury, and frequency ± symptoms of UTI. May be family history of nephrolithiasis. Predisposing factors include dehydration (↓urine volume), exercise, or protein load.

Investigations

Dipstick urine for haematuria, leucocyte esterase and nitrate reductase. Urine microscopy for crystals. U+E, CRP, FBC. If signs of infection, culture blood and urine. Unenhanced CT kidneys to confirm diagnosis, site the stone, exclude obstruction and predict response to lithotripsy. IVU is appropriate if CT unavailable. Plain AXR will reveal radio-opaque stones (± 80%).

▶▶ Infection or obstruction is an indication for urgent intervention.

Treatment

- Opiate analgesia: pethidine 75mg/ morphine 5–10 mg IMI/IVI.
- Anti-emetic: metaclopramide 10mg IMI/IVI.
- Paracetamol 1g 4 hourly po.
- NSAIDs are effective analgesics, and can be used as add-on therapy with *caution* (i.e. good renal function).
- Oral rehydration, or vomiting IVI 0.9% NaCl for UO > 2L/day.
- If stone stone ≤5mm, 90% will pass spontaneously.
- If 5–10mm 50% will pass spontaneously.

10–20% of stones fail to pass. High ureteric (proximal) stones are best treated with shock wave lithotripsy if <15–20mm. Ureteroscopy is an alternative if stone >15mm. Low (distal) stones can be successfully treated by either technique. Percutaneous nephrolithotomy has excellent results for stones >20mm or complicated stones.

If associated infection, IVI antibiotic with good Gram negative cover: cefuroxime 1.5g tds IVI, or ciprofloxacin 500mg po bd. Most stones will be passed in 1–3 weeks. Monitor passage of stone with plain AXR weekly.

⚠ *An infected, obstructed system caused by stones (pyonephrosis) is an emergency. Septicaemia ± shock supervenes rapidly. Commence IVI antibiotics and arrange urgent referral for percutaneous nephrostomy to allow immediate drainage.*

The kidney in systemic disease

Diabetic nephropathy (DN)

Diabetes mellitus (DM) is defined as 'a state of chronic hyperglycaemia leading to long-term organ damage', presenting as two distinct entities:

- Type 1 DM is due to auto-immune mediated islet B-cell destruction, presenting acutely, often in childhood (median age 12). Accounts for 5–15% all DM.
- Type 2 DM is a heterogeneous condition, diagnosed empirically from lack of evidence of type 1 DM, but characterized by insulin resistance and islet failure.
  - Presents >40 years.
  - Peak incidence 60–65 years.
  - ♂ preponderance.
  - Incidence 2% in Caucasian population, and higher in Indo-Asians.

Definition and epidemiology

Diabetic nephropathy is now the most common underlying cause of ESRD in Europe and the USA, with an annual incidence of 140 cases per million population (non-diabetic renal disease has an incidence of 15–42pmp). The incidence depends on the ethnicity of the population: Pima Indians have a 40% incidence of ESRD after ten years of DM and microalbuminuria. There is a higher incidence of DN in men. In type 1 DM, age at diagnosis is predictive of outcome:

- Diagnosis at <12 years: time to overt nephropathy = 14 years
- Diagnosis at 12–20 years: time to overt nephropathy = 8 years
- DN affects 30–40% of type 1 DM after 20 years.

Pathogenesis of DN

Renal hypertrophy, hyperfiltration (initially with ↑GFR to > normal) and intra-renal hypertension leads to glomerulosclerosis and tubulo-interstitial fibrosis. ↑ glucose mediates this through:

- ↑shear stress and changes in glomerular haemodynamics.
- Local ↑angiotensin II release → haemodynamic and fibrotic changes.
- Modification of proteins by glucose-degradation products.
- Activation of mitogens and TGF-β → excess matrix deposition.

In addition, a poorly understood genetic pre-disposition exists in both type 1 and type 2 DM that is associated with progressive renal failure.

Mean HbA_{1C} over time correlates with loss of renal function. In long-term studies in type 1 (DCCT) and type 2 (UKPDS) DM, blood glucose concentration is related to the development of micro-albuminuria and progression to overt proteinuria.

Natural history

For type 1 DM, the evolving renal lesion develops serially:

Stage	
1	Renal hypertrophy with ↑GFR
2	Early histological changes, though still clinically silent
3	Microalbuminuria—BP now starts to rise
4	Overt diabetic nephropathy with declining GFR
5	ESRD

A third of type 1 diabetics develop diabetic renal disease, reaching stage 3 about 10 years after diagnosis—after 20 years, this sub-group will have progressed to overt DN.

Type 2 diabetics follow a similar pattern: as they present in middle age, many will not come to ESRD. *But* enough will to make type 2 DM the most common cause of ESRD in the western world. Type 2 diabetics also present *with* ↑BP, and often microalbuminuria.

The long-term UKPDS studies have demonstrated:
- 2% prevalence microalbuminuria/year (incidence 25% over 10 years),
- 2.8% microalbuminuria to overt proteinuria/year (5% over 10 years)
- 2.3% proteinuria with decline GFR (progression to CKD stage IV–V is 1% at 10 years)—equates to 12 times additional risk of CKD compared to non-diabetic population.

Pathology and indications for renal biopsy

Renal biopsy is rarely required to establish a diagnosis of DN. Consider biopsy if:
- Absence of retinopathy (retinopathy observed in 85–99% of patients with established nephropathy).
- Dysmorphic red cells, red cell casts or frank haematuria (microscopic haematuria is seen in 66% patients with DN).
- Rapidly increasing proteinuria, or the nephrotic syndrome.
- Symptoms suggestive of multi-system disorder.

▶23–37% of diabetics without retinopathy will not have DN at kidney biopsy (membranous GN, IgA nephropathy etc.).

Histology

Mesangial expansion leading to inter-capillary nodule formation (Kimmelstiel–Wilson nodules), with capillary lumen encroachment. There may be variable degrees of interstitial fibrosis or the vascular changes of arteriosclerosis and occlusion.

Other renal disease in diabetic patients

Papillary necrosis (📖 p.410)

Occurs in 1:20 with diabetic nephropathy. May be asymptomatic. Can present as pain (recurrent renal colic) or infection. Haematuria and modest proteinuria (<2g/24hrs) is common. A sterile pyuria is typical.

Renovascular Disease (📖 p.412)

As a result of associated atherosclerotic renal artery stenosis. Suspect if difficult to control BP, fluid retention, or >20% rise creatinine with ACEI.

Autonomic neuropathy of the bladder

40% of longstanding diabetics have bladder dysfunction, with loss of sensation of fullness and incomplete emptying leading to large-volume bladders with significant post-micturition residual urine volume and stasis.

Often presents with UTI or incontinence. Assessment should include a measure of post-micturition volume and urodynamic studies. Interventions include assisted (suprapubic manual pressure) and regular voiding in the absence of urge, or intermittent self-catherisation. This may lead to ↓bladder volume or partial recovery of detrusor function.

Urinary tract infection (📖 p.424)

Women with diabetes have twice the incidence of UTI compared to non-diabetic ♀, a higher incidence of pyelonephritis or renal abcess formation. 90% of cases of emyphysematous pyelonephritis (📖 p.428) occur in diabetics.

Contrast nephropathy (📖 p.132)

Diabetics, probably as a result of intra-renal microvascular disease, are more susceptible ↑Cr following the use of contrast media.

⚠ Stop metformin for 2 days pre- and post-contrast procedure (risk of lactic acidosis).

Management of diabetic nephropathy

Screening patients for proteinuria/ microalbuminuria

Early detection of diabetic nephropathy delays and may prevent progression to ESRD. Annual screening by urinary albumin/creatinine ratio (ACR, expressed in mg albumin/mmol creatinine) should be performed as:

- An early morning sample
- In the absence of overt urinary tract infection
- In patients with stable glucose control.

ACR in a random urine specimen accurately reflects microalbuminuria:

ACR	24hr albuminuria
<2.5	<30mg/day
2.5–30	30–300mg/day
>30	Overt proteinuria

Investigations in DN

- Measure BP and examine peripheral pulses.
- Dipstick urine (?haematuria → if so, microscope for ?casts).
- Quantify proteinuria (as above).
- Check visual acuity and perform fundoscopy.
- Test for peripheral neuropathy (other microvascular disease).
- U+E, Alb.
- HbA$_{1C}$ (or fructosamine), cholesterol.
- USS (kidneys often normal sized despite ↓GFR).

Primary prevention of nephropathy

- Improve glycaemic control:
  - HbA$_{1C}$ <7.5% in insulin-requiring patients.
  - HbA$_{1C}$ <6.5% not on insulin.
- Control BP aiming for target <130/80 or lower if tolerated.
- Stop smoking, lose weight and exercise.

Management of microalbuminuria and proteinuria

- Glycaemic control
  - HbA1C <7.5%
  - Stop metformin when creatinine >150µmol/L eGFR <60ml/min (☞ risk of lactic acidosis).
- Blood pressure control (see opposite).
- Other interventions:
  - Treat dyslipidaemia: HMG-CoA reductase inhibitors significantly reduce cardiac events in diabetics. May also ↓proteinuria and preserve GFR in overt nephropathy (aim fasting LDL <3.0).
  - Dietary protein restriction (0.8g/kg per day, 📖 p.190) may slow decline in GFR by 60–75%.

BP control in DN

- Good blood pressure drastically alters renal prognosis.
  - 30% have ↑BP at diagnosis of type 2 diabetes.
  - 70% have ↑BP at diagnosis of DN.
  - ↑BP is proportional to ↑albumin excretion.
  - Good BP control reduces the decline in GFR associated with DN from ±12ml/min/year to < 5 ml/min/year.
  - ACEI/ARB may restrict progression to as little as −0.3 mL/min/year.
- Emphasize importance of a low salt diet <5g/day (📖 p.190).
- Drug therapy.
- ☛ *Although inhibitors of the renin–angiotensin system (ACEI, ARB) are preferred by consensus, this practice is not always evidence-based.* We still recommend (▶ usually need multi-drug therapy):
  - Start with low-dose long-acting tissue-bound ACEI (e.g. ramipril) or ARB (e.g. irbesartan) and titrate to maximum dose.
  - Step-wise add-on therapy aiming for BP < 130/80 with:
    — Loop diuretic.
    — Non-dihydropyridine calcium channel blockers (e.g., diltiazem).[1]
    — β-blocker (caution with hypoglycaemia).
  - Combination therapy with both ACEI and ARB may have additive effects in ↓proteinuria and slowing progression. May require low K⁺ diet ± furosemide 40mg od.
  - 📖 p.348 for difficult ↑BP.

Summary of recommended interventions to slow progression of renal disease in patients with DM

	Target
BP control	<130/80
Inhibition of RAS[2]	Urinary protein <0.3g/day
Glycaemic control	HbA1C <7%
Correction of dyslipidaemia	LDL cholesterol <2.6mmol/L

---

1 Much has been made of whether dihydropyridine calcium channel blockers are effective (or even harmful) in this group of patients. The evidence is conflicting—in practice, these drugs (e.g. amlodipine) are useful as part of a multi-drug approach to achieving BP targets in DN.

Management of ESRD in diabetes

Diabetic patients should initiate dialysis at an earlier stage than patients with another cause of end-stage renal failure, i.e. GFR 10–15ml/min, or creatinine >500µmol/L, as diabetics are more susceptible to uraemic symptoms, fluid retention and hyperkalaemia.

Survival and causes of death in diabetics on dialysis

Diabetics with ESRD have a 5-year survival rate of 30.2% (compared with 62.2% in non-diabetic dialysis patients). This difference is due to greater co-morbidity, particularly macrovascular disease. There is also a higher incidence of withdrawal from dialysis reported in diabetics.

Outcome of dialysis: peritoneal dialysis versus haemodialysis

A clear difference in outcome between PD and HD has not been observed, and studies from USRDS and Canada have given differing results, which may be explained by age and comorbidity. Overall, there is a suggestion that older diabetic patients survive longer on HD, and younger patients longer on PD.

Renal transplantation in diabetics

Renal transplantation is both safe and effective, offering improved survival and rehabilitation compared to dialysis. Recent studies have shown similar 1- and 5-year graft survival in diabetics and non-diabetic patients, when data is censored for patients dying with a functioning graft. Living donor graft survival is superior to cadaveric donor grafts (80% vs. 64% graft 5 year survival).

Type 1 diabetics should be considered for combined kidney/pancreas transplantation.

The kidney in multiple myeloma

Multiple myeloma (MM) is characterized by an aberrant clone of plasma cells producing an immunoglobulin (IgG or IgA) or immunoglobulin light chain, generally presenting > 60 years, ♂>♀. Median survival after diagnosis is 3 years. In the UK, the incidence is 30–40pmp/year. Proliferation of these plasma cells leads to bone marrow failure, skeletal destruction and ↑Ca^{2+}. Paraproteinaemia (= monoclonal Ig produced by plasma cells) may cause renal failure, recurrent bacterial infections or hyperviscosity.

Diagnosing MM
- Monoclonal immunoglobulin band (M-band) in serum or urine.
- >10% plasma cells on bone marrow.
- Evidence of end-organ damage: ↑Ca^{2+}, Renal impairment, Anaemia or Bone lesions (CRAB).

Renal impairment is a major complication of MM, found at, or preceding diagnosis in 20–30% of patients, and occurring in 50% of patients during the course of the disease. Causes, often multi-factorial, include:
- Hypercalcaemia and dehydration
- Cast nephropathy (myeloma kidney, 30–65%)
- AL amyloidosis (usually lambda subtype light chain, 20%)
- Light-chain deposition disease (usually kappa light chains, 10%).

Symptoms and signs

Think of MM in any patient (esp. if elderly) with unexplained renal impairment, normal sized kidneys and a bland urine deposit.

Bone pain (esp. backache), weakness, fatigue. Symptoms of ↑Ca^{2+} (📖 p.542). Easy bruising, pallor, hepatomegaly (20%).

▶ Urine dipstick may be negative (does NOT detect light chains).

Investigations

FBC (↓Hb), ↑ESR, U+E (↑Cr), Alb, ↑Ca^{2+}, ↑urate/LDH (↑cell turnover). Serum protein electrophoresis and immunoglobulins (?immunoparesis), M-band, β-2 microglobulin (activity monitoring). 24-hr urine for Bence–Jones proteinuria (urinary free light chains). Serum light chains may be useful.

Skeletal survey (?osteolytic lesions, osteoporosis, pathological fractures). Bone marrow aspirate and trephine is diagnostic (>10% plasma cells). If renal impairment, proceed to *renal biopsy*.

What is in an Ig?

Immunoglobulin is made up of 2 heavy chains (with a complement fixing site) and 2 light chains (with an antigen binding site). Plasma cell dyscrasias may produce whole Ig (monoclonal), whole light chains or heavy chains, or parts of either. This leads to the slightly confusing though exact naming of renal and underlying diseases found with each protein.

Pathogenesis and histology

Cast nephropathy—freely filtered light chains bind tubular Tamm–Horsfall protein (📖 p.19) forming proteinaceous casts that obstruct the tubular lumen. Multiple large casts are apparent on LM, particularly in the distal tubule and collecting duct, with a fractured appearance. Casts may be surrounded by multinucleated giant cells, with tubulitis and interstitial inflammation common. Casts are polychromatic with Masson's trichrome, may stain with Congo Red, but are not birefringent under polarized light (see amyloid). The risk of developing renal failure is 5–6 fold greater if Bence Jones proteinuria > 2.0g/day compared to those with proteinuria < 0.05g/day.

AL amyloidosis (📖 p.450), and light chain deposition disease (📖 p.452)

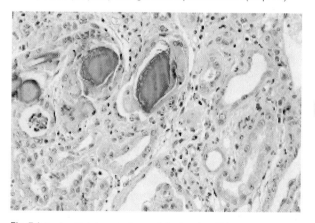

Fig. 7.1 Fractured tubular casts characteristic of myeloma kidney

Reproduced with permission from Davison AMA, Cameron JS, Grunfeld J-P *et al.* (eds) (2005). *Oxford Textbook of Clinical Nephrology*, 3rd edn. Oxford: Oxford University Press

Managing myeloma kidney

▶ Correct associated reversible causes of acute renal failure: dehydration, hypercalcaemia, and hyperuricaemia.
- Rehydrate:
  - 0.9% NaCl IV—may require large volumes (>5L) if ↑Ca^{2+}.
  - Alkaline diuresis does not alter outcome.
  - Monitor lying and standing BP, daily weight, fluid charts.
  - Expect Hb to fall—consider need for transfusion.
- Correct hypercalcaemia (📖 p.542).
  - *Once euvolaemic*, if still ↑Ca^{2+}, consider IV bisphosphonates (📖 p.542).
- Correct hyperuricaemia.
  - Start allopurinol 100mg daily.
- If anaemic, consider for erythropoietin.
Encourage all patients with CKD and MM to drink 3L/day.

Specific treatment for cast nephropathy

Involves reducing Ig or light chain deposition:
- ↓synthesis: most treatment regimes include corticosteroids (either dexamethasone or prednisolone) with alkylating agents. Newer treaments include thalidomide or proteasomal inhibitors. Autologous stem cell transplantation offers hope of complete remission.
- ↑clearance: plasma exchange may offer benefit in ARF by removing circulating light chains. Definitive evidence is still awaited (MERIT trial)

When myeloma isn't myeloma

Finding a paraprotein in serum or urine is not always due to MM!
- *Monoclonal gammopathy of uncertain significance (MGUS)* is characterized by:
  - M-band (monoclonal IgA, IgG, or IgM) <3g/dL.
  - <10% plasma cells in the bone marrow.
  - Minimal Bence–Jones proteinuria.
  - No end-organ damage ('CRAB', 📖 p.446).
The paraproteinaemia tends to remain stable over time—but MGUS may evolve into MM (1% year). Follow up should include 6-monthly testing of SPE and urine light chains.
- *Smoldering MM* refers to asymptomatic patients with M-band >3g/dL and a plasma cell infiltrate, but no end-organ damage. Evolves into MM in 3% patients/ year
- *Plasmacytomas* are solid tumours made up of plasma cells in bone or elsewhere that do not (usually) produce an M-band.

ESRD in MM

Either by HD or CAPD: of patients surviving beyond two months after diagnosis, actuarial survival is approximately 45% at one year, and 25–30% at three years. Patients who respond to chemotherapy with a reduction in light chain burden do much better, with a mean survival rate in one study being as high as 47 months versus only 17 months in non-responders.

Renal amyloid

Amyloidosis is a group of conditions characterized by tissue deposition of degradation-resistant fibrillary proteins as a β-pleated sheet leading to disease. Classically, amyloid appears an apple-green colour on Congo Red staining when viewed under birefringent light. Amyloid is deposited within the kidney in the mesangium and capillary walls: evolving glomerular involvement presents as worsening proteinuria and renal dysfunction.

The amyloids

Primary (AL) amyloid: monoclonal light chains (usually lambda) or light chain fragments produced by a plasma cell dyscrasia form amyloid sheets. More common in ♂ (2:1) >50 years. Prognosis poor.

Reactive (AA) amyloid: reactive amyloidosis results from deposition of fragments of serum amyloid A (SAA) proteins (an acute phase reactant) in patients with underlying inflammatory conditions. Prognosis depends on cause of inflammation.

Familial amyloid: inherited defects of (usually) transthyretin leading to amyloid formation in middle-age. Better prognosis.

Symptoms and signs

Asymptomatic or heavy proteinuria, → nephrotic syndrome ± CRF. Fatigue, weight loss, bruising and easy bleeding (including GI tract). Cardiomyopathy and cardiac failure (AL alone). Autonomic and peripheral neuropathy. Hepatomegaly, splenomegaly, macroglossia (AL alone) ± lymphadenopathy. Adrenal or thyroid involvement.

Causes of reactive (AA) amyloid

- Rheumatoid arthritis (40% of AA amyloid)
- Other arthropathies: ankylosing spondylitis, psoriatic arthropathy
- Inflammatory bowel disease
- Chronic suppurative infections (osteomyelitis, bronchiectasis, leg ulcers)
- TB or leprosy
- Malignancies (renal cell carcinoma, lymphoma)
- Familial Mediterranean fever (FMF).

FMF affects Jews, Armenians, and Turks, and is inherited by autosomal recessive transmission. Periodic acute attacks present before the age of 20, with fever, severe abdominal pain, arthritis and pleurisy (though 25% will have fever alone), lasting 48–72 hours and resolving spontaneously. During the attack, ↑WCC and ↑CRP.

Investigations

Dipstick urine (no or little haematuria). U+E, ↓Alb, ↑CRP, cholesterol. PCR or 24h proteinuria. Consider diagnostic fat pad aspirate for capillary amyloid staining if in doubt. USS kidneys (may be ↑size). Renal biopsy. Radio-labelled serum amyloid protein P component (SAP scan) binds to all types of amyloid fibrils, and allows quantitation of disease load and response to treatment.

▶ Adrenal involvement (↓Na$^+$, ↑K$^+$), cardiomyopathy (echocardiogram).

AL suspected: SPE, M-band (positive in 90%) and immunoglobulins. 24h urine for Bence–Jones proteinuria (73% will have urinary free light chains, usually lambda). Bone marrow aspirate + trephine (56% will have ↑plasma cells, 15% will have true myeloma).

AA suspected: Serum amyloid A protein (useful to monitor response). Search for underlying cause.

Familial suspected: mutant transthyretin in serum, and genetic analysis.

Histology

Amyloid fibrils have characteristic appearance on EM (Fig. 7.2) and bind Congo red (→ apple-green birefringence under polarized light), or thioflavine-T (→ yellow-green fluorescence). Amorphous deposits of pale hyaline material is demonstrated in the mesangium and capillary loops, staining positive with Congo red. IF may be positive (for light chains) in AL, but is negative in AA amyloid. EM will show fibrils.

Management

AL: consider chemotherapy as melphan + prednisolone (± autologous stem cell transplant). In responders (~30%) ↑patient survival, ↓proteinuria and ↓progression to end-stage renal disease. All patients considered 'fit' for therapy are thus treated. In elderly or frail patients with much co-morbid disease, an alternative is pulsed dexamethasone + alkylating agents and interferon.

AA: treat underlying cause. Cytotoxic therapy or monoclonal antibodies (esp to TNF-α) in inflammatory diseases. Antibiotics ± surgery for infections. FMF treated with colchicine 1.2 mg/day reduces acute attacks, and improves renal outcome.

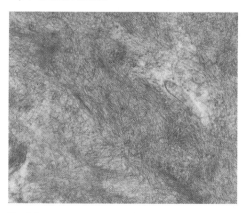

Fig. 7.2 Amyloid fibrils on renal biopsy.

Reproduced with permission from Davison AMA, Cameron JS, Grunfeld J-P *et al.* (eds) (2005). *Oxford Textbook of Clinical Nephrology*, 3rd edn. Oxford: Oxford University Press

Other non-amyloid dysproteinaemias

Light chain deposition disease (LCDD)

Is caused by a plasma cell dyscrasia leading to tissue deposition of monoclonal Ig light chains (kappa [κ] chains in 65%). Differs from amyloid in that the light chain lacks hydrophilic residues, and so cannot organize into fibrils *or stain positive for Congo Red.* May be associated with overt myeloma in 50% (or MM may subsequently develop). Absence of a monoclonal band on SPE (up to 30% patients), or plasma cell expansion in the bone marrow is still consistent with LCDD. Free light chains may be detected in serum.

Patients may present with asymptomatic proteinuria, but more usually with the nephrotic syndrome ± progressive renal failure. May be features of AL amyloid, esp diastolic dysfunction on echocardiography.

On renal biopsy, a nodular glomerulosclerosis is present that is Congo red *negative*. IF is positive for monoclonal light chains in capillary walls and the mesangium. EM demonstrates widespread amorphous, granular deposits without fibril formation.

Heavy chain deposition disease is a rare disorder where abnormal heavy chains deposited in the glomerulus cause similar disease.

Immunotactoid (or fibrillary) glomerulonephritis

Ill-understood disorder(s) characterized by the deposition of non-amyloid (i.e. Congo red *negative*) proteinaceous fibrils derived from Ig. Although two forms are described, they probably represent a spectrum of a single process:

Fibrillary GN (FGN): deposition of polyclonal Ig (and C3) in mesangium and glomerulus.

Immunotactoid GN (ITGN): monoclonal Ig deposits forming rod-like microtubular structures.

There may be an underlying M-band, 📖 p.84, or CLL, B-cell NHL, HCV infection or other auto-immune disease.

▶ There are no extra-renal features of the disease.

Presents with proteinuria (nephrotic range 60%), haematuria, ↑BP, and progressive CRF. No specific diagnostic test, proceed to renal biopsy where fibrils of 21–35nm diameter infiltrate the glomerulus (amyloid is 8–10nm). Always exclude M-band or HCV.

There is no proven effective treatment to slow progression. Small trials of immunosuppressive therapy have been disappointing, except in patients with crescentic changes on renal biopsy(prednisolone 60mg od + cyclophosphamide 2mg/kg/od).

Monoclonal Ig-derived material in the kidney

Can arise from any part of an immunoglobulin (📖 p.447), and on biopsy (EM) can be classified on the appearance of the deposits:

Organized	Crystalline	Cast nephropathy
		Fanconi's (📖 p.564)
	Fibrillar	AA or AL amyloidosis
	Microtubular	Immunotactoid GN
		Cryoglobulinaemia
Disorganized	Granular	LCDD
		HCDD

Immunoglobulin and Ig-derived fragments have an affinity for basement membranes, perhaps explaining the strong association with renal disease (particular as ~20% of cardiac output passes through the kidneys).

Sickle cell nephropathy

Renal involvement affects 4–8% of patients with sickle cell disease, in patients with homozygous sickle cell anemia (HbSS) or combined HbSC disease. HbS carriers (sickle cell trait) can develop milder tubular defects.

Erythrocyte sickling in the low oxygen environment of the medullary capillaries → obstruction and occlusion of capillaries, ischaemia, interstitial fibrosis, and papillary necrosis. The medullary counter-current mechanism is also impaired. Glomerular hypertrophy, hyperfiltration and glomerulosclerosis (≈FSGS, 📖 p.396) evolve, leading to ESRD.

Symptoms and signs

Impaired concentrating ability presents as nocturia or polyuria (occurs early). Asymptomatic haematuria is common. Sloughed necrotic papillae may present with frank haematuria and painful clot colic (and ureteric obstruction). Proteinuria and ↑Cr occur with time (↑BP is less usual: tubular salt wasting may be protective).

Renal medullary carcinoma

An aggressive malignancy found in patients with sickle cell disease occuring at a young age. Presents as abdominal or flank pain, haematuria, weight loss, ± an abdominal mass. Treatment is surgical, but metastasis common at diagnosis—median survival is usually less than 4 months.

Investigations

U+E, Alb, FBC. 24h urinary volume (↑), spot osmolality or specific gravity (SG)—↓concentrating capacity. May be incomplete RTA (ur-pH ↑ with normal bicarb, 📖 p.556). USS if gross haematuria (papillary necrosis, PN ± obstruction, 📖 p.410). IVU may show clubbed calyces from PN, and isotope renography (DMSA) may confirm this. Flank pain and new haematuria may suggest renal vein thrombosis (📖 p.416) or renal medullary carcinoma.

Management

No specific therapy prevents the disease—aim to limit sickle crises, and prevent infection. Encourage fluids for target UO >2L/day.
- Massive haematuria (?PN)
    - Bed rest.
    - Vigourous IV hydration with 0.45% NaCl.
    - In resistant cases, consider transfusion ± tranexamic acid (1g tds po)—consider renal angiography and embolization.
- Progression
    - ACEI (◆ unproven) to maximum tolerated dose to ↓proteinuria (📖 p.150).

ESRD in sickle cell disease

Anaemia may be resistant to EPO, and patients remain transfusion-requiring. Patients may become iron overloaded—desferrioxamine chelation may be useful.

4.2% of patients with sickle cell disease progress to requiring dialysis. Dialysis by either HD or PD is well-tolerated, and survival no different to the non-diabetic population as a whole.

Renal transplantation is successful with graft survival is comparable at one year with the general transplant population. Recurrent disease (usually mild) is likely.

Vasculitis and renal disease

The systemic vasculitides are a group of inflammatory diseases of unknown cause, which are often fatal if untreated. The term 'vasculitis' simply reflects the underlying process: inflammation and leucocyte infiltration of the walls of blood vessels. This may lead to local inflammation (e.g. purpura), vessel wall damage (aneurysm formation or haemorrhage), or vessel occlusion (ischaemia or infarction).

Some vasculitides do not present with renal impairment—however, most of the potentially fatal diseases do. This may present as gradually progressive CRF or oligo-anuric ARF with life-threatening multi-system involvement.

⚠ When considering a diagnosis of vasculitis, 3 important differential diagnoses ALWAYS need to considered:
- ▶ Infective endocarditis
- Systemic or occult infection
- Paraneoplastic states

A brief primer on vasculitides
- Takayasu's arteritis affects the thoracic aorta and its branches in ♀, presenting with ↑BP, pulse deficits, and ischaemic limbs or viscera (brain, heart, lungs, gut).
- Giant cell arteritis (temporal arteritis) presents in older patients with headache, jaw claudication, visual symptoms and myalgia.
- Kawasaki's disease affects children, presenting as a febrile illness with lymphadenopathy, skin rash, conjunctivitis and mucositis (lips, tongue).
- Classical polyarteritis nodosa (🕮 p.464).
- Churg Strauss syndrome (🕮 p.462).
- ANCA-positive small vessel vasculitis (🕮 p.458).
- Henoch–Schönlein purpura (🕮 p.375).
- Cryoglobulinaemia (🕮 p.484).
- Other vasculitides include:
  - In association with other auto-immune diseases (SLE, RA, Sjogren's, Behçet's).
  - Hypersensitivity vasculitis (related to drug reactions).
  - In association with viral infection (hepatitis B+C, CMV, EBV and others).

All vasculitides tend to present with constitutional symptoms (fever, weight loss, malaise)—there is often myalgia ± arthralgia, and may be a skin rash (described as a leucocytoclastic vasculitis on biopsy). Acute phase markers (ESR, CRP, ferritin) are usually elevated. The size of vessel and organ affected will then dictate how the disease presents and evolves.

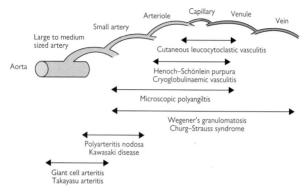

Fig. 7.3 Chapel Hill classification of vasculitis based on the size of vessel

Modified with permission from Jeanette JC, Falk RJ, Andrassy K et al. (1994) Nomenclature of systemetic vasculitides. Proposal of an international consensus conference. *Arthritis Rheum* **37**: 187–92.

ANCA-positive vasculitis

Small-vessel vasculitides characterized by the presence of anti-neutrophil cytoplasmic antibodies (ANCA), a group including Wegener's granulomatosis (WG), microscopic polyangitis (MPA) and renal-limited vasculitis (see below). Churg–Strauss syndrome, often ANCA+, is dealt with elsewhere (📖 p.462). Affects ± 20pmp (in Europe), ♂ = ♀, with an increasing incidence with age (peak 55–70). Wide geographic, ethnic and seasonal differences are described. Untreated, prognosis is poor (90% mortality at 2 years) – with immunosuppression, the outlook is good (70–80% 1 year patient survival). However, aggressive disease remains difficult to treat, and treatment-related morbidity is substantial.

Symptoms and signs

Fever, weight loss, malaise. Myalgia and a flitting polyarthralgia. Other features depend on affected system:

- Upper respiratory tract (► usually WG): nasal discharge, epistaxis, sinusitis, oral or nasal ulcers, otitis media (deafness), cartilaginous involvement (collapse of nasal bridge and tracheal stenosis).
- Lungs: cough, dyspnoea, haemoptysis → pulmonary haemorrhage.
- Kidney: asymptomatic urinary abnormalities to a rapidly progressive GN and ARF.
- Skin: palpable purpura or diffuse fine vasculitic rash.
- Mononeuritis multiplex presenting as peripheral neuropathy.
- Eyes: conjunctivitis, episcleritis, uveitis. Optic tract granulomata and proptosis (WG).
- Gut: abdominal pain and bloody diarrhea.
- Deep vein thrombosis appears to be more common.

Investigations

Urine dipstick, microscopy for red cell casts, 24hr proteinuria or PCR. FBC (↓Hb, ↑Plt). U+E, Alb, LFT. ↑ESR, ↑CRP. ANCA, antiGBM ('double positive ANCA+ and AGBM+ disease occurs, and behaves like Goodpasture's disease). Full GN screen, 📖 p.84. Complement normal.

CXR may show patchy or diffuse alveolar shadowing—cavitation is characteristic of WG. If ↓O_2 saturation, ABG. If able, lung function testing with transfer factor (KCO): free blood (Hb) in alveoli will bind CO artefactually ↑KCO > 100% expected.

Skin biopsy will suggest leucocytoclastic vasculitis without immune deposits. Renal biopsy is important prognostically and diagnostically.

Histology

A focal and segmental necrotizing, crescentic glomerulonephritis is apparent, ± granulomatous small vessel vasculitis. On IF no immune complex or complement deposition is seen, i.e. 'pauci-immune'. The presence of renal (or other tissue) granuloma formation is characteristic of WG.

Renal-limited vasculitis refers to a pauci-immune GN (as above) in patients who are often ANCA-positive, but have no systemic disease.

Does discriminating WG from MPA matter?

Perhaps not—treatment is similar, and the clinical and serological presentation overlaps often enough to conclude they may be a spectrum of disease rather than distinct entities.

	WG	MPA
ENT involvement	Yes	No
ANCA specificity	c-ANCA (PR3)	p-ANCA (MPO)
Granulomata	Yes	No
Likelihood of relapse	High	Lower

A–Z of ANCA

Anti-neutrophil cytoplasmic antibodies are antibodies directed against intracellular antigens, most commonly proteinase-3 (PR3) or myeloperoxidase (MPO). On immunofluorescence, the cytoplasmic or c-ANCA is now known to be PR3, and the perinuclear or p-ANCA is MPO. Antigen-specific ELISA testing has improved assay reliability, and a positive ANCA is 99% specific and 70% sensitive in the right clinical context.

▶ Low titre ANCA–positivity is recognized with other connective tissue disorders, or systemic infection. Higher titre ANCA-positivity is also recognized with drug-induced vasculitis (esp. anti-thyroid drugs).

Does ANCA cause disease?

In mice, evoking ANCA causes a systemic small vessel vasculitis. In humans, we do not yet know if ANCA is pathogenic, or an epiphenomenon. More is known about how ANCA may contribute to disease.

It is thought that ANCA+ vasculitis is a 'two-hit' disease: the release of local or systemic pro-inflammatory cytokines (esp. TNF) in response to infection (nasal *S. aureus* carriage, viral infection) primes neutrophils (→ surface expression of MPO and PR-3) and activates endothelial cells. ANCA binds primed neutrophils, increasing:

- Neutrophil tethering and migration on and across endothelium.
- Neutrophil degranulation → secondary recruitment of monocytes.
- Augmentation of inflammation and endothelial cell injury through free radical generation.

Treatment of ANCA-positive vasculitis

Both the disease and the highly toxic therapy may cause morbidity or death. Balance the risk and benefit in pursuing treatment. For a full discussion on starting immunosuppression, (📖 p.370). (► Preventative and protective measures that should be taken when using immunosuppressants.)

Induction therapy (to achieve remission)

Prednisolone:
- *If rapidly ↑Cr, Cr > 500 or pulmonary haemorrhage,* 'pulse methylprednisolone' as 500mg—1g in 100mL 0.9% NaCl IVI over 30 min x 3days, then po steroid as below.
- Prednisolone at 1mg/kg/day, aiming to taper ↓10–15mg/month (but not less than 7.5mg/day at 6 months).

Cyclophosphamide.
- Oral 1–2mg/kg/day (to a maximum of 150mg) for 3–6 months.
- An alternative is monthly IVI cyclophosphamide as IVI may be less toxic, but associated with higher rate of relapse.
- Toxicity is less usual if total dose <10g (📖 p.370).

Using this regimen, expect 90% clinical improvement and 75% complete remission in 75%—often takes 12 months or longer of therapy. In those who achieve remission earlier (i.e. at 12 weeks), cyclophosphamide may be discontinued, and maintenance therapy commenced.

> ## Plasma exchange
> ❧ The as yet unpublished MEPEX trial apparently recommends PEX if:
> - Pulmonary haemorrhage
> - Dialysis-requiring or Cr > 500
> - Co-existing anti-GBM antibodies.
> Treat for 5–7 consecutive days as 4L plasma exchange (2–3L of 4.5% human albumin with 1–2L FFP) and re-assess for benefit.

Maintenance therapy (to maintain in remission)
- Continue prednisolone at 7.5–15mg/day po.
- Convert cyclophosphamide to azathioprine 1.5–2mg/kg/day po (or perhaps mycophenolate mofetil [MMF] 0.5–1.5gbd po).

The risk of relapse is ± 25–50% within 3–5 years, and is more likely if:
- Wegener's
- Persistently positive high titre ANCA (esp. anti-PR3).

❧ It is not known how long to continue therapy for: most would treat for at least 2 years, and consider discontinuation of immunosuppression in those in prolonged remission. However, many would treat for 5 years or more, esp. if Wegener's.

Monitoring response and predicting relapse

Disease remission may be judged by:
- Clinical assessment (absence of symptoms)
- Urinary abnormalities (↓haematuria, ↓proteinuria)
- ↓CRP
- Improving renal function.

The Birmingham Vasculitis Activity Score (BVAS) provides a good tool for monitoring Wegener's.

A rising ANCA titre may predict relapse, but there is no role for presumptively increasing immunosuppression in the absence of other (clinical) features of ↑disease activity.

Relapse should be treated as for first presentation. Novel therapies are being investigated for resistant or frequently relapsing disease, including rituximab (anti-CD20 antibody) and deoxyspergualin. Etanercept (anti-TNF-α antibody) has not proved useful in maintaining remission, but such therapies may yet have a role in inducing remission in difficult disease.

Churg–Strauss syndrome

CSS is a rare multi-system disorder presenting as allergic rhinitis, asthma, and eosinophilia, with a small- and medium-vessel vasculitis affecting predominantly the lungs and skin. ♂ = ♀, aged 30–50 (unlike Wegener's or MPA, 📖 p.458). The cause remains unknown.

Symptoms and signs

Disease evolves from an atopic prodrome to a life-threatening systemic vasculitis. Allergic rhinitis or other atopic conditions ± late-onset asthma precedes vasculitis by weeks to years. Often steroid-requiring or severe.

Vasculitis presents as fever, malaise, weight loss. Myalgia ± polyarthralgia. Skin rash (urticarial or vasculitic) ± mononeuritis multiplex common.

Visceral involvement includes:
- Lungs: dyspnoea, haemoptysis.
- Kidneys: urinary abnormalities common, though renal impairment usually mild. ↑BP is common (presumably renal ischaemia).
- Gut: abdominal pain and bloody diarrhea ± ischaemic bowel.
- Heart: coronary vasculitis (angina), myocarditis (LVF) or pericarditis (⚠ even tamponade).

Investigations

- Urine dipstick, microscopy for red cells and casts PCR or, 24hr proteinuria.
- FBC (↓Hb) and prominent eosinophilia (>10% total WCC, or absolute count >1.5 x 10⁹/L) or eosinophilic-rich infiltrates on biopsy of affected tissues.

▶ Eosinophilia is exquisitely steroid-sensitive, and may resolve rapidly on treatment.

↑ESR, ↑CRP, immunoglobulins (?↑IgE). U+E, Alb, LFT, CK. CXR (flitting, patchy infiltration) ± ABG. ECG, echocardiogram. ANCA positive in 45% (either specificity, 📖 p.459).

Tissue biopsy may be required: classically shows eosinophil-rich granulomatous inflammation, and if vessels are sampled, a small to medium vessel necrotizing vasculitis. Renal biopsy may show vasculitis ± focal and segmental necrotizing GN, though with an eosinophilic infiltrate and granuloma formation in the interstitium.

Treatment

Prednisolone po 1mg/kg/day for 6–12 weeks or until remission. If full remission achieved, discontinue steroids, and monitor for relapse using:
- Eosinophil count
- Acute phase reactants (ESR, CRP)
- ▶ ANCA positivity does not predict disease activity.

Relapse can be expected in ± 25% of cases. Difficult to control disease may be treated by add-on cyclophosphamide (📖 p.460), interferon-∝.

Classical polyarteritis nodosa

A rare medium-vessel necrotizing arteritis involving principally the skin, nerves, gut and kidney. It is *not* synonymous with microscopic polyangitis, one of the ANCA-positive *small* vessel vasulitides ([□] p.456). It may be associated with hepatitis B infection. ♂ = ♀. Onset 40–60 years.

Symptoms and signs

Fever, weight loss (>4kg), arthralgia, and myalgia. Mononeuritis multiplex (peripheral neuropathy) or livedo reticularis. Medium vessel involvement in the gut presents as abdominal pain, or bloody stool. May be testicular pain (epididymo-orchitis). Renal ischaemia → ↑BP and renal impairment. May be haematuria or loin pain with segmental renal infarcts.

Investigations

U+E, Alb, LFT, ↑CK (muscle injury). FBC, ↑ESR. ANCA negative. Hepatitis B (positive in a minority). Diagnosis is made on angiography: arterial aneurysms in the renal or mesenteric tree. Renal biopsy may show segmental transmural fibrinoid necrosis in medium-sized arteries, but may sample downstream ischaemic changes or frank infarction alone. There should not be any glomerulonephritis.

Management and natural history

Untreated, prognosis is poor. With therapy, 10-year patient survival is approximately 80%. Risk factors associated with poor outcome include:

- Age > 50 years
- Renal impairment
- Gut or coronary involvement.
- Low risk: prednisolone 1mg/kg/day against clinical and biochemical response.
- High risk: as above, + oral cyclophosphamide 1–2mg/kg/day (limit to 150mg daily). See [□] p.370 for starting immunosuppression.
- If HBsAg positive, short-term prednisolone followed by interferon-α and plasma exchange.

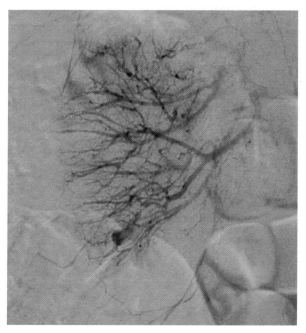

Fig. 7.4 Medium vessel aneurysms in the kidneys at ateriography. Reproduced with permission from Wu K and Throssell D (2006) *Nephrology Dialysis Transplantation* **21**(6): 1710–12

Goodpasture's disease

Also known as anti-GBM disease, a rare pulmonary renal syndrome presenting as a rapidly progressive GN and pulmonary haemorrhage. It has an incidence in Europe of ± 0.5pmp (and is more common in whites), and affects two groups: ♂ aged 20–30, or ♂ and ♀ > 60 years.

Pathogenesis

Pathogenic IgG anti-GBM antibodies against the α3 chain of type IV collagen (found in the basement membranes of the glomerulus and alveolus) cause disease. A trigger (?cigarette smoking, ?other environmental) exposes antigenic epitopes on the normally 'hidden' α3 chain. On binding, anti-GBM antibodies fix complement and cause local injury.

Symptoms and signs

May present gradually (over months–years), or abruptly over days with fulminant lung haemorrhage and renal failure. Severe pulmonary haemorrhage may present with profuse bright red haemoptysis and respiratory failure requiring intubation and ventilation—usually in smokers.

Fever and loss of weight may be present, but few other 'constitutional symptoms'. Dyspnoea and cough (non-productive → flecking or frank haemoptysis). Haematuria and proteinuria on dipstick.

Investigations

Urine for microscopy (red cells, casts), 24h proteinuria. U+E. Alb. LFT. FBC (↓Hb). Complement normal. ANCA (25% 'double positive'—treat as for anti-GBM, but expect better outcome). Anti-GBM and titre: by IF and ELISA. CXR (diffuse alveolar shadowing), ABG (↓pO$_2$). ↑KCO on pulmonary function testing if alveolar blood. Proceed to renal biopsy.

Histology

A focal and segmental necrotizing, crescentic GN. Bowman's capsule may be ruptured. IF shows *linear* capillary wall staining for anti-GBM (IgG) and C3 deposition in a similar pattern.

Treatment

⚠ Oligo-anuria (<200mL/day) or Cr >500 implies severe crescentic glomerular damage and a poor renal outlook. Once dialysis requiring, renal recovery is very unusual. Therapy should include:
- Pulsed methylprednisolone 0.5–1g daily in 100mL 0.9% NaCl over 30 min x 3days. Then prednisolone 1 mg/kg/day (to a maximum 60mg)
- Cyclophophamide 1–2mg/kg/day (to a maximum of 150mg)

Continue prednisolone + cyclophosphamide for 3–6 months.
And *unless* dialysis-requiring (when it offers little *renal* benefit):
- Plasma exchange as 8–10 treatments in < 2 weeks of 4L (by volume, $^2/_3$ 4.5% human albumin solution, $^1/_3$ FFP). Check anti-GBM titre weekly to confirm efficacy of therapy.

Treating pulmonary haemorrhage

▶ Differentiating pulmonary oedema from pulmonary haemorrhage can be difficult. Always aim to dry such patients out.

- Transfer to ITU for invasive monitoring.
- May (often do) require intubation, ventilation.
- Institute early plasma exchange as above in *all* cases.

Treatment is continues until anti-GBM titre negative: this may take up to 12 weeks (but may be very rapid with plasma exchange. The disease does not usually recur, and immunosuppression can be discontinued. Cigarette smoking should be discouraged, as it may be related with rare relapse.

Renal transplantation is the best treatment for ESRD 2° Goodpasture's—it should be deferred until six months after anti-GBM is negative. *De novo* anti-GBM disease can cause graft loss in ESRD patients transplanted for Alport's syndrome (📖 p.382).

Lupus nephritis

Systemic lupus erythematosus is a heterogenous multi-system disease characterized by autoantibody production and impaired immune complex clearance. SLE is more common in Afro-Caribbean, Hispanic, or Asian ♀ (10♀:1♂) presenting in youth/young adulthood (although autoantibodies pre-date disease). ~50% patients will develop renal involvement within 3 years of diagnosis, and ~10% progress to ESRD by 10 years.

How do autoantibodies arise in SLE?

Genetic and environmental factors influence risk for developing lupus. Loss of tolerance to self-antigens is the primary driver in the aetiology of SLE—a wide range of interacting immune defects has been described as resulting from this. *Part* of the explanation goes thus: apoptosis (programmed cell death) is part of normal cell replacement.

Faulty phagocytosis/clearance of apoptotic waste → nucleosomal (and other) proteins being engulfed by circulating B cells. Processed peptides are presented to histone-specific CD4+ T cells, which in conjunction with appropriate co-stimulation (📖 p.240) → cytokine-dependent autoreactive B cell activation with auto-antibody production. Usually, IL-2-mediated pathways are responsible for the elimination of these autoreactive lymphocytes: patients with SLE have low T cell IL-2 production.

Diagnosing SLE

The American College of Rheumatology offer clinically useful criteria: ▶ >3 criteria is diagnostic, but many with 2–3 criteria will evolve over time to develop full-blown SLE.

Malar rash	Fixed erythematous ('butterfly') rash
Discoid rash	Raised erythematous patches that may scar
Photosensitivity	
Oral ulcers	Painless (may be nasopharyngeal)
Arthritis	Non-erosive, x 2 more peripheral joints
Serositis	Pleural or pericardial (pain), rub or effusion
Renal disease	Urinary red cell casts or proteinuria > 0.5g/day
CNS disease	Psychosis or seizures
Blood disorder	Haemolysis, ↓WCC, ↓Plt or lymphopaenia
Immunology	Positive anticardiolipin, anti-dsDNS or anti-Sm antibodies, or false positive syphilis serology
Anti-nuclear factor	

Other clinical features include constitutional symptoms (fever, weight loss, fatigue), lymphadenopathy, Raynaud's phenomenon, scleritis or sicca symptoms, polyarthralgia, myalgia, pneumonitis, interstitial lung disease (or pulmonary hypertension), sterile (Libman–Sacks) endocarditis, or vascular thrombosis (► antiphospholipid syndrome).

Investigations

FBC (Hb↓, ↓Plt, lymphopaenia), ↑↑ESR. Screen for haemolysis (including Coombs' test). U+E, Ca^{2+}, LFT, CK.
► CRP is *normal* in active lupus, but may ↑ if infection complicates SLE. A clinically useful tool for differentiating infection from flare!
ANF, dsDNA (may be useful to monitor response to treatment), anti-Ro and –La, anti-Smith, anticardiolipin antibodies. Complement (active disease → ↓C3/C4).
  Urine dipstick, microscopy for dysmorphic red cells or casts (📖 p.12), 24h proteinuria. USS kidneys ± renal biopsy: indicated if haematuria (esp. PCR or if rbc casts), >300mg proteinuria/day ± ↓ GFR.

Pathogenesis and histology of lupus nephritis

Circulating (or locally derived) immune complexes fix within the glomerulus, activating (and consuming) complement. Recruited monocytes and leucocytes → pro-inflammatory cytokines, neutrophil-induced oxidant injury and activation of the coagulation cascade. The histology that results is often varied. Characteristic deposition of IgG- and complement-rich (C3 and C1q) immune deposits in the mesangium or subendothelial space. A lupus membranous-like lesion is characterized by deposits in the subepithelial space. The histological lesion has important therapeutic and prognostic implications.

ISN/RPS classification of lupus nephritis

I	Normal light microscopy (but mesangial deposits → EM)
II	Mesangial proliferation (hypercellularity)
III	Focal involvement: affecting < 50% of glomeruli
IV	Diffuse involvement affecting > 50% of glomeruli, either segmentally (IV-S) or globally (IV-G)
V	Membranous change (subepithelial deposits)
VI	Advanced sclerosis with > 90% glomeruli obsolescent

Class III or IV is further subclassified as active or chronic (e.g. Type IV-GA is an active global diffuse proliferative lesion)

Management of lupus nephritis

✒ How to treat LN is mired in controversy, and poorly directed by good clinical trials. Only the aims of treatment are clear:
- Identify those most at (renal) risk.
- Induce (renal) disease remission (only 80% will achieve remission).
- Maintain (renal) disease remission (relapse can be expected in 30%).
- Prevent CKD → ESRD.
- Minimize drug toxicity (in the short- and longer-term).

Those at risk

▶ Type I (and some say type II) LN is rarely an indication for treatment in its own right (may be required for other involved organs). Types III–V require treatment. Predictors of ↑renal risk include:
- Afro-Caribbean or Hispanic (esp. if male).
- Poor socio-economic status.
- Renal impairment, neuropsychiatric, or other severe extra-renal disease.
- High activity or chronicity index on biopsy.
- Poor response to therapy or frequent relapse.

Inducing remission (⚠ 📖 p.370 for using IVI cyclophosphamide)

- Type II LN ± risk factors:
  - Prednisolone 1mg/kg/day for 4–8 weeks ↓ to 7.5mg od over months against activity
  - If no response or progressive disease add in *either* azathioprine 1.5–2mg/kg/day *or* mycophenolate mofetil 0.5–1.0g bd.
- Type III or IV (or mixed type III or IV with V):
  - *either* pulsed methylprednisolone 0.5–1g in 100 mL 0.9% NaCl for three days followed by prednisolone as below,
  - *or* prednisolone 1 mg/kg/day od for 4–8 weeks tapering *slowly* to 7.5mg od over months against disease activity
  - If no response, or severe disease, *add in* one of 4 regimes:
    1. IVI cyclophosphamide 750mg/m^2 in 250mL 0.9% NaCl over 30 min monthly for 6 months (check WCC at day10–14). ↑dose to 1g/m^2 if possible. If GFR < 60 mL/min, ↓ dose to 500 mg/m^2.
    2. IVI cyclophosphamide regimen monthly 500mg fixed dosing rather than /m^2 as above.
    3. ▶ Oral cyclophosphamide to induce remission at 1.5–2 mg/kg/day. Patients showing prompt response can transfer to maintenance therapy after as little as 4–8 weeks (▶ MMF) avoiding the higher toxicity seen with prolonged oral cyclophosphamide. The need to achieve remission often outweighs risks, and much longer periods of oral cyclophosphamide may be required.
    4. ▶ Mycophenolate mofetil 0.5–1g bd is a real alternative for induction to cyclophosphamide, though *perhaps* with ↑ relapse risk.
- Type V:
  - Prednisolone 1mg/kg/day for 4–8 weeks ↓ to 7.5mg by 6 months
  - Depending on severity, or lack of response, *add on either* azathioprine 1.5–2mg/kg/day, ciclosporin 5mg/kg in two divided doses, MMF or cyclophosphamide as above.

Maintaining remission

If signs of remission, consider switching from intermittent (or oral) cyclo-phosphamide to *either*:

- Azathioprine 1.5–2mg/kg/day.
- *or* mycophenolate mofetil 0.5–1.0g bd.
- *continue* lower dose (± 0.15mg/kg/day) prednisolone.

Prevent CKD → ESRD

- Stop smoking, limit salt and exercise.
- Control BP <130/80.
- If proteinuric >1g/day, use ACEI ± ARB.
- Treat dyslipidaemia with statins.

Minimize toxicity see 📖 p.370

Monitoring disease activity

- Symptoms
- Urinary sediment (↓proteinuria <0.5g/day, ↓rbc/hpf <10)
- Cr
- ESR (and CRP to exclude infective complication)
- Anti-dsDNA antibody titre
- Complement.

More experimental therapies

- ▶ Rituximab is increasingly used for resistant disease and even as initiation therapy. No trial data yet though.
- Immunoablative cyclophosphamide and rescue GCSF.
- Abatacept (CTLA4Ig).
- Interferon-α.
- Watch the literature, as much is expected of clinical trials using these agents.

Antiphospholipid syndrome

Antibodies directed against the phospholipid components of coagulation factors → recurrent arterial and venous thrombosis. Initially described in association with SLE, unrelated primary APS is an increasingly recognized entity, and frequently found in conjunction with renal disease.

Described antibodies may directed against:
- Cardiolipin (a phospholipid)
- β2 glycoprotein I (binds to cardiolipin)
- Prothrombin

Often found in conjunction with the lupus anticoagulant.

Symptoms and signs
- DVT, spontaneous superficial thrombophlebitis ± pulmonary emboli
- Arterial thrombosis: TIA, RIND or stroke
- Livedo reticularis (~ 20%)
- Recurrent miscarriage
- ↑BP (~ 30%)
- Features of SLE (📖 p.468) or other connective tissue disorder
- Sterile (Libman–Sacks) endocarditis.

The renal lesion tends to be an ischaemic nephropathy (i.e. small vessel renovascular disease, 📖 p.412, with ↓GRF and bland urine). Less commonly, the APS may present acutely with a thrombotic microangiopathy (📖 p.400).

Investigations
- FBC (↓Hb, ▶ ↓Plt), evidence of haemolysis (↑LDH, ↑Bili). Clotting (↑APTT). U+E.
- ANF, dsDNA, complement, RhF. False positive syphilis serology.
- Testing for antibodies:
  - Positive IgM anticardiolipin antibodies at titre > 50
  - Positive IgG anticardiolipin antibodies at tire > 80
  - Positive lupus anticoagulant (failure to correct prolonged APTT after mixing with normal plasma)
  - Positive anti-β2 glycoprotein I antibodies

A single positive test is insufficient to make the diagnosis—needs repeating after 6 weeks (and can be done on warfarin)

Treatment

20–30% of untreated APS patients will have a further thrombotic event. Evidence is modest, but consensus suggests:
- Lifelong warfarin for INR 2–3.
- If new event on warfarin, aim for target INR 3–4.
- In those with positive antibodies, but no (diagnostic) thrombotic event, prophylactic aspirin seems sensible

Anti-phospholipid antibodies in ESRD
- May be found at a high prevalence in haemodialysis patients.
- Appear to predict increased AVF stenosis and failure.
- Increase the risk of early transplant failure due to graft renal artery or vein thrombosis, a risk only partly ↓ by anticoagulation.

Scleroderma renal crisis

Systemic sclerosis (SS) or scleroderma frequently involves the kidneys—scleroderma renal crisis, however, affects far fewer (5–10%). SS characteristically causes sclerosis of the skin and subcutaneous tissue, and an obliterative vasculopathy. It may be diffuse (traditional scleroderma), or limited (used to be 'CREST' syndrome). Other skin-limited varieties are also described.

- Diffuse: ↑skin fibrosis score (sclerosis beyond the hands and face), frequent solid organ involvement, positive anti-scl-70 antibodies, anti-RNP).
- Limited: ↓skin fibrosis score (hands and face affected), unusual solid organ involvement, positive anti-centromere antibodies.

Symptoms and signs of SS

Patchy skin oedema → fibrosis and calcinosis ± digital ulceration. Peri-orbital tethering and microstomia, nasal beaking, and tapering of the fingers (sclerodactyly). Raynaud's phenomenon, facial and limb telangiectasia, non-erosive arthritis, and myalgia. Oesophageal (and intestinal) dysmotility. Pulmonary fibrosis and pulmonary hypertension.

Scleroderma renal crisis

Severe and life-threatening renal disease develops in 12% of patients with diffuse disease, but only 1% of those with limited SS. Characterized by:

- Acute renal failure
- ↑BP (can be *normotensive* though with marked vessel changes)
- Bland urine

May be accelerated ↑BP (📖 p.350) with hypertensive encephalopathy or acute LV failure, ± thrombotic microangiopathy (📖 p.400).

Investigations

- Immediate:
  - FBC (↓Hb, ↓Plts), blood film (?fragments), ↑LDH, ↓haptoglobins.
  - U+E, Alb, LFT. Urine microscopy, 24h urine protein.
  - USS kidneys (proceed to renal biopsy once BP controlled).
- Evaluate end-organ hypertensive damage:
  - Fundoscopy for hypertensive retinopathy.
  - ECG (LVH ± strain), echocardiogram.
- To confirm systemic sclerosis:
  - Nail-fold capillaroscopy (dilated capillaries).
  - ANF, anti-topoisomerase I (also called anti-Scl70), anti-centromere antibody, anti-RNA polymerase antibodies.

Renal histology

Within vessels, fibrinoid necrosis and fibrin thombi, with 'onion-skin' intimal thickening. Varying degrees of collapsed and ischaemic glomeruli or ATN.

Management

Admit high dependency unit
- Cardiac monitor.
- Strict input and output (indwelling catheter).
- Arterial line for invasive BP monitoring if severe ↑BP.
▶ BP control with ACEI is the mainstay of therapy.
ACEI have reduced mortality in renal crises from 80% to 15%. Good BP control can prevent further renal deterioration, or even aid renal recovery and dialysis-independence. Progression to ESRD occurs in 20–50%.
- Start captopril (short-acting) 12.5–50mg po tds.
- Add in calcium-channel blockers.
- Aim BP reduction 10–15mmHg/day.
- Target diastolic BP 85–90mmHg.
- Avoid β-blockers.

Unproven interventions include IVI prostacyclin infusion for 24–48h or fish oils (as for IgAN, 📖 p.374).
⚠ If ACEI do not provide adequate BP control, or if complicated hypertensive emergency (seizures, acute LVF), haemofiltration is effective at controlled BP reduction.

All SS patients should have urine dipstick and BP measured 3-monthly. ↑BP should be treated with ACEI as a first-line.

Rheumatoid arthritis

Renal conditions complicating RA
- Secondary membranous nephropathy (MN)
- Renal amyloidosis (AA amyloid)
- Analgesic nephropathy (NSAIDs)
- Rheumatoid vasculitis
- Other glomerular lesions.

2° MN (📖 p.394)
Presents with proteinuria (less commonly nephrotic syndrome), usually due to disease-modifying drugs (gold, penicillamine), timed with starting therapy (6–12months). Stopping the drugs → remission (may take up to 1 year).

Renal amyloidosis (📖 p.450)
Presents with nephrotic range proteinuria, often normotensive. Long history of poorly-controlled active RA, often sero-positive (RhF+)

Analgesic nephropathy (📖 p.410)
May present as papillary necrosis, or insidious renal impairment with bland urine.

Rheumatoid vasculitis
A small and medium vessel vasculitis affecting sero-positive patients, often with rheumatoid nodules. Presents as a skin leucocytoclastic vasculitis and mononeuritis multiplex (peripheral neuropathy). The renal lesion is a pauci-immune necrotizing glomerulonephritis. ↑ESR, ↑↑RhF. ↓C_3, ↓C_4. ANCA may be positive.
⚠ It is an aggressive and life-threatening complication—treat as for ANCA positive small vessel vasculitis with corticosteroids and cyclophosphamide (📖 p.460).

Glomerular lesions
A mesangio-proliferative GN (≈ IgAN, 📖 p.374) may also occur, presenting with an active urinary sediment, and less commonly, renal impairment.

Other connective tissue disorders associated with renal disease

- Sjogren's syndrome may present with:
  - Type 1 renal tubular acidosis (📖 p.556)
  - Impaired concentrating ability (nephrogenic DI, 📖 p.527)
  - Acute interstitial nephritis (📖 p.406).
- Mixed connective tissue disorder is associated with:
  - Membranous nephropathy (📖 p.392).
  - MCGN (📖 p.380).
- Polymyositis and dermatomyositis.

Myositis and myoglobinuria may lead to false-positive haematuria (📖 p.12), or less commonly, ARF 2° rhabdomyolysis.

Almost all connective tissue disorders may have a degree of overlap, or present atypically—renal disease is not uncommon, and kidney biopsy is often indicated in patients with urinary abnormalities, ↑ BP or renal impairment.

Sarcoidosis

Sarcoidosis is a multi-system granulomatous disease of unknown cause, usually affecting the chests of young men. It is characterized by non-caseating granulomata. Renal disease complicates sarcoidosis in up to 40% of cases (although often subclinical).

Symptoms and signs

Sarcoid is the great mimicker of the post-syphilis era, involving anything and everything.

- Lymph adenopathy, fevers, loss of weight, malaise.
- Chest: bilateral hilar lymphadenopathy, infiltrates, pulmonary fibrosis.
- Eyes: uveitis, keratoconjunctivitis sicca.
- Skin: pigmentary changes, lupus pernio, erythema nodosum.
- Cardiac: conduction defects, arrythmias (▶ VT), cardiomyopathy.
- CNS: mononeuritis multiplex, aseptic meningitis, pituitary infiltration (cranial DI, 📖 p.527), or neurosarcoidosis presenting like multiple sclerosis.
- Liver: granulomatous hepatitis.
- Kidney: granulomatous tubulo-interstitial nephritis, ↑Ca^{2+}.

Investigations

- Dipstick urine (often bland), urine microscopy (?crystals) and 24h proteinuria (<1g/day). FBC (↓Plt, lymphopaenia), ↑ESR.
- U+E, Alb, LFT. ↑Ca^{2+}, ↑urinary Ca^{2+}.
- Consider intact PTH (↓), calcitriol. Polyclonal ↑Ig, ↑serum angiotensin converting enzyme, ACE (produced by granulomata).
- CXR (?bilateral hilar lymphadenopathy, diffuse nodular infiltrates), pulmonary function tests ± high resolution CT chest.
- Lymph node, salivary gland, skin or kidney biopsy.

Calcium homeostasis in sarcoidosis

Activated macrophages within granulomata convert 25-(OH) vitamin D_3 to its active metabolite, 1,25-$(OH)_2$ vitamin D_3, particularly during sunny months. This leads to increased gut calcium uptake, resulting in:

- Hypercalciuria (50%)
- Hypercalcaemia (10–20%)
- Calcium-containing renal calculi or nephrocalcinosis (📖 p.432).

In the renal tract, sarcoidosis may also be associated with:

- Diffuse nephrocalcinosis (▶ cause of ESRD)
- Retroperitoneal lymphadenopathy and obstruction
- Glomerulonephritis.

Granulomatous tubulo-interstitial nephritis

Presents as mild → progressive renal impairment with mild proteinuria or bland urine. Other features of sarcoidosis might suggest it as a cause, but biopsy often provides the diagnosis—histology shows a lymphocytic tubulo-interstitial infiltrate with non-caseating epitheloid granulomata. Differential diagnosis may include:

- TB (caseating granulomata!) or other infections
- Drug hypersensitivity (esp. NSAIDs).

↑Ca^{2+} may contribute to renal impairment, and rehydration is always sensible prior to therapy.

Management

- Rehydrate if ↑Ca^{2+} with 0.9% NaCl.
- Prednisolone 1mg/kg daily: renal fuction often improves rapidly.
- Taper once Cr stabilized: there are few accurate predictors of remission or relapse, so maintain high index of suspicion, and regular follow-up.

HIV and renal disease

Almost 40 million people worldwide are infected with the human immunodeficiency virus-1 (HIV). HIV is associated with almost every described renal lesion, but HIV-associated nephropathy (HIVAN) has been the most common renal lesion identified in such patients in the developed world. The renal complications of HIV elsewhere (and esp. in Africa) remain poorly described.

HIVAN

HIVAN results from direct HIV infection of renal proximal tubular cells and podocytes, causing the so-called collapsing variant of focal and segmental glomerulosclerosis (🕮 p.396) with cystic tubular dilatation. As HIV infection has burgeoned globally, HIVAN has become a significant cause of ESRD, particularly in black adults. It occurs once HIV infection is advanced (↓CD4 <200), often in the context of AIDS-defining illness.

Symptoms and signs

Oedema, nephrotic-range proteinuria and renal impairment (often due to super-added ATN) is common. BP is often normal.

Investigations

Microscopy may show broad, waxy casts, PCR or 24h proteinuria. U+E, ↓↓Alb, LFT. ↓CD4 count. Hepatitis B and C. USS kidneys (large echogenic kidneys). Renal biopsy shows FSGS (🕮 p.398). Characteristically, the glomerular tuft is collapsed with a wrinkled basement membrane and microcystic tubular dilatation. Tubular atrophy, interstitial infiltrates and fibrosis and oedema is common.

Management of HIVAN

Highly active anti-retroviral therapy (HAART), a three-drug regimen of 2 reverse transcriptase inhibitors and a protease inhibitor, has completely transformed the outlook in HIV-infected individuals. HAART appears to have similar effects on HIVAN:

- ↓proteinuria ± induce full/ partial remission of nephrotic syndrome
- Delay progression of renal impairment
- Promote renal recovery and dialysis-independence

ACEI may reduce proteinuria and delay progression.

⚫ Prednisolone has been used, but evidence to support its use is poor.

Other renal lesions found with HIV infection

In HIV+ patients with renal disease, 40% of lesions are *not* due to HIVAN, with wide ethnic and geographical variations.

- Other glomerulonephritis, often a diffuse proliferative GN (🕮 p.378)
- Thrombotic microangiopathy (🕮 p.400)
- Acute interstitial nephritis (🕮 p.406).

HAART-related renal side-effects

Common problems include:

- Indinavir (and acyclovir): crystalluria, stones, interstitial nephritis—consider change to another protease inhibitor?
- Cidofovir, adefovir, tenofovir: proximal tubular cell injury causing a Fanconi-like syndrome. Tenofovir is the least toxic nucleotide reverse transcriptase inhibitor
- *All* reverse transcriptase inhibitors may cause lactic acidosis, often severe, thought to occur through mitchondrial DNA damage.

HIV-infected patients with ESRD

Standard universal precautions—do not require isolation on haemodialysis. Survival on either HD or CAPD seems comparable. Renal transplantation is increasingly thought to improve patients survival compared to dialysis, but patient selection is important. Those with stable disease, compliant on medication, with low viral load and preserved CD4 counts can be referred for consideration—drug interactions and toxicities are a major challenge.

Hepatitis B-related renal disease

Hepatitis B (HBV) affects 350 million people world-wide, especially in Africa and SE Asia. It is a DNA virus transmitted from mothers to children, or between close (family) and sexual contacts.

In adults, an acute sero-conversion illness (with appearance of HBV surface antigen, HBsAg) follows 1–6 months after exposure. 90% of adults clear the virus (and develop immunity)—chronic carriers then remain at risk for hepatic and extra-hepatic complications.

▶ If acquired in childhood, chronic carriage is usual.

Chronic HBV (i.e. HBsAg positive) carriage is associated with renal disease—viral antigen (usually HBe antigen, HBeAg) and host antibody form immune complexes depositing in the kidney, causing injury. Three common nephropathies are described:

Membranous glomerulonephritis (MN)

Common in children between 2–12 years old (♂>♀), presenting with proteinuria. Usually HBeAg positive. Tends to remit spontaneously with clearance of HBeAg and development of anti-HBe antibodies.

Adults present with a chronic nephrotic syndrome, viral liver disease and progressive renal impairment. (📖 p.394).

Mesangiocapillary glomerulonephritis (MCGN)

Common in adults (>MN). Presents with ↑BP, heavy proteinuria, haematuria and progressive ↑Cr. HBsAg and anti-HB core antibody positive. Renal histology is similar to type 1 MCGN (📖 p.380). Unlike hepatitis C-associated MCGN, cryoglobulins are not detected.

Classical polyarteritis nodosa (PAN)

Occurs within 4 months of infection in adults, presenting as a medium vessel vasculitis (📖 p.464).

Investigations

Full hepatitis B serology (surface, e and core antigen and antibody), and if indicated HBV DNA load. Hep C ± HIV. U+E, alb, LFT. 24h proteinuria. Full GN screen. FBC, INR, cholesterol. USS liver and kidneys. Proceed to renal biopsy.

A brief primer: treatment of HBV-related liver disease

- Chronic HBeAg-, anti-HBe antibody+ carriers with normal ALT should be monitored 6 monthly for reactivation.
- HBeAg+ patients with >10^5 copies/mL HBV DNA and ↑ALT should have a liver biopsy.
- Treatments include oral lamivudine, interferon-α, or newer agents such as adefovir: combination therapy may provide the best option.

Treatment of HBV-associated GN in adults

Aim to clear the virus (HBsAg negative, undetectable viral DNA) and promote sero-conversion to immune status (anti-HBs antibody positive). Significant renal disease tends not to remit without treatment (and may progress)—liver disease may require treatment on its own merits. Response rates are higher in MN (than MCGN). Remission tends to follow clearance of HBeAg and the appearance of anti-HBe antibodies.

- Interferon-α_{2b} 5million U sc 3x/week for 4/12 (or longer) results in ± 50% response
- Lamivudine 100mg od (lamivudine-resistance develops in ~15%/year) *may* offer benefit, but trials are awaited

⚠ Avoid corticosteroids: ↑viral replication, and at withdrawal may be associated with hepatic failure. However, in classical PAN steroids ± plasma exchange is required, (📖 p.464).

The best means of controlling HBV-related renal disease is to prevent it. Offer vaccination against HBV to high risk individuals.
▶ Household contacts and family members of HBsAg positive patients should be vaccinated. Avoid alcohol and sharing blood-contaminated items (toothbrushes, etc). Use condoms.

Hepatitis B-infected patients with ESRD

Require isolation on haemodialysis units in addition to standard universal precautions. Dedicated machines should be used, and dialyzer re-use avoided. There is no contra-indication to CAPD in well patients. Transplantation is thought to offer a survival benefit over remaining on dialysis, but selecting appropriate patients requires full HBV serology testing, viral load, and may require liver biopsy to predict risk.

Yearly screening for hepatocellular carcinoma, with serum α-fetoprotein and USS liver should be performed in high risk patients (▶ ♂>45)

Hepatitis C-related renal disease

HCV is a RNA virus with 6 different genotypes, causing hepatitis, cirrhosis and hepatocellular carcinoma. It is transmitted parentally, affecting IV drug users and those accidentally infected through needle-sharing or blood products (prior to screening). Infection is mild and often subclinical after a long incubation period (6–9 weeks). 70–85% fail to clear acute infection and become chronic carriers. Chronic HCV and its associated mixed cryoglobulinaemia is now known to be the principal cause of type 1 MCGN (previously thought to be idiopathic).

HCV-related type 1 MCGN (🕮 p.380)

Cryoglobulins deposited in medium and small vessels in the skin, joints and glomeruli, fixing complement and causing local inflammation and injury leading to GN.

Symptoms and signs

Fatigue, weakness, weight loss. Episodic palpable purpuric rash on legs (leucocytoclastic vasculitis on biopsy), arthralgia, myalgia, and mononeuritis multiplex. Hepatosplenomegaly and Raynaud's phenomenon. May present as an acute and disseminated vasculitis. Renal manifestations include haematuria, proteinuria (often nephrotic range), ↑BP, renal impairment (may be progressive, or even present as ARF).

Investigations

Microscopy for red cells, casts, 24h proteinuria. U+E, Alb, LFT (↑ALT). FBC, ↑ESR. Rheumatoid factor (often positive, see below), cryoglobulins, serum immunoglobulins (polyclonal ↑), complement (normal C3, ↓C4). ANF, anti-smooth muscle antibodies (?auto-immune disease). USS liver and kidneys. Anti-HCV antibody ± PCR for HCV RNA. HCV genotyping. Hepatitis B and HIV. Renal biopsy (🕮 p.636).

Cryoglobulins

Are immunoglobulins which precipitate at <37°C, and dissolve once again on warming.

- Type I cryoglobulinaemia: a monoclonal immunoglobulin (IgG or IgM), associated with lymphoproliferative disease (myeloma, lymphoma, CLL, Waldenstrom's macroglobulinaemia).
- Type II: or mixed essential cryoglobulinaemia. Monoclonal IgM with polyclonal IgG, associated with hepatitis C infection or autoimmune disease. Hepatitis C enters host cells (hepatocytes and CD5+ B cells) via the LDL receptor—infected B cells are resistant to apoptosis, and increase production of auto-antibodies. This monoclonal IgM autoantibody is a *rheumatoid factor*, i.e. directed against the Fc portion of other immunoglobulins.
- Type III: polyclonal IgM directed against IgG (as above), found in low concentration and associated with viral infection and autoimmune disease. It is thought that type III evolves into type II with HCV over time.

Management

Most HCV-infected patients have evidence of liver disease, and seemingly normal hepatic function does not exclude the presence of HCV. Patients with HCV infection are generally treated with pegylated interferon-α and the oral anti-viral agent ribavirin (if renal function good) for 24–48 weeks. Of the 6 known HCV genotypes, types 2 and 3 are more responsive to therapy than types 1 or 4, with sustained virological response rates of 80% v 45%. Side-effects are common—haemolysis related to ribavirin is common.

▶ No known therapy specifically alters renal outcome in MCGN: although IFN may clear HCV and have modest effects on proteinuria and renal function, on cessation of treatment, HCV RNA and cryoglobulins return. Consider:

- EPO to maintain Hb >11g/dL (ribavirin induces red cell fragility)
- ACEI to limit proteinuria
- HMG-coA-reductase inhibitors if LFT normal.

Also recommend:

- Avoid alcohol
- Avoid sharing blood-contaminated items (toothbrushes, etc.)
- Use condoms.

Hepatitis C-infected patients with ESRD

- Standard universal precautions—do *not* require isolation on haemo dialysis (unlike Hep B). Check ALT 6-monthly.
- Yearly screening for hepatocellular carcinoma ± cirrhosis by USS liver and serum α-fetoprotein should be performed.
- Renal transplantation offers superior survival to maintenance HD or CAPD, but HCV+ transplant recipients do less well over the long-term than HCV- patients. A sub-group of HCV+ ESRD patients may benefit from anti-HCV treatment with pegylated-IFN prior to transplantation.

The kidney in infective endocarditis

Bacterial infection of any valve on either side of the heart may be complicated by renal disease, including:

- Post-infectious immune complex-mediated GN.
- Aminoglycoside-induced ATN.
- Renal emboli (off infected valves).
- Drug-induced AIN.

IE should be suspected in patient with a fever, new murmur, splenomegaly and haematuria, especially if known to have a valvular abnormality or prosthesis. Careful examination may reveal splinter haemorrhages, although classical stigmata of IE are often absent.

Common causes include *S. aureus* in acute IE, or viridans streptococci or coagulase negative staphylococci in more chronic IE.

▶ Repeated cultures and sensitivity testing are the key to management

The severity of the glomerulonephritis is related to the duration of infection prior to the institution of antibiotics. Control of infection usually leads to rapid resolution, with return of renal function to or near the previous baseline. However, irreversible renal failure can occur if appropriate therapy is delayed.

Symptoms and signs

- Urinary abnormalities and ↑Cr *at presentation* suggest GN, especially if improving with antibiotics. ↑Cr over time on antibiotics with bland urine → aminoglycoside toxicity. A new and persisting fever ± 10 days after starting antibiotics, especially if timed with a rash ± eosinophilia → AIN (📖 p.406). Check for historic aminoglycoside levels (?toxic).
- Renal emboli present as acute (unilateral) flank pain ± frank haematuria.
- May be peripheral emboli in other beds (▶ feet). May occur months after bacteriologic cure.

Investigations

- Repeated blood cultures, urgent echocardiography (?TOE).
- Dipstick, urine for microscopy (if sterile pyuria or eosinophiluria, ?AIN), 24h urinary proteinuria (>1g/day → GN). FBC (eosinophilia → AIN), ESR↑, U+E, Alb, CRP↑. Aminoglycoside levels.
- ↓C_3, ↑CICs, positive cryoglobulins, positive RhF if GN.
- USS kidneys ± DMSA for focal perfusions deficits (if emboli suspected).
- May require kidney biopsy if diagnosis unclear.

Histology

The histologic findings are similar to post-streptococcal glomerulonephritis (📖 p.378), AIN (📖 p.406), or ATN (📖 p.96).

Treatment

- If GN, cure IE using appropriate antibiotics against sensitivities ± valve surgery if indicated. No role for adjunctive treatments, even if crescentic change on biopsy.
- If ATN, tailor aminoglycoside doses to levels, or change antibiotic.
- IF AIN, change antibiotic. No role for steroids.

Renal tuberculosis

Tuberculosis is caused by *Mycobacterium tuberculosis*, affecting 8–10 million people every year, usually presenting as pulmonary disease. The global burden of TB has risen sharply as a result of HIV infection—in the developed world, TB is a disease of the elderly and those from ethnic minorities. Extra-pulmonary disease (in HIV-negative patients) presents in 15% of active cases (of which 27% is due to renal tract TB).

Genito-urinary TB

Due to direct infection of the GU tract, either as a sole site of infection or with disseminated (miliary) disease. Both kidneys are usually infected, and disease tends to spread along the entire urinary tract (▶ ureteric strictures). The renal medulla is preferentially affected, but subsequent papillary and pelvic involvement causes scarring and calcification over time. Other sites infected by TB include the epidiymus and prostate.

Symptoms and signs

⚠ May be asymptomatic (25%): maintain a high index of suspicion in those at risk. Lower abdominal pain, dysuria and frequency, back and flank pain—often presents as recurrent UTI unresponsive to antibiotics. Haematuria (may be frank). Longer term bladder fibrosis may present with urgency or incontinence. 2° bacterial infection is common.
▶ Fever, weight loss, and nightsweats are rare. Pulmonary symptoms may be absent (30% will have an abnormal CXR). Foci in the urinary tract may remain dormant indefinitely—or activate with immunosuppression. Chronic TB may cause AA amyloid, with renal involvement (📖 p.450).

Investigations

* Sterile pyuria on microscopy and negative culture is characteristic.
* 3 consecutive early morning urine samples: microscopy on centrifuged urine for acid-fast bacilli (Ziehl–Nielson stain) and culture (takes 2–4 weeks).
* PCR for mycobacterial DNA may be helpful (but false positives). U+E, CRP, FBC, ESR, CXR, plain KUB (?renal tract calcification).
▶ Consider HIV testing
   Skin tuberculin tesing is of limited use (false positive results).
* IVU: abnormal (70–90%), with calyceal tip erosions, filling defects and distortion. Ureteric strictures ± obstruction. May demonstrate absent kidney. USS if obstruction suspected.

Tuberculous interstitial nephritis

May be an underestimated worldwide cause of renal failure. TB causes a parenchymal reaction with (caseating) granuloma formation containing giant cells and chronic tubulo-interstitial inflammation. Usually presents with ↑Cr in at risk populations (South Asians). Dipstick is bland, and USS confirms ↓renal size with a smooth contour. EMU for AFBs are usually *negative*. CXR may demonstrate prior or active pulmonary TB, and skin tuberculin testing is often strongly positive. Diagnosis is made at renal biopsy (M tuberculosis may be identified on tissue stains).

Anti-tuberculous treatment → ↑improved renal function (and even recovery from advanced CRF).

Management

Cure requires combination, fixed-dose therapy for 6 months. Compliance may be problematic and should be reinforced by good patient education.

- *Initial phase*: once daily rifampicin, isoniazid, pyrazinamide for 2 Months (available as combination preparations, e.g. *Rifater®*).
  Add-on ethambutol (15mg/kg po) or streptomycin (15mg/kg IMI) if immunocompomised, or previously treated for TB (⚠ isoniazid resistance).
- ▶ Confirm sensitivity of cultured M tuberculosis.
- Continuation phase: isoniazid and rifampicin for further 4 months.
  If drug resistance is suspected, ethambutol (800–1200mg od) may be added for the initial 2 months.
  - Check local protocols for drug selection and dosing.
  - Check LFT before and 3-weekly during initial phase.
  - Add pyridoxine 10–20mg od if using isoniazid (prevents peripheral neuropathy).
  - Check visual acuity if using ethambutol.
  - Dosing in renal failure: ↓dose for ethambutol and streptomycin.
  - If HIV positive, may require prolonged multi-drug treatment.

Schistosomiasis

Infestation with schistosomes (a water-borne trematode) affects as many as 200 million people worldwide, and may lead to urinary tract disease or glomerulonephritis. *S. haematobium* is endemic in most of Africa and the Middle East, and preferentially migrates to the venous plexus surrounding the bladder. *S. mansoni* (additionally found in Latin America) and *S. japonicum* (found in Asia alone) establish in the mesenteric vessels or portal tree.

Acute infestation tends to occur in childhood in residents in endemic areas, but afflicts travelers of any age. This is characterized by dermal invasion ('swimmer's itch'), a later systemic serum-sickness like syndrome (Katayama fever) and eventual maturation of a worm in blood vessels. Lodged eggs released from mature worms evoke granulomatous inflammation in local tissues.

Although worms have strategies to evade immune recognition, if incomplete, an antibody response may result in circulating immune complexes. These may become trapped in glomeruli (esp. if liver fibrosis → poor immune complex clearance), leading to schistosomal glomerulonephritis.

Urinary schistosomiasis

Caused by *S. haemotobium* infestation. Chronically, urinary tract infestation presents with terminal haematuria (frank blood at the end of micturition), dysuria, and frequency as a result of an inflammatory cystitis. Bladder fibrosis may be asymptomatic, or lead to detrusor failure. Ureteric stricturing and obstruction is common (10%). Recurrent bacterial infection, bladder calculi, and ↑risk of bladder cancer may complicate chronic disease.

Diagnosis:

* Typical ova on urine microscopy (centrifuge sample to improve yield)
* FBC (eosinophilia), U+E.
* Anti-schistosomal antibodies (serological testing) may be helpful in excluding infestation (positive one month after exposure).
* Plain KUB may demonstrate calcification.
* USS to exclude obstruction.
* Cystoscopy may show a nodular, polypoid, and ulcerating haemorrhagic cystitis.

Treatment

Praziquantel 40mg/kg po stat (80–90% cure rate). If *S. japonicum*, ↑dose to 60mg/kg in 2 divided doses 3 hours apart. Can repeat treatment if need be.

* May be some resolution of urinary tract lesions (esp. if little fibrosis)
* Strictures may require surgical intervention.

Schistosomal glomerulonephritis

Occurs in 10% patients with *S. mansoni* (less commonly *S. haemotobium*). Most commonly a MCGN-like lesion on kidney biopsy presenting as nephrotic range proteinuria, haematuria, and impaired renal function. Other investigations show ↑Igs, ↓C3, ↓chol, false positive syphilis serology, ± ova on faecal microscopy. Tends to carry a poor renal prognosis, progressing to ESRD. No treatment is of proven benefit (including praziquantel).

Other histological variants also occur, esp. in association with hepatitis C virus co-infection (acquired as part of unsterile treatment programs in the 1980s) and acute salmonella infection (▶ good prognosis with treatment).

Malaria

Malaria is caused by *Plasmodium* parasites transmitted via *Anopheles* mosquitoes. It is endemic to large parts of the globe, and is responsible for 1–3 million deaths/year. Species causing disease:
- *P. falciparum*—sub-Saharan Africa, Indian subcontinent
- *P. vivax*—central America
- *P. malariae* and *P.ovale*—rare outside Africa.
▶ Only *P. falciparum* and *P. malariae* cause renal disease.

Transient glomerular abnormalities (≈ post-infectious GN, 📖 p.378) occur in up to 18% of infected individuals, presenting with haematuria and proteinuria (may be heavy). Renal dysfunction is unusual. Biopsy shows mesangial matrix expansion with hypercellularity, with IgM and C3 in granular deposits in capillary walls. Prognosis is good, with complete recovery after treatment of malaria.

Acute malarial nephropathy

ARF complicates severe *P. falciparum* malaria in 1–4% cases in endemic areas, but is more common in non-immune travelers. The renal lesion is always due ATN associated with circulatory collapse (as a result of 'malignant' parasitaemia, haemolysis, and a cytokine and oxidant 'storm'). If severe > 50% will require dialysis—mortality can be as high as 10%.

Symptoms and signs

Malaise, headache and confusion, fevers and chills often explosive myalgia (→ rhabdomyolysis). (Profound) ↓BP, peripheral vasodilatation, oliguria (haemoglobinuria = 'Blackwater fever'). Nausea, vomiting, diarrhea, and jaundice (75%). Hepatosplenomegaly and anaemia.

Investigations

FBC (haemolytic anaemia), ↓Plt (70%). Thick and thin blood film for parasitaemia (usually > 5%). ↓Haptoglobins. DIC (↑APTT, ↑TT, D-dimers↑). U+E (severe ↑K^+, ↓Na^+, ↑Cr), ↑LFT (↑ALP) and ↑lactic acidosis. Mild proteinuria (<1g/24h).

Management

- Manage in high care setting and initiate CVVHF or HD early.
- Supportive blood products as required.
- Culture blood and empirical broad-spectrum antibiotics (bacterial superinfection is not uncommon).
- IV quinine loading dose as 20mg/kg (no more than 1.4g) over 4h
  - 10mg/kg IVI over 4h 8 hrly for 7days, with cardiac monitoring (not > 700mg/dose).
  - Convert to po therapy once appropriate.
  - ⚠ If G6PD deficient, consult local pharmacy.

- IVI quinidine is an alternative—confirm local protocols for oral completion therapy depending on chloroquine-resistance patterns.
  ⚠ Monitor for hypoglycaemia (quinidine/quinine ↑insulin release)
- Artemether/lumefantrine (Malarone®) or proguanil/atovaquone (Riamet®) are alternatives.
- Exchange transfusion may be useful if heavy parasitaemia (>10%)

Chronic malarial nephropathy

Caused by *P. malariae*, affecting African children (~5 years old). Presents as proteinuria (may be nephrotic range) ± haematuria. Oedema (co-existant malnutrition), ↓Hb and hepatosplenomegaly. Renal biopsy shows a MCGN with subendothelial deposits (📖 p.380). The disease runs a progressive course to ESRD despite eradication of the infection.

Urinary tract obstruction

Approaching obstruction

Obstruction of the urinary tract is a not uncommon and often silent cause of renal impairment or disease. It leads to delayed urinary transit, and over time, increased intra-tract pressures → renal impairment. Obstruction tends to present in infants and young children (as a result of anatomical abnormalities) or in older people, particularly men (tumours, stones and prostatic disease). The key to diagnosis rests on siting the level of obstruction correctly.

Normal physiology

Urine reaches the bladder as a result of three inter-related mechanisms:
- Glomerular filtration pressure
- Renal tract peristalsis
- Gravity.

Co-ordinated smooth muscle contraction in the ureters directs urine toward the bladder, with maximum intraluminal pressures of ~25mmHg.

Classification

- *Upper or lower:*
  - Upper tract ≈ obstruction at the level of the ureter or higher.
  - Lower tract ≈ bladder or lower.
- *Unilateral or bilateral:*
  - Lower tract obstruction affects both kidneys.
  - Upper tract obstruction may affect one or both.
  - Bilateral obstruction will cause renal impairment, as will unilateral obstruction of a single functioning kidney.
- *Complete or partial:*
  - Complete obstruction is the commonest cause of anuria. It may be easy to diagnose and imaging is often clear cut in confirming this.
  - Partial obstruction may be more difficult to diagnose, as the patient's urine output may vary.

Causes

Table 8.1 Causes of urinary tract obstruction

Level of obstruction	Obstruction within the lumen	Obstruction within the wall	Extrinsic compression
Kidney	Stones Sloughed papillae	Cysts Tumours Anatomical abnormalities e.g. PUJ obstruction	Lower polar renal vessels crossing at PUJ
Ureter	Stones	Tumours Stricture (malignant, post surgery or post-radiotherapy), tuberculous, schistosomiasis) Anatomical abnormalities e.g. VUJ obstruction	Tumours Retroperitoneal fibrosis Retrocaval right ureter (congenital) Pancreatitis, inflammatory bowel disease (rare)
Bladder/ bladder neck	Stones Clot retention	Tumours Functional obstruction (diabetes, neurological damage to bladder, drugs)	Pelvic tumours
Urethra	Stones Blood clots (after catheterization or surgery)	Stricture (post infective, or post surgical) Congenital urethral valves Tumours	Prostate enlargement

Imaging urinary tract obstruction

History and examination can often make a diagnosis in acute obstruction (📖 p.3). ► A palpable bladder is an important finding → lower tract obstruction, but imaging is always required to diagnose upper tract obstruction.

Ultrasound (USS)

- Portable, non-invasive and quick.
- May demonstrate dilated ureters.
- The upper (but not always the lower) ureter may be visualized.
- Imaging of choice in patients with renal impairment, pregnancy.

However, USS is operator-dependent, and (early) obstruction can occur without a dilated system in some circumstances. Moreover, a dilated system does *not* necessarily imply obstruction is present (see box below).

How good is ultrasound at diagnosing obstruction?

► Do not rely on imaging alone to diagnose obstruction.

Obstruction without a dilated system
- Hydronephrosis may not be apparent in early (2–3 days) obstruction.
- Dilatation may not occur if tumour or fibrous tissue encases a kidney.
- Chronically obstructed kidneys fail → anuria ∴ no hydronephrosis.
- Partial obstruction may not show a hydronephrosis (but ↑Cr).

Dilated system without obstruction
- Anatomical variants: extra renal pelvis, megaureter (possible secondary to vesicoureteral reflux).
- Pregnancy: hormonal changes cause dilated ureters and renal pelvis.
- Post obstruction: a 'baggy' system may remain long after relief of chronic obstruction. Review previous imaging and compare.
- If doubt exists then consider (but not in pregnancy):
  - IVU.
  - Diuretic renography.

CT KUB (kidneys, ureters, bladder)

- Has superceded plain X-ray (still useful to identify radio-opaque stones).
- If clinical findings and USS unclear, CT KUB is most likely to provide the most information on the site and cause of the obstruction.
- Particularly useful in stone disease—esp. renal colic (📖 p.436)
- Useful to diagnose cause of extrinsic compression, staging of tumours and retroperitoneal fibrosis.
- Beware contrast nephropathy if renal impairment is present (📖 p.132)

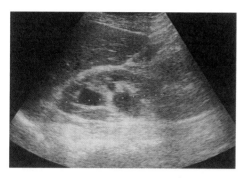

Fig. 8.1 Renal ultrasound appearances of acute obstruction with pelvicalyceal dilatation. Reproduced with permission from Warrell D, Cox T, Firth J, and Benz EJ (eds) (2004) *Oxford Textbook of Medicine*, 4th edn, p.451. Oxford University Press, Oxford.

Intravenous urography (IVU)

More difficult to perform than CT, and requires contrast. But useful if:

- CT fails to demonstrate the level of obstruction.
- Suspected obstruction and complicated staghorn calculi or multiple renal cysts (CT, USS cannot differentiate hydronephrosis from cysts).

Obstructed nephrogram of unknown cause

Occasionally in the context of acute unilateral loin pain, IVU shows evidence of obstruction but no stone. Consider:

- Recent passage of radio-opaque stone.
- Radiolucent uric acid stone (→ CT).
- Acute PUJ obstruction (distended pelvis may be seen).
- Sloughed papilla (🕮 p.410)(?clubbed calyces on IVU). Consider:
  - Diabetes
  - Analgesic abuse
  - Sickle cell disease and trait.
- Blood clot (*always* with macroscopic haematuria).

Isotope renography

A DTPA or MAG-3 renogram (🕮 p.43) may show delayed excretion with obstruction. Helpful in diagnosing unilateral obstruction (compare excretion with the normal side) or partial (with furosemide, increased urinary flow may reveal a partially obstructed system). Estimates split function.

MRI

Has a growing role in tumour staging and extrinsic compressive lesions.

Acute obstruction (see □ p.3)

Clinical features

Complete bilateral obstruction presents with anuria and progressive ARF. Partial or unilateral obstruction may present with localized pain or signs of sepsis, or may be asymptomatic and diagnosed late with a non-functioning kidney.

Features resulting from the underlying cause include:

- *Prostatic disease* may present with symptoms of difficulty, dribbling or poor stream (□ p.514). Examine for a palpable bladder and perform PR.
- *Retroperitoneal fibrosis* is suggested by backache ± AAA (□ p.506).
- *Stones* present with pain (acute obstruction secondary to stones is usually painful), haematuria (macro or microscopic) (□ p.432).
- *Tumours* rarely present with acute obstruction. Intrinsic and extrinsic tumours compression → partial obstruction, haematuria or pain (□ p.512). ♀ may require a vaginal examination if cancer suspected.
- *Papillary necrosis* may present with pain ± haematuria (□ p.410).
- *Clot colic* is usually accompanied by frank haematuria.

⚠ Pain, fever, or systemic signs of sepsis are important features of an obstructed infected system(s). Proceed to *urgent* decompression.

Investigations

⚠ Always exclude obstruction in cases of unexplained renal impairment.

- If the bladder is palpable, then the diagnosis may be made at the bedside. If not, then USS almost always leads to the diagnosis.
- Microscope urine for red cells, crystals. U+E, Ca^{2+}, CRP, FBC, ESR, culture blood, and urine if febrile. *PSA* in ♂.
- Further imaging may be (and often is) required (□ p.34) Once the nature and extent of obstruction is known, direct investigations appropriately.
- Cystocopy ± ureteroscopy may eventually be required to make a definitive diagnosis when the cause is within the lumen.

Management of acute obstruction

The quicker obstruction is relieved the better: chronic obstruction → irreversible decline in renal function.

- Do not delay: time = nephrons.
- *An obstructed urinary system is an emergency.*
- If bladder outflow obstruction: *catheterize*. If insertion is difficult, insert a suprapubic catheter—don't traumatize the urethra.
- If ureteric: a *nephrostomy* or retrograde ureteric stenting is needed. If ARF with fluid and electrolyte abnormalities are present, then a nephrostomy to one kidney should be enough to secure the patient until definitive drainage is performed.

Further management depends on the cause:

- Before removing a nephrostomy, do a nephrostogram (injection of contrast via the nephrostomy to examine ureteric flow).
- Ureteric stents can be inserted from above (via nephrostomy) or from below (cystoscopically—can be technically difficult/impossible if the ureteric orifices are diseased and difficult to cannulate).
- Stones and tumours should be managed by the relevant experts.

Organizing a nephrostomy

Is it necessary?

- *Pros*: relieves ureteric obstruction and corrects renal failure and its associated electrolyte abnormalities.
- *Cons*: invasive, has serious potential complications (bleeding, infection), and is temporary. If it is possible to relieve the obstruction from below, this may be preferable.

How urgent is it?

- Infection → emergency nephrostomy required. Often only clinical signs may suggest infection (pain, systemic signs of sepis).
- If K^+ >6.0, pulmonary oedema or severe uraemia (limiting patient cooperation), then it may be safer to dialyse the patient first.
  ▶ *Dialysis is not risk-free* (lines etc.).
- Otherwise a delay of *hours* to ensure an expert operator may be justified.

What blood tests should I send?

U+E, FBC, clotting screen, G+S

What about consent?

Must be obtained by the person doing the procedure, as always. Bleeding or trauma to the kidney are rare but occur.

Which kidney?

In an emergency, relieve the one kidney most likely to work (i.e. the larger kidney with the thicker cortex). Otherwise both.

Post procedure care

- *Exact* fluid balance: there is likely to be a brisk post-obstructive diuresis. Often >5–10L UO/day.
- May require IVI 0.9% NaCl replacement (as urine output + 50 ml/hour initially).
- Watch for ↓K^+ or ↓Na^+ with diuresis.
- Make sure the nephrostomy is well strapped in or sutured!

Chronic obstruction

▶The presentation may be insidious.

Importantly, unilateral obstruction may not present with renal failure (if the other kidney is functioning), but may cause ↑BP (renin–angiotensin activation). Symptoms and signs are similar to those described with acute obstruction (🕮 p.3), though pain is infrequent. More chronic features may include local feelings of fullness or pain, nocturia or urinary frequency, other prostatic symptoms (🕮 p.514), or symptomatic uraemia. Always examine for a palpable bladder, enlarged prostate or other pelvic masses.

Renal consequences of obstruction

- Acute obstruction causes an acute reduction in the GFR, which is *fully* reversible if relieved within a few days.
- In chronic obstruction, the renal parenchymal changes may never fully recover despite relief. The longer obstruction has been present, the longer renal function takes to recover. With severe renal failure (Cr >600μmol/L) recovery to <300μmol/L is unusual.
- Chronic tubular damage may lead to:
  - Salt losing nephropathies (🕮 p.408)
  - Type 1 or 4 renal tubular acidosis (🕮 p.556)
  - A persistent 'baggy' renal pelvis on imaging.

Management

Aim to relieve obstruction as for the patient with acute obstruction (🕮 p.500).

Further management depends on the cause:

- Whenever possible remove stones, treat tumours, treat prostatic enlargement, dilate strictures, offer surgery if anatomical abnormalities.
- In some circumstances, a long-term catheter, a prostatic stent, or ureteric stents may be the most practical and sensible option (e.g. for inoperable tumours or frail patients with advanced disease).
- Urethral catheters and ureteric (JJ) stents require long term follow up:
  - Change the catheter or stent at appropriate intervals (depending on catheter/stent, can be weeks–months if well-tolerated).
  - Watch for infection (may require exchange or removal if antibiotics ineffective) or blockage (▶ deterioration of renal function).

Mechanism of renal damage in chronic obstruction

Not fully understood, but likely important mediators are:
- Back pressure: ↑proximal tubular pressure leads to ↓filtration pressure.
- Vasoconstriction in response to ↑intra-tubular pressure. Mediated locally by angiotensin II and thromboxanes (a physiological response redirecting blood away from non-functioning nephrons).
- Ischaemic nephrons release mediators of inflammation, leading to local injury, interstitial fibrosis and irreversible atrophy of the disused nephrons.

PUJ and VUJ obstruction

Both obstruction at the pelvi-ureteric junction (PUJ) and vesico-ureteric junction (VUJ) are thought to be congenital in origin, perhaps arising from urinary tract adhesions or persisting foetal folds → mechanical and structural changes.

- PUJ obstruction: failure of normal urine flow from the renal pelvis into the ureter, resulting in a 'baggy' high-pressure pelvis
- VUJ obstruction: urine cannot pass from the ureter into the bladder, with a resultant megaureter. Ureteric reflux may mimic it, or co-exist.

Symptoms and signs

PUJ obstruction is increasingly diagnosed ante-natally, when it is often bilateral. Older children present with flank pain, a palpable mass, urinary tract infection, or haematuria after trauma. However, 20% of cases are diagnosed as adults, and presumably a large number are never diagnosed at all. Characteristic flank pain after drinking alcohol, coffee or taking diuretics (i.e. anything that promotes diuresis). VUJO presents with a similar constellation of symptoms, but often later in childhood or as an adult.

Diagnosis

USS to confirm structural changes. IVU or isotope renography (with furosemide) will describe functional consequences. MCUG (micturating cystoureterogram) may demonstrate reflux in ?VUJ obstruction.

Management

- Generally managed conservatively unless:
  - Impaired renal function
  - Recurrent infection
  - Calculi
  - Persistent pain.
- PUJ obstruction can be managed by open Anderson–Hynes pyeloplasty, laparoscopic pyeloplasty or endopyelotomy (antegrade or retrograde). Balloon dilatation is usually unsuccesful
- VUJ obstruction can be managed by re-implantation of the ureter. If + reflux into ureter (on MCUG), consider antibiotic prophylaxis against UTI. See 📖 p.430 for full discussion on vesico-ureteric reflux.

Posterior urethral valves

The commonest form of lower tract obstruction in ♂ infants. Valves in the posterior urethra obstruct urinary flow with sequential dilatation of the proximal urethra, bladder wall hypertrophy, bilateral megaureters and hydronephrosis, → (if uncorrected) obstructive uropathy.

- Often diagnosed during pregnancy.
- Reflux is often present as well.
- When diagnosed late, tends to present with CKD or UTI.

Standard fetal USS often makes then diagnosis. MCUG in infancy can be used to confirm features. Management includes immediate bladder catheterization followed by endoscopic resection of valves as early as possible. Bladder dysfunction may persist after correction.

Retroperitoneal fibrosis

Obstruction at the mid- to lower-third of the ureter by an encasing inflammatory fibrous tissue → impaired ureteric contractility. This leads to a chronic obstructive uropathy, often presenting with unexplained renal impairment. It is caused by the leakage of pro-inflammatory lipid-derived material across the wall of an atheromatous (and sometimes aneurysmal) aorta. This in turn → a ureteric inflammatory response which, over time, heals as fibrosis. RPF is also, and perhaps more appropriately, known as peri-aortitis. 3♂:1♀, usually occurring in patients > 50.

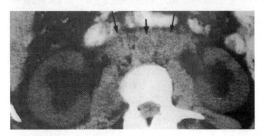

Fig. 8.2 Retroperitoneal fibrosis—CT appearances. Note the peri-aortic mass and aortic calcification. Reproduced with permission from Warrell D, Cox T, Firth, and Benz EJ (eds) (2004) *Oxford Textbook of Medicine*, 4th edn, p.454. Oxford University Press, Oxford.

Causes

- Idiopathic. Underlying mechanism as above.
- Drug induced: classically methysergide, but also some beta blockers.
- Lymphoma and other lympho-proliferative disorders.
- Prostatic and pelvic malignancies may have similar radiological features, but represent a different disease.

▶ Establish tissue diagnosis in all patients if possible. *Needle biopsy* may miss this by sampling error, *so open biopsy preferred.*

Clinical features

Often found on investigating impaired renal function with bland urine and ↑BP. Rarely, abdominal mass or backache.

Investigations

U+E, Ca^{2+}, (↓Hb), ↑↑ESR (a consistent marker of inflammation, and useful for monitoring disease). CT or MRI are investigations of choice to:
- Make or confirm the diagnosis.
- Image the aorta (and assess any aortic aneurysm).
- Characterize any lymphadenopathy.

CT-guided biopsy can be performed unless surgery and excision biopsy is planned (see above).

Management

If fit, patients are best managed with a combination of immunosuppression and surgery.

Medical management

- Corticosteroids ↓inflammatory tissue encasing the ureter(s), and may restore ureteric patency.
- Start prednisolone 30mg/day for 12 weeks. Taper the dose, titrating down against ESR and serial imaging.
- Longer term, azathioprine, and mycophenolate have been used in patients unsuitable for surgery. ☞ Controlled trials are needed.

Surgery

- Insertion of bilateral retrograde JJ ureteric stents may obviate the need for nephrostomies to relieve obstruction.
- Definitive surgery is best if preceded by a course of steroids to shrink the mass
- Ureterolysis and omental wrapping is the definitive surgical procedure. The ureters (with JJ stents in situ) are identified, freed and moved laterally, wrapped in a protective layer of omentum.
- Aortic aneurysm repair may also be required
- Steroids can be stopped after surgery, but relapse can occur

Follow-up should be lifelong (U+E, ESR)

Investigation of a renal mass

Renal masses may be asymptomatic or symptomatic, single or multiple, cystic or solid:

	Solid	**Cystic**
Single	Tumour	Simple cyst
	Angiomyolipoma	
	AV malformation	
Multiple	Congenital syndromes e.g. von Hippel-Lindau syndrome, tuberous sclerosis	Polycystic kidney disease
		Acquired cystic disease (□ p.422)

When is a cyst not a simple cyst?

Diagnosis by USS—criteria for a simple renal cyst are that it be:
- Round
- Smooth walled
- Anechoic
- With good transmission of ultrasound through the cyst.

If all these are present, then it is almost certainly benign. If not, then proceed to contrast-enhanced CT KUB. On CT, simple cysts have:
- Smooth thin walls
- A density similar to that of water
- No enhancement with contrast.

Uncertain cases should be followed up 6–12 monthly with repeat scanning. The differential diagnosis and investigation of cystic disease is discussed elsewhere (□ p.422).

The solid renal mass

May be benign (angiomyolipoma) or malignant. No imaging technique can completely reliably say a solid lesion is benign, although MRI may detect small quantities of fat, highly suggestive of an angiomyolipoma. Worrying features of a solid lesion are:
- Diameter >3cm
- Enhancement with contrast
- Thick or irregular wall
- Necrotic areas (implying rapid growth).

Removal is usually advocated. Consider nephron-sparing surgery (i.e. partial nephrectomy) especially if there is reduced renal function or a problem with the other kidney. Borderline cases or indeterminate lesions should receive serial CT with or without ultrasound. MRI may be useful in evaluating the internal contents of the cyst. Even small lesions may progress.

Renal cell carcinoma

RCC are adenocarcinomas accounting for 80% of 1° malignant tumours of the kidney. They may be slow growing and hence commonly present as an incidental finding. 4♂:1♀, with bilateral lesions occurring in up to 50% of cases. Smoking has been strongly implicated in development of RCC.

Clinical features

The classic presenting triad is pain, haematuria, and a palpable mass. In reality, other features are often as common. Flank or back pain (capsular stretch) radiating into the groin occurs with large tumours, as with cystic tumours complicated by haemorrhage or infection. ↑BP occurs. Haematuria is common and may be macroscopic. Tumour may obstruct a kidney. 25% present with distant metastases (lung, liver, bone, nodes, the other kidney) or extensive local disease. Some develop scrotal varicoeles due to occlusion of the testicular vein (always arouse suspicion if found). Paraneoplastic symptoms (see box below).

Differential diagnosis

⚠ Most solid lesions in the kidney are renal cell carcinomas.
- Oncocytoma—benign, and not reliably distinguishable on CT.
- Angiomyolipoma—has a fat density < water on CT. If bilateral, then likely to a feature of tuberous sclerosis.
- Xanthogranulomatous pyelonephritis (🕮 p.428).

Paraneoplastic syndrome with RCC

- Fever (up to 20%, often with night sweats)
- Cachexia
- Erythrocytosis (the tumour may make erythropoietin)
- Anaemia (may be disproportionate)
- Hypercalcaemia (due to bony metastases, or due to production of PTH related protein). Poor prognostic sign
- Hepatic dysfunction without liver metastases
- 2° amyloid deposition (AA amyloid)
- Polymyalgia
- Other hormonal effects (production of ACTH-like substance, gonadotrophins, renin, and insulin have all been reported).

Investigations

Urine cytology. U+E, Ca^{2+}, alk phos, LFT. FBC, ↑↑ESR. CT kidneys (or US + IVU). MRI if unable to tolerate IV contrast. May need bone scan.

Preoperative work up

Evaluate local spread of disease by CT. Invasion of the renal vein is best assessed by MRI (important if planning nephron-sparing surgery). MAG 3 renogram and estimation of GFR to assess differential renal function. Look for metastases—CT of the chest and a bone scan.

▶ Avoid needle biopsy of the renal mass: low reliability, risk of seeding.

Staging

Using the TNM classification, prognosis is related to staging at diagnosis:

- If T1 lesion, five year survival >90%.
- If metastatic disease, five year survival <10%.

The grade of tumour or the presence of paraneoplastic features also influences prognosis.

Treatment

Resection of the primary tumour is treatment of choice (reports of metastases shrinking after removal of the primary exist). Radical nephrectomy has been the standard, but nephron-sparing surgery is increasingly used to preserve renal function.

High dose immunotherapy with interleukin-2 ± interferon in addition to debulking surgery has given promising results, and sometimes cure.

☞ Other more experimental therapies including anti-angiogenic factors have been tried but data is lacking.

Wilms' tumour (nephroblastoma)

The most common malignant tumour of the urinary tract in children, with a peak incidence at 3–4 years. Of mesodermal origin it presents as a well demarcated solid lesion in the kidney in the context of ↑BP. 15% of affected children have other congenital abnormalities.

Urothelial tumours

Bladder cancer

Over 90% of bladder cancers are transitional cell cancers (TCC), affecting $3\sigma':1\varphi$ over the age of 60. Exposure to urothelial carcinogens → malignant transformation, with environmental factors playing a key role in tumour genesis. Squamous cell cancers are seen in areas of chronic schistosomiasis infection.

Risk factors

- ► Cigarette smoking
- Aniline dyes, aromatic amines, diesel fumes (lorry drivers) and hair dyes (hairdressers) have all been linked to TCC
- Significant levels of arsenic in drinking water
- Long term exposure to laxatives or phenacetin (+ ?other analgesics)
- Previous radiotherapy to the pelvis
- Previous chemotherapy—especially with cyclophosphamide (📖 p.371).

Pathogenesis

N-acetylation detoxifies potential carcinogens (such as arylamines)—an ↑ risk of bladder cancer is found in those with mutations → slower acetylation kinetics.

Clinical presentation

Occupational history is important. Haematuria (microscopic → frank) is the cardinal presenting feature. Pain is a feature of advanced disease. Urinary frequency, a feeling of incomplete emptying and urge incontinence may occur. Weight loss, fatigue, and anorexia occur late.

Investigations

Repeat urine cytology (×2) for cancerous cells. U+E, Ca^{2+}, alk phos, FBC. Proceed to cystoscopy if at risk: allows visual inspection of the bladder ± ureters, collection of urine for cytology and biopsy.

IVU allows examination of the upper tracts and detection of small lesions of the ureter or renal pelvis, and USS may pick up renal parenchymal disease or hydronephrosis.

Staging

CT abdomen and pelvis (or MRI) if locally invasive disease is suspected. CXR (if abnormal then chest CT). Bone scan if invasive disease, bone pain, ↑Ca^{2+}, or ↑alkaline phosphatase.

If tumour is superficial the prognosis is good, though recurrence is common and surveillance with regular cystoscopy is necessary. Advanced tumours have a poor prognosis.

Management

Briefly, non-invasive superficial tumours are removed by trans-urethral resection of bladder tumour (TURBT). Because of recurrence, especially with high-grade tumours, adjuvant treatment with intravesical BCG may be recommended and reduce this risk by up to 40%. Invasive tumours require radical surgery ± radiotherapy and chemotherapy.

Tumours of the renal pelvis and ureter

- The urothelium of the renal pelvis and ureter may also develop transitional cell carcinomas (often multifocal). Such tumours are usually uncommon: <1% urinary tract neoplasms, ± 8% of renal tumours. May occur in association with Balkan endemic nephropathy (📖 p.409).
- Occurs in 2♂:1♀ between 50–60 years. Investigate as for bladder TCC, though emphasis should be on IVU or CT, proceeding to flexible ureteroscopy ± brush biopsies. Careful evaluation for synchronous or multifocal urothelial tumours is required. Treatment is surgical (nephroureterectomy).

Benign prostatic hypertrophy (BPH)

BPH is a common and important condition in ♂, and a major cause of bladder outflow obstruction and renal impairment. The incidence rises steadily after the age of 50, affecting >50% of ♂ over 60. BPH is thought to be multifactorial in cause, with sex hormones and growth factors interacting with prostatic stromal epithelium → unbalanced cell proliferation and extra-cellular matrix production. Of the many implicated factors, age is clearly important, as are androgens (eunuchs do not get BPH). BPH is *not* an independent risk factor for prostatic carcinoma.

Clinical features

BPH classically presents with lower urinary tract symptoms (LUTS):
- Urinary frequency, hesitancy, and a poor stream.
- Urgency, nocturia and dribbling.

Chronic BPH may complicate as:
- Long-term bladder outflow obstruction (BOO) → bladder wall hypertrophy with ↑ post-void residual volumes and irreversible bladder dysfunction, UTIs, or bladder stones.
- Acute urinary retention ± obstructive uropathy

On PR examination, the prostate is characteristically enlarged, smooth and symmetrical. Always exclude a palpable bladder (and obstruction).

Differential diagnosis
- Carcinoma of the prostate or bladder
- UTI or prostatitis
- Bladder stones
- Neurogenic bladder.

Investigations

Urine dipstick (⚠ haematuria may occur with BPH—*but* always assess the bladder and upper tracts for other lesions). Urine for MC+S. U+E, PSA. Other tests which may be useful include:
- Frequency volume chart
- Urine flow rate measurement
- Post-micturition residual volume assessment
- Urodynamics if bladder dysfunction suspected.

Management

Symptom scoring systems exist to assess the severity of disease. Many ♂ benefit from conservative management ('watchful waiting') if symptoms are mild (the cost and side-effects of drugs outweigh potential benefit).

If in acute urinary retention → indwelling catheter. After catheterization for acute retention, treat with α–blocker (e.g. tamsulosin MR 400µg od) for 48 hours prior to trial without catheter to improve chance of success.

Active therapies for BPH

Indications for further intervention include:

- More severe symptoms
- Large prostate volume
- ↑PSA (reflecting ↑prostate volume rather than cancer)
- Low maximal flow rate
- High post-voiding residual volume.

Alpha-blockers (e.g. tamsulosin, alfuzosin)

Cause bladder neck and prostatic smooth muscle relaxation. Provide effective symptomatic relief, ↑quality of life, ↑maximum flow rate, ↓risk of acute urinary retention and may also ↓need for surgery. Side effects (15%) are usually mild. Include postural hypotension, headaches and dizziness. Long acting preparations are a significant advance.

5-α reductase inhibitors (e.g. finasteride, dutasteride)

Inhibit conversion of testosterone to dihydrotestosterone (more active in the prostate). They have a slow onset of action (3–6 months), but long-lasting effects. Most effective in ♂ with large prostates, they improve symptoms, quality of life, flow rate, with ↓prostate volume, ↓risk of urinary retention and ↓need for surgery. Side effects include impotence.

Combination of an α–blocker with a 5-α reductase inhibitor

Appears to be more effective than either class of drug alone. Stopping the α–blocker after several months may be possible.

Surgery

Is recommended for severe symptoms, or complications of BOO:

- UTI
- Persistent retention of urine
- Renal failure.

Flow rates and urodynamic studies help patient selection. Surgery is more successful in ♂ with proven BOO (flow rate <10mL/s), and less successful in ♂ with symptomatic detrusor overactivity (frequency, urgency)

- *Transurethral resection of the prostate* (TURP) is usually the operation of choice.
- For small glands, a bladder neck incision may be all that is required.
- Very large glands may require a retro-pubic approach.

Acute complications of surgery include haemorrhage, sepsis and the TUR syndrome (systemic absorption of glycine from the irrigated bladder leading to ↓ Na^+). Longer term complications may include impotence, retrograde ejaculation, urethral stricture, and urinary incontinence.

▶ Laser prostatectomy, thermotherapy, microwave therapy, transure-thral needle ablation of the prostate (TUNA) and transurethral ethanol ablation of the prostate (TEAP) are promising treatments in the pipeline.

Prostate cancer

The most common malignancy in ♂ after skin cancer, with an incidence of 50/100 000 ♂, rising with age (rare <45). Race (more common in black population), genetics (more common in 1st degree relatives of affected people) and diet (animal fats, dairy products) are implicated in the aetiology.

Clinical features

LUTS (📖 p.514), erectile dysfunction, haematuria, or haematospermia, symptoms of BOO or metastatic disease may lead to a digital rectal examination, with characteristic irregularity, nodules or asymmetry. An abnormal-feeling prostate should always be investigated, even if PSA normal (20% of such patients have a normal PSA).
⚠ In early disease the prostate may feel normal!

Investigations

Urine for MC+S, U+E, PSA, Ca^{2+}, LFT. Trans-rectal ultrasound (TRUS). USS pre- and post-micturition + kidneys if BOO. Further investigations depend on stage and grade (see below)

Staging and grading

TRUS-guided prostate biopsy of nodules or abnormal areas for tissue diagnosis. Other areas are also sampled ('sextant biopsy'). Up to 25% of cancers may be missed, and re-biopsy may be required.
- A Gleason score is calculated to grade the tumour: the degree of glandular differentiation and gland architecture are graded 1–5 (1 = well differentiated). These are combined to give a score out of 10.
- The TNM classification is used to stage the tumour (see below)
  - Patients with stage cT2 or less, PSA <10 and Gleason <6 do not need a bone scan as yield is low for these patients.
  - Similar criteria are used for CT abdomen/pelvis, unless external beam radiotherapy is planned.
  - Endo-rectal coil MRI has best sensitivity at diagnosing extracapsular spread and seminal vesicle invasion (but *not* routine).

TNM staging of prostate cancer

The c stage is based on clinical and ultrasound findings:
- cT1: clinically inapparent
- cT2: confined to the prostate
- cT3: extension through the capsule
- cT4: adjacent structures involved.

The p stage depends on the findings at the time of radical prostatectomy:
- pT2: organ-confined
- pT3: extra-prostatic extension
- pT4: invasion of bladder/rectum.

Nx: nodes not examined.
N0: regional nodes not affected.
N1: regional nodes affected.
M0: no evidence of distant metastases.
M1: distant metastases present.

Screening with PSA

PSA is a glycoprotein produced by both normal and malignant prostate tissue. It rises with age after the age of 40. There is considerable overlap in PSA measurements between benign and malignant prostate disease. Causes of an elevated PSA:
- Carcinoma of the prostate
- BPH (🕮 p.514)
- Prostatitis
- Trauma (prostatic biopsy, TURP: avoid measuring PSA for 6 weeks).

Digital rectal examination causes a *clinically insignificant* rise in PSA. The normal range is *age-specific*, but as general rules:
- If PSA <4ng/mL, cancer is possible though diagnostic yield is lower, and disease is more likely to be confined to the gland.
- If PSA 4–10ng/mL, ~20% chance of malignancy. Biopsy usually recommended but depends on individual circumstances.
- If PSA >10ng/mL, probability of Ca prostate is >50%. Biopsy usually recommended.

Rate of rise of PSA (>0.75 ng/ml/year may prompt biopsy), PSA density (PSA corrected for prostatic volume on USS), and the ratio of free to bound serum PSA (↓ fraction of free PSA in malignancy) may become useful tools in enhancing specificity. Not yet useful in clinical practice.

Controversies

- Many older ♂ have asymptomatic prostate cancer, and will go on to die of something else. They ∴ do not benefit from investigation, the associated anxiety, or the possible treatments offered.
- PSA is not sensitive or specific for cancer when normal or moderately raised (<10ng/mL). More invasive tests (biopsy) and potentially needless anxiety may be generated.
- We do not yet know what the optimal treatment for early prostate cancer is: watchful waiting may be better management than radical prostatectomy and/or radiotherapy.
- Screening tests are only valuable if they allow earlier and more beneficial treatment to be instituted.

Management of prostate cancer

Early disease

The options are watchful waiting, radical prostatectomy, or radiotherapy: no good trial data separates these therapies. The general health of the patient, clinical stage, and grade are all important in the decision making process, but it may boil down to the choice of the patient. Newer alternatives include brachytherapy, cryoablation or androgen ablation, though not yet well-tried or widely used.

- 5-year survival was 67% in 1970s. It is 98% today. So earlier and aggressive treatment has ↑survival (in early disease).
- ▶ Radical prostatectomy may → erectile dysfunction and incontinence.

Follow-up

Watchful waiting: some have disease which advances. Monitor as:

- Regular physical examination (? urinary retention or incontinence).
- PSA 3–6 monthly.
- Surveillance CT or bone scans are not justified.
- Repeat prostatic biopsy may be helpful with ↑PSA.

Post radical prostatectomy/radiotherapy:

- Regular PSA ± rectal examination, usually every 6 months.

Recurrence and late disease

Local recurrence after radical prostatectomy → radiotherapy. Local recurrence after initial radiotherapy treatment → salvage prostatectomy, with an increased risk of post-operative complications.

Metastatic disease is treated with palliative (*not* curative) androgen deprivation therapy. Measure PSA every 6 months. Patients who 'escape' (↑PSA, usually after ~2 years) on anti-androgens have a poor prognosis (median survival = 12 months).

Androgen deprivation therapy

Prostate cells are androgen sensitive, and malignant cells respond to androgen manipulation. Androgen production can be ↓ by bilateral orchidectomy (produced in testes) + anti-androgen treatment (to block adrenal production), or oestrogens (e.g. diethylstilboestrol) or LHRH agonists (e.g. goserelin). Competitive androgen-receptor blockers (bicalutamide, flutamide, cyproterone acetate) can contribute to combination therapy and are thought to improve survival marginally.

Fluids and electrolytes

Sodium: salt and water balance

The human body is made up of 50–60% water by weight. More accurately, total body water (TBW) in litres can be estimated as weight (kg) x a correction factor as below:

	♂	♀
<65 years old	0.6	0.5
>65 years old	0.5	0.45

So in a 70kg ♂, TBW = 0.6 x 70 = 42L. Water is contained in specific compartments,
- Intracellular space (~ $^2/_3$ TBW, or 28L in a 70kg ♂)
- Extracellular fluid is then ~ $^1/_3$ TBW, or 14L in a 70kg ♂. This includes,
  - Interstitial fluid (~ $^2/_3$ ECF water, or 9.4L in a 70kg ♂)
  - Plasma (~ $^1/_3$ ECF water, or 4.6L in a 70kg ♂).

The hydrophobic cell membrane acts as a barrier between intra- and extra-cellular fluid, and the capillary wall separates plasma from the interstitium. Every compartment maintains osmotic pressure through an actively retained, specific solute.
- Intracellular: K^+ (pumped inwards by Na^+/K^+-ATPase)
- ECF: Na^+ (see below)
- Plasma: proteins (esp. albumin, impermeable through the normal endothelial barrier).

Extracellular volume is controlled by Na^+ retention and excretion (water will passively follow salt). The body ignores the ECF as a whole, and 'samples' a portion of it: the effective arterial blood volume (EABV)[1].
- Amounts to ~ 700mL (blood in the arterial tree at any one time).
- Is a function of cardiac output (CO) and systemic vascular resistance (SVR).

Changes in EABV (due to hypovolaemia, ↓CO, or ↓SVR) are sensed by:
- Systemic baro-receptors (carotid sinus, aortic arch)
- Intra-renal volume sensors (juxtaglomerular apparatus).

With ↓EABV, these volume sensors activate the sympathetic nervous system, with Na+ then retained by the kidney (often to u-Na^+ < 10 mmol/L). Conversely, with ↑EABV, salt-wasting (> 100 mmol/L) takes place with appropriate changes in TBW. This requires intact renal salt handling (and kidney function) for such homeostasis.

Low-pressure volume sensors sited in the atria and the great veins (*NOT* contributing to EABV sensing) are also important: ↑ ECF leads to increased atrial natriuretic peptide (ANP) release and renal salt-wasting, as well as suppressing sympathetic tone. These receptors may control non-osmotic ADH release if the ECF is under-filled.

---

1 Schrier RW (1988) *N Engl J Med*, **319**: 1065

Falling EABV increases sympathetic tone
- ↑ circulating catecholamines, leading to ↑CO and ↑SVR.
- Activated renin–angiotensin system, improving renal haemodynamics, and salt-retention through 2°hyperaldosteronism.
- ↑ non-osmotic ADH (vasopressin) release.

Rising EABV (including low pressure whole ECF sensing)
- ↑ANP (atrial natriuretic peptide, a potent natriuretic).
- Suppressed renin production, and thus angiotensin and aldosterone.

Water handling

TBW is mainly regulated by hypothalamic osmoreceptors (*not* volume sensors) capable of sensing changes in ECF osmolality: ↑osmolality triggers thirst, and pituitary ADH (vasopressin) release. Relatively dilute urine arrives at the collecting duct, as Na^+ reabsorption in the ascending limb of the loop of Henle occurs without water (this is the basis for the counter-current mechanism, leading to a hypertonic medullary interstitium).

Without ADH, this fluid is passed little-modified as urine (and explains the polyuria of DI, 🕮 p.527). ADH binds V2 (vasopressin) receptors on the basolateral aspect of the principal cells in the collecting duct, leading to translocation of aquaporins to the apical membrane, where these water-channels allow free water absorption along an osmolar gradient into the hypertonic interstitium.

With water-loading, osmoreceptors sense a falling osmolality. Thirst and ADH release are suppressed → dilute urine is formed, rapidly (within 6 hr) restoring normal osmolality (~ 285mOsm/kg)

With water depletion, osmoreceptors sense ↑osmolality, trigger ADH release, retain water with (highly) concentrated urine. Increased thirst eventually corrects the absolute water deficit.

So, for normal water homeostasis an individual needs:
- An intact thirst centre
- Access to water
- The ability to secrete ADH (vasopressin)
- A responsive collecting duct

Abnormalities in one or more of these components → abnormal water homeostasis

Hyponatraemia

As with many electrolyte disorders, $\downarrow Na^+$ is relatively common in hospitalized patients—symptomatic hyponatraemia is associated with a mortality of 10–50%. Hyponatraemia usually occurs as a result of altered water balance, making clinical assessment of body water the key to management. The NR for Na^+ is 135–145mmol/L. Causes include:

With depleted ECF (Na^+ loss > water loss)

- Renal losses:
  - Diuretics
  - Osmotic diuresis (glucose, urea in recovering ATN)
  - Salt-wasting nephropathy (due to chronic tubular dysfunction)
  - Addison's disease.
- Non-renal losses:
  - Diarrhoea or vomiting
  - Sweating
  - 'Third space' losses (burns, bowel obstruction, pancreatitis).

▶ Severe volume depletion causes a state of appropriate ADH secretion: although initially suppressed as $Na^+\downarrow$, hypovolaemia over-rides osmoreceptor-induced inhibition, and is a potent stimulus for ADH release, despite the Na^+ concentration.

With excess ECF (water retention > Na^+ retention)

- CCF
- Nephrotic syndrome or CRF
- Cirrhosis.

With a normal ECF

- Syndrome of inappropriate anti-diuretic hormone secretion (SIADH).
  - Pneumonia, COPD, TB, other lung diseases (usually with $\downarrow pO_2$)
  - Malignancy (usually small cell lung ca, occ head and neck tumours)
  - Drugs (anti-psychotics, NSAIDs, anti-depressants)
  - Neurological disease (eg, CVA, trauma, acute psychosis, tumours)
  - Pain, opiates, stress (⚠ surgery).
- Hypothyroidism.

Psychogenic or drug-induced (ecstasy) polydipsia

Pseudohyponatraemia results when Na^+ is corrected for a falsely large volume, rather than the actual aqueous phase: occurs with ↑lipids, ↑plasma proteins (▶ myeloma) or hyperglycaemia (▶ for every 5mmol/L above the normal range for glucose, correct ↓ by 1.7mmol/L). Glycine-or sorbitol-containing bladder irrigants may also be absorbed, esp. after prostatectomy, falsely $\downarrow Na^+$.

Symptoms and signs

Rare if chronic, or Na^+ >125mmol/L. Common if acute, or Na^+ <110mmol/L. Headache, apathy, confusion (esp. in elderly) → seizures and coma. Symptoms due to cerebral swelling as osmolality falls: the encephalopathy is exacerbated by ↓pO_2 of any cause.

If ↑ ECF (overloaded) or ↓ ECF (dry), the diagnosis is usually apparent.

Investigations

Re-check an abnormal result (⚠ 'drip-arm' Na^+ in patients on 5% dextrose infusions).

- U+E, plasma osmolality (normal/↑ if pseudohyponatraemia).
- ↓ K^+ and ↓ Mg^{2+} potentiate ADH release (⚠ diuretics).
- Urine osmolality (u-Osm *should* be < 100 mOsm/kg, and will be if ADH suppressed [e.g. psychogenic polydipsia]).
- Urine Na^+ (if <20mmol/L = non-renal salt losses, if >40mmol/L = SIADH [unless salt intake low])—⚠ diuretics may confound interpretation of urinary electrolytes.
- Urine dipstick for SG and protein.
- TSH and 9am cortisol if indicated.
- Ca^{2+}, albumin, glucose, LFT. ↓s-urate is common with SIADH.

▶ Consider Addison's if ↓Na^+, ↑K^+ and volume depletion—check random cortisol and ACTH, and if unwell, treat with vigorous 0.9% saline replacement and IMI hydrocortisone.

Diagnosing SIADH

- ↓ Na^+ in patients not on diuretics
- Euvolaemic (i.e. no oedema)
- Normal renal, adrenal and thyroid function
- Urine osmolality >100mOsm/kg, often >300mOsm/kg
- Urine Na^+ >20mmol/L (unless salt-restricted).

▶ ADH may be released inappropriately from the pituitary, or from cells of neuro-endocrine origin in the lungs.

Cerebral salt-wasting

Brain injury of any cause (SAH, trauma, tumour) → brain natriuretic peptide (BNP, ≈ ANP 📖 p.521) release, resulting in salt wasting and volume depletion. ↓ECF → appropriate ADH release and ↓Na^+.

Is probably over-diagnosed. Confirm if:

- Volume deplete.
- With volume resuscitation, u-Osm rapidly rises (with ADH suppression).

Management of hyponatraemia

In all cases

- Identify those at risk for neurological complications:
  - Thiazide-induced ↓ Na$^+$
  - Pre-menopausal ♀ (?oestrogen, ↑responsiveness to ADH)
  - Malnourished or alcoholic patients
  - Even if well, ↑ surveillance as for symptomatic patients with repeated Na$^+$ checks (see below).
- *Assess the volume status correctly* (📖 p.91). The key to correct diagnosis and management.
- Stop contributing drugs ± fluids (⚠ 5% dextrose)
- Correct ↓K$^+$ (📖 p.534) and ↓Mg^{2+} (📖 p.544) if present.

Managing hyponatraemia without encephalopathy

- Unless encephalopathic, manage conservatively as:
  - If volume overloaded, *fluid restrict* <1L/day (≈ 5 cups/day)
  - If euvolaemic, *fluid restrict* as above. An alternative is give po NaCl as 600 mg 4–8 tablets daily (contains 10mmol/tab Na$^+$, e.g. Slow sodium$^®$) ± furosemide 20–40 mg/daily.
  - If volume deplete, *resuscitate* with 0.9% saline.
- Specific points for managing asymptomatic SIADH:
  - Demeclocycline 150–300mg 6 hourly induces nephrogenic diabetes insipidus, reversing ADH's effects. Use with caution if chronic hyponatraemia, as diuresis may be brisk.
  - Newer aquaretics act by inhibiting ADH's V2-receptor-mediated actions—still experimental, but offer real promise.

☞ The brain and ↓Na$^+$

The skull limits the brain's capacity to increase in size: with ↓Na$^+$, a falling osmolality → ↑intracellular water and symptomatic brain swelling. In response, the cerebral ECF is rapidly reduced (to allow more room), and intracellular organic solutes exported (lessens the osmolar gradient that causes water influx) over days. If too rapid correction of chronic ↓Na$^+$ occurs, osmotic or *central pontine myelinosis* (CPM) may occur. As the brain cannot restore the solute contribution to intracellular tonicity quickly, when the ECF osmolality is rapidly normalized, water leaves cells, causing cerebral dehydration and demyelination (affecting the whole brain, not just the pons as in the original description).

Managing hyponatraemia with encephalopathy

1. Manage in high-dependency setting.
2. ↑ Na^+ by as little as 3–7mmol/L will usually treat symptoms
3. Repeat Na^+ every 2 hours initially, and then 4 hourly.

- IF **acute** <48 hours duration (often post-operative):
  - Aim for ↑Na^+ by 2mmol/L/hr or until asymptomatic.
  - **Do not correct by** >10mmol/L/24 hours.
- IF **chronic** >48 hours duration:
  - **Always consider CPM.**
  - Aim for ↑Na^+ by 0.5mmol/L/hr or until asymptomatic.
  - **Do not correct by** >10mmol/L/24 hours.
- Other measures:
  - Add in furosemide to prevent volume overload (as 20mg IVI 8 hourly). The diuresis caused will be hypotonic (i.e., water in excess of salt), adding to sodium correction.
  - In volume overloaded patients intolerant of salt-loads, 20% mannitol may be useful to allow use of 3% saline.
  - *Do not correct by >10mmol/L/24 hours.*
- Calculate Na^+ deficit and select appropriate mode of administration.
- Na^+ deficit = total body water x [desired Na^+ - actual Na^+]
  - TBW = 60% body weight in ♂ and 50% body weight in ♀
  - If age >65, use 50% BW in ♂ and 45% BW in ♀
  - For example, aiming for a safe Na^+ of 125 mmol/L in 53-yr-old 70kg ♂ with Na^+ 115, deficit = 0.6 x 70 x 10 = 420 mmol Na^+.
- Generally use 2.7% or 3% (hypertonic) saline, containing 462mmol and 513mmol NaCl respectively per 1L.
- Deliver via a central line.
- Estimate effect of infusion by calculating change in Na^+:
  - Change in Na^+ = $\dfrac{\text{infusion fluid } Na^+ - Na^+}{TBW + 1}$ for 1000mL infusion
  - For example, in the above patient, using 3% hypertonic saline 1L over 24 hours, change in Na^+ = $\dfrac{513 - 115}{42 + 1}$ = 9.25mmol/L

  If a rapid increase was required (e.g., if fitting), and a target of >120mmol/L was desired, over 3 hours (see below) aim to infuse [5/9.25 x 1L] = 540mL of 3% saline at 180mL/hr.

Hypernatraemia

Serum Na^+ >146mmol/L is usually due to a water deficit, and is associated with significant mortality (±50%). With ↑Na^+, ECF osmolality ↑, increasing osmotic drag on the intracellular compartment. This leads to cellular dehydration, most importantly in the brain: loss of volume creates vascular shear stress, resulting in bleeding and thrombosis. As in hyponatraemia (📖 p.522), compensation begins with cellular retention of salts and organic solutes in the brain, increasing cellular tonicity and lessening water losses to the hyperosmolar ECF (occurs over days). Over-zealous correction leads to too-rapid intracranial expansion of the brain, with potential tentorial herniation. Causes include:

Excess hypertonic fluids

- IVI infusions (▶ antibiotics), TPN or enteral feeds.
- Rarely, salt ingestion or sea water drowning.

Excess water loss

- Renal
  - Diabetes insipidus (see opposite) with/out altered thirst
  - Diuretics
  - Osmotic diuresis (glucose in DKA, urea in recovering ATN)
- Gut
  - Diarrhoea (and laxatives such as lactulose)
  - Vomiting, NG losses or fistulae
- Skin
  - Sweating, burns.

Decreased thirst

In the unwell and elderly, esp. if on psychotropic drugs

Symptoms and signs

Reflect cerebral dehydration. Thirst, apathy, weakness, confusion → ↓consciousness, seizures and coma. Cause often apparent clinically. Investigations: U+E, plasma osmolality, glucose. Urine Na^+, osmolality. With osmotic diuresis, u-Osm is always >300mOsm/kg.

Treatment

- ▶ Treat underlying cause.
- Aim for Na^+ 145mmol/L
- Calculate water deficit (and include ongoing losses in calculations):

$$\text{Change in } Na^+ = \frac{\text{infusion fluid } Na^+ - Na^+}{\text{TBW} + 1} \text{ for 1000 mL infusion}$$

TBW = 60% body weight in ♂ and 50% body weight in ♀
If age > 65, use 50% weight in ♂ and 45% weight in ♀

For example, in a 53-yr-old 70 kg ♂ with Na^+ 170 mmol/L, TBW = 42L. Using 5% dextrose (no Na^+), [0–170]/43 = –3.95 mmol/L. So 1L 5% dextrose will reduce Na^+ to 166mmol/L. Aiming to correct only 0.5 mmol/L/hr will require 1L/8h, or 125mL/h *if no ongoing fluid losses*. As a rule of thumb, allow for 1.5L insensible loss/day.

- *Re-assess patient repeatedly*
- If ↑Na^+ is acute (<24 hours), can be reversed quickly. Usually occurs with infusion of hypertonic solutions, but also with rapid loss of hypotonic fluid (sweating, burns).
  - Correct at 1 mmol/L/h.
  - Measure Na^+ 2 hourly initially, then 4 hourly.
- If chronic (>24 hours), correct more slowly to prevent rehydration injury to the brain:
  - Document neurological status.
  - Correct at not >0.5mmol/L/hr, or <10mmol/L/day.
  - Correct 50% of the water deficit in first 12–24 hours.
  - Correct remaining water deficit over next 24–48 hours.
  - Measure Na^+ 2 hourly initially, then 4 hourly.

Choice of fluid:
- Water po if orientated, or per NG if able.
- 5% dextrose or 0.45% (half-normal) saline IVI if cannot use the gut. May require insulin to control hyperglycaemia if using 5% dextrose.

Diabetes insipidus
ADH (also called arginine vasopressin) binds the V2 receptor on collecting duct cells, leading to surface expression of free water channels, or aquaporins, through which water is rapidly taken up. DI can be cranial (i.e. impaired release of ADH):
- Trauma
- Tumours or infiltrative processes (sarcoid, TB)
- Infective (meningitis, encephalitis)
- Cerebral vasculitis (SLE, Wegener's).

More commonly, DI is nephrogenic (resistance to ADH). Causes include:
- Congenital
- Drug-induced (lithium, amphotericin B, foscarnet, demeclocycline)
- Hypokalaemia or hypercalcaemia
- Tubulo-interstitial disease (medullary cystic disease, 📖 p.422).

Diagnosis rests on finding ↑UO (>3L/day) with dilute urine (<300mOsm/kg). Exclude osmotic diuretics, ↓K^+ or ↑Ca^{2+}. A fluid deprivation test ± DDAVP (synthetic analogue of ADH) is diagnostic (▶ seek expert advice).

Treatment depends on cause. Cranial DI is treated with intranasal DDAVP 10–20 µg bd. Nephrogenic DI is treated with thiazide diuretics (hypovolaemia → ↑Na^+ absorption proximally, ∴ reduced water delivery to the collecting duct) and NSAIDs (such as indometacin antagonize effect of ADH).

⚠ Simultaneous use of DDAVP and 5% dextrose should be used with extreme caution (analogous to pouring water into a closed box).

Oedema and its treatment

Oedema occurs with interstitial expansion of the ECF, becoming clinically apparent if >2L fluid excess in this compartment. It is most obvious in the dependent areas (ankles), but if may affect the face and eyelids, especially in the morning. Anasarca refers to severe oedema progressing from the peripheries to the trunk. Oedema may occur with other extravascular signs of salt and water retention (pleural effusions, ascites). Causes include:

- Congestive heart failure
- Liver failure
- Nephrotic syndrome ((📖 p.386)
- Acute or chronic renal failure ($\downarrow$GFR→ $\downarrow$salt excretion)
- Drug-induced (NSAIDs, calcium channel blockers)
- Pre-menstrual or pregnant ♀ (oestrogen effect)
- Venous insufficiency (localized oedema).

Development of oedema

For oedema to develop, salt and water retention must occur (to expand the ECF), and/or capillary permeability must increase (to allow fluid shifts into the interstitium).

The *'overfill'* hypothesis suggests that Na^+ retention is the primary factor in the development of oedema: any state that leads to $\downarrow$EABV (📖 p.520) → 2° hyperaldosteronism, sympathetic over-activity, and non-osmotic ADH release. This then causes salt and water retention, an increase in ECF volume, and oedema.

The 'underfill' hypothesis explains oedema associated with $\downarrow$albumin as a fall in plasma oncotic pressure (provided largely by albumin) with unchanged hydrostatic pressure resulting in fluid movement into the extravascular space. This then leads to 2° fluid retention.

Oedema and hypoalbuminaemia in the nephrotic syndrome

Experimental evidence suggests the 'underfill' hypothesis to be incorrect with $\downarrow$s-albumin: the transcapillary oncotic gradient is maintained with hypoalbuminaemia, as interstitial colloid osmotic pressure (COP) is reduced in tandem with falls in the plasma COP (the interstitial fluid not only maintains a COP countering plasma COP, but can be varied). Rather, inflammatory cytokines impair capillary permeability, a falling EABV → salt retention, ↑urinary albumin modifies Na^+ handling directly in the nephron and renal resistance to ANP develops. The net effect is one of salt retention, with equilibration of the expanded ECF into the interstitium.

Diuretics

All diuretics block the re-uptake of Na^+, and thus Cl^- and water. All circulate highly protein-bound, and are thus not well-filtered by the glomerulus. This complex is taken up from the peritubular fluid by proximal tubular cells, and the diuretic released prior to excretion to act in the urinary space (except for spironolactone and other mineralocorticoid receptor antagonists). For use in hypertension, (📖 p.332).

Commonly used diuretics include
Loop diuretics
- Site of action: blocks Na^+ uptake at the $Na^+K^+2Cl^-$ (NKCC) co-transporter in the thick ascending limb of the loop of Henle.
- Specific side-effects: ↑u-$Ca^{2+,}$ ototoxicity.
- Examples: furosemide, bumetanide, torasemide.

Thiazide diuretics
- Site of action: blocks Na^+ uptake at the Na^+Cl^- co-transporter in the distal tubule.
- Specific side-effects: ↓u-Ca^{2+} (may cause hypercalcaemia).
- Examples: bendroflumethiazide, hydrochlorothiazide, metolazone, indapamide.

Amiloride/triamterene
Site of action: blocks Na^+ uptake at the apical Na^+ channel (ENaC) in the collecting duct.

Mineralocorticoid receptor antagonists
- Site of action: blocks Na^+ uptake by downregulating apical Na^+ channel (ENaC) expression in the collecting duct. Spironolactone enters cells from the circulation rather than the urinary space, and binds the intracellular mineralocorticoid receptor (MR).
- Specific side-effects: ↑K^+, antiandrogenic effects (not eplerenone).
- Examples: spironolactone, eplerenone.
- General side effects include ↓K^+ (*not* with spironolactone), ↓Na^+, ↓Mg^{2+}, ↑uric acid, skin rashes, interstitial nephritis, dyslipidaemia, (☀insulin resistance, impotence).

Using diuretics in oedematous states
⚠ Always institute appropriate salt restriction when using diuretics, and consider fluid restriction to <1000mL/day.
- Assess volume status daily.
- Measure weight daily to assess response.
- Strict input/output charts may be helpful.
- Measure serum electrolytes regularly.
- Monitoring u-Na^+ excretion may be helpful in diuretic resistance.

Nephrotic syndrome

Often requires high doses of loop diuretics (furosemide 160–1000mg daily), as ↑urinary albumin binds free diuretic. Consider add-on thiazide diuretics (e.g. metolazone 2.5–5mg/day po), but beware rapid-onset ↓Na^+, and titrate dose against daily weight loss.

◆ Furosemide and albumin infusions are frequently used in an attempt to improve drug delivery—probably without real benefit. *May* be of use if s-Alb <20g/dL. Administer as 100mL 20% human albumin solution with 40–160mg furosemide IVI over 2–4 hours.

Renal failure

Loop diuretic if GFR <50mL/min. May require 250–1000mg po daily, in 2–3 divided doses. Best response with IVI loop diuretic (furosemide 200mg), or as continuous infusion (furosemide 10–50mg/h to a maximum of 1000mg/day to prevent ototoxicity). Bumetanide is better absorbed, and should be considered in diuretic resistance (up to 8mg/day). If poor response, consider add-on thiazide as above.

Congestive cardiac failure

Loop diuretics better than thiazides, eg furosemide 40 mg od. Evidence from RALES and EPHESUS trials has confirmed a role for mineralocorticoid receptor blockade, so this class often used as first line. Hyperkalaemia is a real concern, as such patients are often on ACE inhibitors or β-blockers (📖 p.533).

Cirrhosis

Spironolactone (50–200mg od) prevents 2° hyperaldosteronism, with add-on thiazide (*not* loop–too marked a diuresis may precipitate ARF) if required. Resistant ascites is best treated with paracentesis under albumin cover.

Potassium

K^+ is the second most abundant cation in the body (~3.5mol). Dietary K^+ amounts to 80–150 mmol/day. Once absorbed K^+ is rapidly buffered by removal from the ECF into the intracellular compartment: insulin and β-adrenergic catecholamines stimulate membrane Na^+/K^+-ATPase to pump K^+ into cells. This electrochemical gradient (the cell membrane potential) is critical to nerve conduction, muscle contraction and normal cell function. Total body K^+ balance is regulated by renal excretion: K^+ is freely filtered at the glomerulus. It is reabsorbed by the PCT (75%), the loop of Henle (15%), and the α-intercalated cells of the collecting duct. K^+ secretion is tightly controlled by aldosterone in the DCT and the principal cells of the collecting duct. Aldosterone secretion is increased directly by hyperkalaemia, and suppressed by hypokalaemia, controlling K^+ in the normal range (3.5–5.0 mmol/L).

Hyperkalaemia see 📖 p.102 for full discussion

▶ $\uparrow K^+$ is often spurious: *always re-check result*. Traumatic venopuncture → cellular K^+ leakage and false hyperkalaemia. More common with $\uparrow$WCC or $\uparrow$platelet count (so-called 'pseudohyperkalaemia').

True hyperkalaemia is either due to increased release from cells, or decreased excretion by the kidney. Since the release of important trials using spironolactone or eplerenone (in addition to ACE inhibitors) in the treatment of heart failure, dangerous hyperkalaemia has become more common in those with normal renal function.

Common causes include
- CRF
- Drug induced (esp. combinations of the following)
  - ACE inhibitors/ARB
  - K^+-sparing diuretics (spironolactone, eplerenone, amiloride)
  - NSAIDs
  - Heparin and LMW heparins (inhibit normal aldosterone release)
  - Ciclosporin
  - High-dose trimethroprim
  - Digoxin *toxicity* (but not therapeutic levels of digoxin)
- Hypoaldosteronism (incl. type 4 RTA, 📖 p.556).
- Addison's
- Increased release from cells
  - Acidosis
  - Insulin deficiency (DKA)
  - Rhabdomyolysis, strenuous exercise or tumour lysis.

Rare causes of hyperkalaemia include

- *Hyperkalaemic periodic paralysis:* mutations in skeletal Na^+ channel lead to episodic paralysis, $\uparrow K^+$, and $\downarrow Na^+$ in response to varied triggers, as Na^+ and water are pumped into cells in exchange for K^+.
- *Type 1 pseudohypoaldosteronsim:* Presents in infancy as salt-wasting, $\downarrow Na^+$ and collapse. Either due to resistance to the actions of aldosterone (defect in type 1 mineralocorticoid receptor, with $\uparrow K^+$), or defects in ENaC (📖 p.628).
- *Gordon's syndrome* (type 2 pseudohypoaldosteronism): The clinical inverse of Gitelman's syndrome (📖 p.536). Presents as $\uparrow BP$, $\downarrow renin$ and aldosterone, $\uparrow K^+$ and acidosis. Mutations in genes encoding WNK-1 and –4 (negative regulators of NCCT, 📖 p.626) are responsible.

Hyperkalaemia since RALES and EPHESUS

These two trials demonstrated a 15–30% reduction in mortality due to CCF in patients treated with agents that block the action of aldosterone (spironolactone, eplerenone). Widespread use (occasionally inappropriate) has followed. Since ACE inhibitors/ARB are also indicated to treat CCF, serious hyperkalaemia may occur. If using such combination therapy:

- Calculate GFR (📖 p.30)—caution if abnormal.
- Stop NSAIDs .
- Advise about dietary K^+ restriction (📖 p.190).
- If $\downarrow GFR$ <60mL/min, add in loop diuretic to waste K^+.
- If acidotic (s-HCO_3 <21mmol/L), add $NaHCO_3$ 500–600mg bd.
- Do not increase spironolactone above 25mg/day if + ACE inhibitor.
- Check K^+ regularly. If K^+ >5.5mmol/L, discontinue either ACEI/ARB or sprinolactone/eplerenone.

⚠ Hyperkalaemia arises when dehydration, concurrent illness or deteriorating renal or cardiac function supervenes in patients on combination therapy. *Always check K^+. Those with K^+ >5.0 are at risk.*

Hypokalaemia

One of the most common electrolyte abnormalities seen, esp. in patients on diuretics. Although K^+ of 3–3.5mmol/L is generally well tolerated, hypokalaemia of <2.5mmol/L can be life-threatening.

Symptoms and signs

See list of causes for specific associations—usually picked up on U+E. Fatigue, constipation, weakness and ↓tone (progressing to ascending paralysis as K^+↓). Cardiac arrythmias, esp. if underlying heart disease.

Investigations

U+E, Mg^{2+}. CK (may have spontaneous rhabdomyolysis). Digoxin level if on drug. If not drug-related, or obviously associated with an underlying illness, consider: urine pH and electrolytes (if urinary K^+ < 20 mmol/day, K^+ losses are extra-renal), renin, aldosterone. May need urinary laxative and diuretic screen if suspecting abuse. Alkalosis suggests long-standing hypokalaemia.

ECG: small T waves, U wave (after T), PR interval ↑, ST segments ↓

Treatment

❶ Is the patient on digoxin? Will potentiate digoxin's arrythmogenicity. Note that diuretic-induced hypokalaemia is exacerbated if dietary Na^+ intake is high. Always aim to treat the underlying cause over time.
Mild (>2.5mmol/L):

- Oral slow-release potassium chloride 50–150mmol/day in divided doses (treatment limited by GI intolerability).
- Check K^+ regularly.
- Rule-of-thumb is to treat until *alkalosis* resolves
- ↑ dietary K^+ and ?switch to/add in K^+-sparing diuretic
- Common options include Sando-K® (12mmol/tab), Kloref® (6.7mmol/tab) or Slow-K® (8mmol/tab). If acidotic, rather use $KHCO_3$.

⚠ Severe or symptomatic hypokalaemia (K < 2.5mmol/L, arrythmias, liver failure or extreme weakness):

- Cardiac monitor.
- Check Mg^{2+} and correct if need be (📖 p.544).
- Avoid glucose-containing solutions or sodium bicarbonate.
- IVI 0.9% saline 1L with 20–40mmol KCl at no more than 10–20 mmol KCl/h through peripheral cannula. If ↓K^+ with hyperchloraemic acidosis (RTA, 📖 p.556, or gut losses) avoid 0.9% saline, and rather use KCl as below.
- ▶ *Danger of rapid onset hyperkalaemia.* Re-check K^+.
- In volume-restricted patients, or those with profound and ongoing hypokalaemia, KCl can be given into a central vein as 20–40 mmol/100 mL 0.9% saline at not >40mmol/h using a volumetric pump. Must be in high dependency surroundings.

Causes
- Inadequate intake <25mmol/day (either dietary or IV).
- Increased gut losses.
  - Vomiting (actually, ↑Na^+ loss in vomitus → 2° hyperaldosteronism).
  - Diarrhoea or laxative abuse.
  - VIPoma, Zollinger–Ellison syndrome.
  - Ileostomy or enteric fistula, colonic villous adenoma.
- Redistribution into cells.
  - β-agonism (any cause of ↑sympathetic drive, eg delirium tremens).
  - β-agonist drugs (bronchodilators, decongestants, tocolytics).
  - Insulin, theophyllin or caffeine (activate Na^+/K^+-ATPase pump).
  - Alkalosis.
- 1° hyperaldosteronism (Conn's syndrome).
- 2° hyperaldosteronism (📖 p.310).
  - Liver failure, heart failure, nephrotic syndrome.
- Renal losses.
  - Diuretics (esp. thiazides, loops) including abuse of diuretics.
  - Acquired renal tubular disease (📖 p.564) or RTA (📖 p.556).
  - Bartter's, Liddle's, and Gitelman's syndromes (📖 p.536).
- Other drugs.
  - Amphotericin and aminoglycosides (tubular toxicity).
  - Glucocorticoids (esp. at high dose) or mineralocorticids.
  - Carbenoloxone and liquorice (have a mineralocorticoid effect).
- Familial hypokalaemic periodic paralysis.
- Thyrotoxicosis.
- Correction of vitamin B_{12} deficiency.

Bartter's, Gitelman's, and Liddle's

Bartter's syndrome

Autosomal recessive inheritance. Caused by impaired NaCl reabsorption in the ascending limb of the loop of Henle. Mutations in a number of channels (including NKCC2 and ROMK) are responsible for salt wasting and mild volume depletion. It is in effect what is seen with *loop diuretic use*. Subsequent 2° hyperaldosteronism (and juxtaglomerular apparatus hyperplasia) leads to a hypokalaemic metabolic alkalosis. ↑ luminal Na^+ impairs Ca^{2+} absorption, leading to ↑u-Ca^{2+}.

Diagnose in children (or adolescents) with failure to thrive, polydipsia, polyuria and cramps. Normal BP, ↓K^+, mild metabolic alkalosis, ↑u-Na^+, ↑u-K^+, ↑u-Ca^{2+}, ↑u-prostaglandin E2 (ill-understood reasons), ↑renin, ↑aldosterone.

Treatment: Aim to normalize K^+. Start with amiloride 5–40 mg day(large doses may be needed!). Add on oral potassium supplementation as potassium chloride 25–100mmol/day (for drugs, 📖 p.534). ⚠ *Re-check* K^+ after 5–7 days to ensure that the dosing is appropriate. NSAIDs (indometacin) if ↑u-PGE2. ACEI may help normalize K^+. Often difficult to treat, and demanding of patient (children) compliance.

Gitelman's syndrome

Autosomal recessive inheritance. Caused by loss of function mutations to the thiazide-sensitive sodium: chloride co-transporter (NCCT) in the DCT, resulting in impaired Na^+ reabsorption. ↑Na^+ loss leads to 2 hyperaldosteronism and a hypokalaemic metabolic alkalosis. It is in effect what is seen with *thiazide diuretic use*. Increased calcium reabsorption leads to increased urinary Mg^{2+} loss, with significant hypomagnesemia.

Diagnose in young adults with usually symptomatic ↓K^+ (2.0–3.0 mmol/L). ↓ Mg^{2+}. Mild metabolic alkalosis. ↑renin, ↑aldosterone. Urinary Ca^{2+} is low (unlike Barrter's). Genetic testing is available, though not widely so.

Treatment: Generally good prognosis. Amiloride 5–40 mg od ± K^+ supplementation (see above).

Liddle's syndrome

Autosomal dominant inheritance. Caused by gain of function mutations in ENaC (epithelial sodium channel expressed on the apical surface of collecting duct cells), resulting in increased sodium retention. ↑Na^+ reabsorption leads to ↓BP ± oedema, and a hypokalaemic metabolic alkalosis, with appropriately suppressed aldosterone.

Diagnose in young hypertensives (often +ve family history) with ↓K^+ (may be mild) and mild metabolic alkalosis. ↓renin, ↓aldosterone.

Treatment: low salt diet ± amiloride 5–10 mg od (or triamterene - directly inhibits ENaC).

Differentiating inherited channelopathies

	Bartter's	Gitelman's	Liddle's
BP	N	N	↑
K	↓	↓	↓
Mg	N or ↓	↓	N
u-PG E2	↑	N	N
Aldosterone	↑	↑	↓
u-Ca	↑ or N	↓	N
Age	Infancy	Early adulthood	Childhood

Calcium, magnesium, and phosphorus

Calcium

99% of total body Ca^{2+} (~1kg) is stored in bone. Extracellular Ca^{2+} accounts for a small fraction: of this, ~50% is bound to albumin, with 40% available as physiologically active, free (or ionized) Ca^{2+}. Ca^{2+} is important in skeletal health, membrane function, cell signalling, neuromuscular integrity and coagulation.

The serum normal range is 2.1–2.5mmol/L (~1.2mmol/L ionized), with Ca^{2+} available from both the gut and bone stores. Gut Ca^{2+} absorption is controlled by calcitriol (active form of vitamin D). The ionized fraction is freely filtered, and mainly re-absorbed in the PCT and loop of Henle. Falling Ca^{2+} activates parathyroid calcium-sensing receptors, leading to parathyroid hormone (PTH) release. PTH increases renal tubular Ca^{2+} reabsorption and hydroxylation of vitamin D_3 to the active metabolite, increasing intestinal uptake. PTH also enhances bone osteoclastic activity.

Magnesium

Magnesium (Mg^{2+}) is the fourth most common cation in the body, and is found largely in the intracellular compartment, or stored in bone. It is a key component of ATP-requiring reactions, and is necessary for the synthesis of protein, and maintaining membrane function, nerve conduction and muscle contraction.

The kidney dominates the control of Mg^{2+} homeostasis. The normal range is 0.75 – 0.95mmol/L in plasma. Mg^{2+} is absorbed from the gut, and renally exreted. Filtered Mg^{2+} is reabsorbed in the loop of Henle and DCT, and modifying uptake allows Mg^{2+} levels to maintained in the normal range. As Mg^{2+} passively follows Na^+ uptake in DCT, inhibiting Na^+ absorption will result in Mg^{2+} wasting.

Phosphorus

Phosphorus occurs largely as the inorganic fraction, phosphate, in the circulation. Organic phosphorus exists as protein-bound phospholipids and is not measured in clinical practice. Phosphate is essential to almost all biochemical systems. Absorbed from the intestine by passive and vitamin D_3-dependent transport, 80% is found in bone. The normal range for plasma phosphate is 0.8–1.4mmol/L (higher in children). Freely filtered in the kidney, it is largely reabsorbed in the PCT depending on oral intake (parathyroid hormone inhibits tubular reabsorption).

Hypocalcaemia

Total serum Ca^{2+} is low with ↓albumin, though the free fraction may be normal. Always correct for albumin:

$$\text{Corrected } Ca^{2+} = \text{measured } Ca^{2+} + [40 - \text{s-Alb}] \times 0.025$$

Symptoms and signs

Depression and anxiety, (peri-oral) paraesthesia, carpo-pedal spasm, tetany, respiratory depression, convulsions, and arrythmias. Examine for Chvostek's sign (tap over the parotid for facial muscle twitching as CN VII excited) and Trousseau's sign (occlude brachial artery with BP cuff inflated > SBP, observe wrist and finger flexion). If chronic, cataracts, dental changes, bone pain and muscle weakness ± skeletal deformities.

Investigations

► ECG: prolonged QT interval. U+E, Ca^{2+}, phosphate, Mg^{2+}, alk phos. If appropriate, amylase, CK, urate. Consider PTH, 25-(OH) vitamin D_3 and 1, 25-(OH) vitamin D_3. Consider X-ray long bones, hands.

Treatment

► Only treat if symptomatic ± acute.
If mild (>1.9): increase dietary Ca^{2+}. Add in oral Ca^{2+} (e.g. calcium carbonate) 0.5–1.5g tds 2 hours after meals. If vitamin D-deficient, oral ergocalciferol (inactive vitamin D) or cholecalciferol 10μg–1mg od, usually in a preparation with Ca^{2+}. If ↓, Mg^{2+}, supplement as on 📖 p.545.
⚠ If acute or symptomatic, infuse Ca^{2+} at 2mg/kg/hr: start IVI 10% calcium gluconate 60mL in 500mL 5% dextrose or 0.9% saline at 125 mL/hr. Re-check Ca^{2+} at + 4 hours and adjust infusion rate accordingly.
⚠ If tetany, give 10mL 10% calcium gluconate 10mL (2.2mmol) IVI over 3 minutes (⚠ extravasation). Repeat if necessary, or infusion as above.

Causes of hypocalcaemia

- Vitamin D deficiency
  - Malnutrition
  - Malabsorption (gastrectomy, short bowel, coeliac disease)
  - CRF
  - Vitamin D-dependent rickets.
- Hypoparathyroidism
  - Post-parathyroidectomy - 'hungry bone syndrome', 📖 p.182.
    ⚠ inadvertent after thyroidectomy!
  - Inherited, pseudohypoparathyroidism.
- Hyperphosphataemia (↑ phosphate increases bone Ca^{2+} deposition)
  - Tumour lysis (📖 p.134)
  - Rhabdomyolysis (📖 p.128).
- Acute pancreatitis
- ↓Mg^{2+}.

Hypercalcaemia

Usually the result of increased absorption from gut, bone resorption, or both. Due to increased PTH or analogues, or osteolytic metastases. Mild $\uparrow Ca^{2+}$ (2.6–2.9mmol/L) is usually asymptomatic, but rapidly evolving $\uparrow Ca^{2+}$ >3.5 may be fatal.

Symptoms and signs

'Bones, stones, groans, and psychic moans'. Nausea, abdominal pain, anorexia, constipation, depression, confusion, polydipsia, and polyuria. Dehydration (?postural drop), renal calculi, nephrocalcinosis. Signs from associated malignancy. Full medication history.

Causes

- 1°hyperparathyroidism (10–20%)—less commonly 3° with CRF.
- Malignancy:
  - Local osteolytic bone lesions.
  - Humoral hypercalcaemia (tumour-derived PTH related protein, PTHrP, has similar actions to PTH).
  - Common cancers include breast, lung, myeloma, lymphoma, oesophagus, renal, prostate, and head and neck primaries.
- Granulomatous diseases (sarcoidosis, TB).
- Drugs (vitamin D, vitamin A, thiazide diuretics).
- Immobilization, thyrotoxicosis, (phaeochromocytoma), milk-alkali syndrome (antacids, calcium carbonate therapy).

Investigations

- U+E, Ca^{2+}, phosphate, alk phos, albumin.
- PTH ± PTHrP, 25 (OH)- and 1, 25 (OH)$_2$ vitamin D$_3$. If indicated, serum ACE, protein electrophoresis, PSA. CXR. Plain KUB.
- ▶ ECG: short QT interval.

Treatment

- Treat the underlying cause:
- Stop thiazide diuretics.
- 1° hyperparathyroidism: surgery if Ca^{2+}>2.75, or if end-organ damage. Cinacalcet (a calcimimetic activating the calcium sensing receptor, providing negative feedback on PTH synthesis) is an alternative.
- Malignancy: surgical resection, radiotherapy, bisphosphonates.
- Corticosteroids (prednisolone 30mg od) is effective when $\uparrow Ca^{2+}$ is driven by increased extra-renal 1,25-(OH)$_2$ vitamin D$_3$ synthesis (granulomatous diseases, myeloma or lymphoma.

Mild hypercalaemia (<3.0): increase salt intake (promotes u-Ca^{2+} loss). Aim to maintain hydration, and treat underlying cause.

⚠ Severe $\uparrow Ca^{2+}$ (>3.0):
  - Vigorous rehydration with 0.9% saline, initially at 250–500mL/h aiming for + 2L positive balance (and giving 3–5L/day).
    ▶ Assess fluid balance regularly
  - Furosemide (increases renal $\uparrow Ca^{2+}$ wasting) 10–20mg 4 hourly, or as IVI infusion (5–40mg hourly). *Do not dehydrate.*

- If urgent control required (and volume resuscitated), calcitonin 4–8IU/kg sc/IM (inhibits osteoclast activity). Repeat 12 hourly. Must add on bisphosphonate therapy, as tachyphylaxis develops.
- Bisphosphonates are powerful and prolonged inhibitors of osteoclasts. Options include zoledronic acid (4–8mg in 100mL in 0.9% saline over 30min, duration of effect 30days) or pamidronate (60–90mg in 500mL 0.9% saline over 4h. Effect ~7 days). Monitor Cr.
- Treat $\downarrow K^+$ or $\downarrow Mg^{2+}$ with IVI supplements.

▶ Hypercalcaemia in ESRD may need treatment by haemodialysis. Will rapidly lower Ca^{2+}, and should be considered if Ca^{2+} >3.5 or depressed level of consciousness. Cinacalcet may offer an alternative.

Distinguishing 1° hyperparathyroidism from malignancy

	1°HPT	Humoral $\uparrow Ca^{2+}$ of malignancy	Metastases to bone
Phosphate	$\downarrow$	$\leftrightarrow$ or $\uparrow$	$\leftrightarrow$ or $\uparrow$
PTH	$\uparrow$	$\downarrow$	$\downarrow$
PTH-rP	$\downarrow$	$\uparrow$	$\downarrow$
Albumin	$\leftrightarrow$	$\downarrow$	$\downarrow$
Chloride	$\uparrow$	$\uparrow$	$\leftrightarrow$
pH	$\downarrow$	$\downarrow$	$\leftrightarrow$

Hypomagnesemia

Occurs in up to 12% of hospitalized patients. Often exacerbated by under-nutrition, chronic diarrhoea, diuretics, nephrotoxins. Causes include:

Renal:
- Diuretic use (loop or thiazide) or prolonged natriuresis
- Nephrotoxins (aminoglycosides, cisplatin, ciclosporin, amphotericin, foscarnet, pentamidine)
- Hypercalciuria or phosphate depletion
- Gitelman's syndrome (📖 p.536) or familial hypomagnesemia-hypercalciuria.

Gut:
- Gut losses due to diarrhoeal disease, prolonged NG suction or malabsorption states
- Pancreatitis (saponification in necrotic fat)
- Alcohol abuse.

Symptoms and signs

↓ Mg^{2+} occurs in conjunction with ↓K^+ (50% of cases), ↓Ca^{2+} and a metabolic alkalosis. Weakness, cramps, carpo-pedal spasm, positive Chvostek's and Trousseau's signs (📖 p.540), tetany, and convulsions may occur.

Investigations

↓Mg^{2+}, ↓K^+ (<3.0mmol/L). Hypokalaemia is often resistant to K^+ supplementation until Mg^{2+} is normalized. ↓Ca^{2+} (if Mg^{2+} <0.5mmol/L), with inappropriately low/normal PTH.

⚠ ECG changes: ↑QRS width, ↑PR interval, flattened T waves. Fatal ventricular arrythmias in context of underlying heart disease (esp. acute coronary syndromes and CCF).

24h urinary Mg^{2+} (NR <10–30mg/day) or fractional excretion of Mg^{2+} will distinguish renal losses from other causes of ↓Mg^{2+}, but is not usually required for diagnosis.

Treatment

Asymptomatic with modest ↓ Mg^{2+} (>0.4 mmol/L): oral slow-release Mg^{2+} 6–18mmol/day in four divided doses. Preparations include Mg glycerophosphate or Mg oxide.

Symptomatic, or with hypocalcaemia or hypokalaemia: 10mmol $MgSO_4$ IVI bolus over 5 minutes, then 20mmol $MgSO_4$ in 100 mL 0.9% saline IVI over 4 hours. Repeat as required. ▶ Can be given as a *painful* IMI.
Oral supplementation once Mg^{2+} >0.5mmol/L with 18 – 24mmol Mg^{2+}/day in 4 divided doses. Diarrhoea may limit use of oral Mg^{2+}.

▶▶ *With arrhythmias* (e.g. Torsade de pointes): IVI $MgSO_4$ 4–8mmol stat, then 20mmol/12 hourly against plasma Mg^{2+}. Aim for >0.4mmol/L.

50% of administered Mg^{2+} will be lost in the urine, so prolonged therapy may be needed. The total body deficit in symptomatic ↓Mg^{2+} may be 0.5 –1 mmol/kg body weight, so up to 150mmol may be required over 5 days (with urine losses). In diuretic-induced chronic Mg^{2+} wasting states, add-on amiloride 5mg od may limit Mg^{2+} losses.

Hypermagnesemia

Urine losses of Mg^{2+} can compensate for rising plasma Mg^{2+}, so $\uparrow Mg^{2+}$ is unusual. Occurs usually if excess Mg^{2+} administered IVI (as in treating pre-eclampsia), or in patients with impaired renal function given exogenous Mg^{2+}. Mg^{2+} containing preparations include: antacids (Mg^{2+} hydroxide or carbonate), $MgSO_4$ enemas.

Clinically

Paraesthesiae, hyporeflexia, weakness, and respiratory depression (Mg^{2+} >2.0mmol/L). Bradycardia and $\downarrow$BP with severe toxicity (>3.5mmol/L). ECG: $\uparrow$PR and QT interval

Treatment

If good UO and normal renal function, stop Mg^{2+} containing preparation and monitor. Excess Mg^{2+} will be rapidly excreted.

▶ If Mg^{2+} >5 mmol/L with bradycardia, consider IVI calcium gluconate 10% 10 mL as slow IVI bolus. May require repeated doses.

In patients with impaired renal function, haemodialysis provides rapid and effective normalization of Mg^{2+}.

Hypophosphataemia

Important hypophosphataemia occurs in ± 1% of hospitalized patients, particularly chronic abusers of *alcohol, diabetics* and those on *TPN*.

▶ Becomes clinically meaningful <0.4mmol/L.

Causes include:
- Redistribution:
  - Re-feeding in malnourished (alcoholic) patients[1]
  - Respiratory alkalosis (↑ pH intracellularly stimulates glycolysis)[1]
  - Exogenous insulin administration (DKA, critical care)[1]
  - Hungry bone syndrome (massive Ca^{2+} and PO_4^- deposition).
- ↑Renal losses:
  - Hyperparathyroidism
  - Impaired vitamin D metabolism
  - Renal tubular disorders, ATN, or resolving obstructive uropathy.
- Gut uptake:
  - Malnutrition or vitamin D deficiency
  - Chronic diarrhoea or malabsorption
  - Antacid abuse.

Symptoms and signs

Proximal muscle weakness → spontaneous rhabdomyolysis (± diaphragmatic weakness and underventilation), ileus, myocardial depression (even heart failure), altered mental state and fits. If prolonged, osteomalacia.

Investigations

Urine pH, U+E, bicarbonate, Ca^{2+}, phosphate. If indicated, PTH, u-phosphate (<16mmol/day = non-renal cause), s-calcitriol.

Treatment

If phosphate >0.4mmol/L, ↑dietary phosphate (milk and dairy products). Oral phosphate (e.g. Phosphate-Sandoz®) 1 g tds (3g = ~100 mmol).

▶ If <0.4mmol/L or if critically unwell, IVI phosphate (eg Addiphos®) 0.15mmol/kg in 500 mL 5% dextrose or feed over 12 hours. Calcitriol po or IVI may reduce urinary phosphate losses. Check Ca^{2+} repeatedly (as phosphate may precipitate sudden hypocalcaemia and tetany).

---

1 *(glycolysis = intracellular shift of phosphorylated glucose metabolites)*

Hyperphosphataemia

Almost always occurs in patients with renal impairment. Calcium and phosphate are at the limits of solubility in plasma, so ↑ calcium:phosphate product leads to precipitation, and ectopic calcification. Over time this leads to vascular calcification (and ↑mortality in CRF?). 2° hyperparathyroidism will attempt to ↑renal losses as compensation.

Usually asymptomatic, causes include:
- CRF
- Tumour lysis (📖 p.134) and rhabdomyolysis (📖 p.128)
- Hypoparathyroidism
- Phosphate-containing enemas (usually with renal impairment).

No treatment is usually required in the acute setting, though if with ↓Ca^{2+} (tumour lysis, rhabdomyolysis), can be life-threatening.

▶ If so, give 10IU actrapid insulin in 100mL 50% dextrose over 30 minutes. This works by redistributing PO_4 into cells. Promote diuresis through volume resuscitation (0.9% NaCl).

If chronic, aim to restrict dietary phosphate, use oral phosphate binders to limit uptake, and in those with ESRD, dialysis.

Acid–base

Understanding normal physiology

pH is tightly controlled within and without cells, in various tissues and fluid compartments of the body. pH is simply the negative logarithmic expression of the concentration of hydrogen ions, or $[H^+]$ in any fluid. In the ECF, pH is maintained at a normal range of 7.38 – 7.42, where $[H^+]$ at pH 7.40 is 40nmol/L – at pH 7.0 (the intracellular pH), $[H^+]$ = 100 nmol/L. Remember the pH of water is 6.8 – this emphasizes the role of buffers in biological fluids.

Intake and generation

Amounts to 1mmol/kg acid/day in adults, largely derived from ingested protein breakdown (sulphur-containing amino acids → H_2SO_4) and a by-product of cellular metabolism.

Buffering

To prevent rapid changes in pH with ↑dietary intake of, or excess production of, $[H^+]$, a system of local (tissue) and systemic buffers has evolved. These buffers include:

- Bicarbonate (HCO_3^-)
- Bone salts (calcium carbonate and calcium phosphate)
- Blood proteins (haemoglobin).

In the short term, bicarbonate is by far the most important, though bone buffers play a more significant role in chronic acidosis.

Acid maths

$$H^+ + HCO_3^- \rightarrow H_2CO_3 \rightarrow CO_2 + H_2O$$

Adding H^+ (acidosis) consumes bicarbonate and generates CO_2 as the reaction is driven rightwards. Removing CO_2 (hyperventilation) returns the pH toward normal according to the Henderson-Hasselbach equation:

$$pH = pK \quad \frac{\log [HCO_3^-]}{[H_2CO_3]} \quad \text{where pK = 6.1, the disso ciation co-efficient of carbonic acid}$$

This does *not* generate more bicarbonate, so the kidney has to ↑H^+ excretion to balance the system.

Excretion: the kidney in acid–base

Preventing bicarbonate loss

80–90% of filtered HCO_3^- is actively reabsorbed in the proximal tubule:

- Proximal tubular cell Na^+ is pumped baso-laterally into the interstitium, creating an inward gradient → Na^+ movement from the lumen.
- Na^+/H^+ antiporter allows Na^+ entry from the lumen, exchanged for H^+.
- In the lumen, $H^+ + HCO_3^- = H_2CO_3$ (carbonic acid).
- Luminal carbonic anhydrase then → CO_2 and H_2O, taken up into cells.
- Intracellular carbonic anhydrase then → $H^+ + HCO_3^-$.
- Intracellular HCO_3^- then passes into the peritubular capillaries.
- The remaining H^+ is available for recycling.

Excreting proton

- Almost all H^+ in the proximal tubule is re-absorbed with HCO_3^-.
- Acid excretion occurs in the collecting duct.
- Na^+ absorbed under the influence of aldosterone (in the principal cells, 📖 p.628) means the tubular lumen becomes increasingly electro-negative.
- K^+ is secreted from principal cells, *and* H^+ is secreted from α-intercalated cells into the lumen (aldosterone acts directly on this cell's H^+-ATPase to effect this) to maintain electrical neutrality.

Buffering urinary proton

The luminal pH rapidly falls to <4.0, inhibiting α-intercalated cell H^+-ATPase. For ongoing net acid excretion, urinary H^+ is buffered (to keep u-pH >4.0) by:

- Titratable acids (H^+ incorporated into phosphoric acid, H_3PO_4 or sulphuric acid H_2SO_4).
- Ammonium (NH_4^+).

In health, titratable acids and ammonium carry ± 50% of the dietary H^+ load, but with metabolic acidosis more ammonium is needed for acid excretion.

Ammonium

Proximal tubular cells deaminate glutamine to form ammonia (NH_3), then released and acidified in the lumen as NH_4^+.

- NH_4^+ is absorbed into the medullary interstitium from the ascending limb of the loop of Henle, where it dissociates to form NH_3 and H^+ once more.
- NH_3 can now move down a concentration gradient into the lumen of the collecting duct, available to buffer H^+, and is then excreted as NH_4Cl in the urine.
- Ammonia synthesis is enhanced by acidosis, and $\downarrow K^+$.

The urine anion gap = u-$[Na^+ + K^+]$ – u-$[Cl^-]$. This difference is urinary NH_4^+. If the kidney responds normally to acidosis (non-renal acidosis), it will $\uparrow NH_4^+$ excretion to waste H^+ into the urine. The UAG will then be *negative* (as $\uparrow Cl^-$ will accompany $\uparrow NH_4^+$). If the renal response is inappropriate (e.g. RTA, 📖 p.556), the UAG will be 0 or *positive*.

Metabolic acidosis

Acidosis occurs if the systemic pH falls <7.35, and is considered metabolic in origin if ↓[HCO_3^-]. Due to excessive acid production, retention, or by ↑ bicarbonate losses. With pure metabolic acidosis, compensation occurs through increasing ventilation and blowing off CO_2 (∴↓pCO_2).

In assessing metabolic acidosis, it is helpful to estimate the anion gap. In health, the difference between cations and anions is made up of organic (negatively charged) acids. An ↑AG occurs if acids other than carbonic acid (→ phosphate, lactate or sulphate), or ↑exogenous acids in plasma.

> ## Calculating the anion gap
>
> • AG = [$Na^+ + K^+$] - [$Cl^- + HCO_3^-$] = 8–16 in health.
> • Albumin is negatively charged: ↓Alb → *Underestimates* the AG.
> • To correct for hypoalbuminaemia, add 0.25 x (44 – s-Alb) to the AG.

Normal AG acidosis

Due to retained H^+ or HCO_3^- losses—as Cl^- is increased with H^+, such acidoses are also called 'hyperchloraemic':
• Non-renal losses of bicarbonate (► *negative UAG*)
  ‣ Diarrhoea, ileostomy, or ureterosigmoidostomy.
• Renal bicarbonate losses (UAG > 0)
  ‣ Proximal RTA (📖 p.556) or Fanconi-like syndromes (📖 p.557).
  ‣ Hypoaldosteronism or mineralocorticoid receptor blockers.
• Failure of renal acid excretion (UAG >0)
  ‣ RTA (distal or type 4, 📖 p.557).
• Increased acid production/load
  ‣ Toluene poisoning, lysine-HCl or NH_4Cl administration.

Increased AG acidosis ('hypo-' or 'normo-chloraemic' acidosis)

Due to ↑organic acids in plasma.
• Renal failure
• Lactic acidosis
• Ketoacidosis (acetoacetate or β-hydroxybutyrate)
  ‣ Diabetic, alcoholic or starvation
• Toxic
  ‣ Salicylate, ethylene glycol or methanol poisoning.

Clinically

Systemic effects of severe metabolic acidosis (pH <7.1)
• Air hunger (Kussmaul's breathing) and hyperventilation.
• ↓myocardial contractility (↓ Ca^{2+} release from sarcoplasmic reticulum), arteriodilatation and venoconstriction (central blood pooling).
• Resistant arrythmias (esp. VF).
The diagnosis is usually apparent. Investigations might include U+E, venous pH (in a blood gas syringe) or ABG, and glucose. Urinary dipstick, pH, electrolytes and ketones. Microscopy for crystals. Toxicology screen

Treatment

▶*Involves treating the underlying cause.*

Refer to pages listed opposite for specific conditions—in cases of renal failure, treating acidosis has important benefits, including preventing:

- Bone demineralization (bone buffers any chronic acidosis)
- Muscle wasting
- Anorexia and malnutrition
- Progression of renal failure (◆).

Using bicarbonate

If mild and prolonged, consider oral $NaHCO_3$ 1.5–4.5 g/day in 3 divided doses if normal AG acidosis.

Treating acidosis with IVI $NaHCO_3$ is rarely indicated:

- Corrects the intravascular pH, not the 'treatable body water' (∴ treats the numbers, not patient).
- Generates CO_2 that must be blown off (⚠ fixed or ↓respiratory rate).
- *May* worsen intracellular pH, as CO_2 rapidly enters cells → acidosis.
- Na^+ load is substantial (150mmol in 500mL 1.26% $NaHCO_3$, and 1 mmol Na^+/mL of 8.4% $NaHCO_3$), and poorly tolerated in volume-overloaded patients.

Newer non-CO_2 generating buffers (such as Carbicarb®) are promising.

Managing severe and life-threatening acidosis

Consider $NaHCO_3$ if pH <7.0 in patients with impaired cardiac performance. If correcting, aim to correct to pH >7.1 or $[HCO_3^-]$ >10, at which pH life-threatening complications of acidosis would be unusual.

$$HCO_3^- \text{ deficit} = (\text{target} - \text{measured } [HCO_3^-]) \times \text{bicarbonate space}^1$$
$$\text{Bicarbonate space} = (0.4 + 2.6/[HCO_3^-]) \times \text{weight (kg)}$$

eg, in a 70kg ♂ with pH 6.9 and $[HCO_3^-]$ = 4mmol/L and cardiac instability: deficit = $(10 - 4) \times ([0.4 + 2.6/4] \times 70)$ = 420mmol HCO_3^- Note that the target bicarbonate is 10mmol/L and NOT normal (24mmol/L).

Aim to give as 1.26% $NaHCO_3$ (1000 mL = 150mmol HCO_3^-) IVI over 4–6 hours. 50mL 8.4% $NaHCO_3$ contains 50mmol HCO_3^-.

Respiratory acidosis

Occurs if pH <7.35 and ↑pCO_2 – may be metabolic compensation if chronic (↑$[HCO_3^-]$). Causes include advanced pulmonary disease, respiratory muscle fatigue, impaired central ventilatory control (drugs or stroke) or as a result of mechanical ventilation.

Treatment (if warranted) usually involves mechanical ventilation.

---

1 the intra- and extracellular volume contributing to buffering

Renal tubular acidosis

A group of disorders characterized by impaired renal handling of acid, usually with normal renal function. The basis for the often confusing terminology used for RTA revolves around physiology: almost all filtered bicarbonate (HCO_3^-) is reabsorbed in the proximal tubule, with no net acid excretion. All net acid excretion occurs in the distal nephron (📖 p.626).

Distal RTA (type 1)

Disordered excretion of acid (H^+) from the α-intercalated cell in the collecting duct leads to acidosis. Presents as a hyperchloraemic, hypokalaemic metabolic acidosis with hypophosphataemic metabolic bone disease, renal stones, or diffuse nephrocalcinosis. Is (rarely) inherited, or more commonly acquired secondary to:

- Sjogren's syndrome, RA, SLE, and other auto-immune diseases.
- Nephrocalcinosis (dRTA is confusingly *both* a cause and result of nephrocalcinosis) of any cause.
- Drugs (analgesic nephropathy, ifosfamide, amphotericin B, lithium).
- Chronic tubulo-interstitial disease (of any cause, 📖 p.408).
- Dysproteinameias (hypergammaglobulinaemia, amyloidosis).

Investigations: ↑u-pH (>5.3 in the face of acidosis), ↓K^+, ↓ HCO_3^- <12 mmol/L, normal AG (↑Cl^-), positive urinary AG (📖 p.553), ↑u-Ca^{2+} (chronic acidosis ↑bone turnover), ↓u-citrate (absorbed to buffer acidosis). Plain KUB or USS. ANF, anti-Ro/La, rheumatoid factor. If partial RTA suspected, *do acid loading test.* Give 0.1 g/kg NH_4Cl po and do u-pH hourly, s- HCO_3^- at + 3 hrs. If s- HCO_3^- <21, and u-pH >5.3, diagnose RTA.

Treatment: potassium citrate 3–10 g/day in 3 divided doses (citrate generates 2 bicarbonate molecules) or sodium bicarbonate 4 – 12g/day in 4 divided doses, aiming for s- HCO_3^- >22mmol/L.

Proximal RTA (type 2)

Impaired retention of HCO_3^- in the proximal tubule leads to bicarbonate wasting and a systemic acidosis. Presents as a hyperchloraemic metabolic acidosis, usually with other features of proximal tubular dysfunction (so-called Fanconi syndrome, see overleaf). Commoner causes include:

- Myeloma and amyloidosis
- Cystinosis, Wilson's disease, or heavy metal toxicity
- Drugs (acetazolamide, anti-retroviral drugs, aminoglycosides).

Investigations: ↓u-pH <5.3 (► if IVI $NaHCO_3$ 1mmol/kg/hr given, distal reabsorption is overwhelmed and u-pH ↑ >7), ↓K^+, ↓ HCO_3^- (12-20 mmol/L), normal AG (↑Cl^-), negative u-AG (📖 p.553). Findings of Fanconi's.

Treatment: ⚠ high-dose bicarbonate merely ↑ HCO_3^- wasting and increases Na^+ delivery to the distal nephron (and so worsens ↓K^+). Aim to allow mild acidosis: potassium bicarbonate 1.5 – 3g/day in 3 divided doses (K HCO_3^- is less calciuric, replenishes K^+ and Na^+ load). Thiazide diuretics may also be helpful.

Fanconi's syndrome

A descriptive term for generalised proximal tubular dysfunction. It is marked by failure of proximal reabsorption of many filtered substances, and classically by phosphate wasting.

- May present with bone pain ± osteomalacia. Causes as for proximal RTA.
- Investigations: metabolic acidosis, ↓s-phosphate, ↓s-urate. Glycosuria and proteinuria (amino acids), ↑u-phosphate and ↑u-citrate.

Hyperkalaemic distal RTA (type 4)

Is much more common than pRTA or dRTA, and is due to hypoaldosteronism, usually hyporeninaemic hypoaldosteronism. Aldosterone promotes urinary K^+ loss, so its absence → hyperkalaemia. ↑K^+ impairs NH_3 secretion, limiting net acid excretion → acidosis. Causes include:

- Diabetes mellitus (often with mild renal impairment)
- Drugs (NSAIDs, ciclosporin, heparin, co-trimoxazole)
- Obstructive uropathy
- Chronic tubulo-interstitial disease of any cause (□ p.408) ± CRF
- Addison's or selective aldosterone deficiency.

Investigations: ↑K^+, ↓ HCO_3^- (rarely <16mmol/L), normal AG (↑Cl^-), negative u-AG (□ p.553), ↓u-citrate (see above). Urine pH variable, but often <5.3.

Treatment: if due to hypoadrenalism, mineralocorticoid replacement (fludrocortisone 100 – 300µg/day) will rapidly reverse the problem.
⚠ Often revealed in patients taking ACEI and increasingly spironolactone for treatment of heart failure. Advise low K^+ diet (□ p.190). Mineralocorticoids rarely useful because of significant Na^+ retention in at risk patients (CRF, heart failure). Trial of furosemide 40–120 mg od. Review drugs.

RTA by numbers

Table 9.1

	Distal RTA	Proximal RTA	Hyperkalaemic distal RTA
Defect	Impaired net acid excretion	Impaired HCO_3 uptake	↓ aldosterone
s-K^+	↓	↓	↑
s-HCO_3^-	<10	12–20	>16
Urine pH	>5.3	<5.3, ↑ with bicarbonate	Variable, (<5.3)
u-AG	Positive	Negative	Positive
u-citrate	↓	↑ or N	↑ or N
Nephrocalcinosis	Yes	No	No

Lactic acidosis

L-lactate is an end-product of anaerobic glucose metabolism: glucose is metabolized to pyruvate. In hypoxic tissue, oxidative regeneration of NAD^+ cannot occur, so pyruvate is used with NADH and H^+ by lactate dehydrogenase to produce NAD^+ (crucial earlier for glycolysis) and lactate. In health, lactate is usually rapidly oxidised by the liver for a plasma concentration of 0.5–1.5mmol/L. Causes include:

- Shock and impaired oxygen delivery
  - Cardiogenic
  - Septic
  - Hypovolaemic
- Localized tissue or organ ischaemia (infarcted gut, muscle)
- ↑energy-dependent work (usually in skeletal muscle)
  - Seizures
  - Extreme exercise
  - Malignant hyperthermia
- Respiratory failure and hypoxaemia
- Metabolic derangements involving oxidation
  - DKA
  - Carbon monoxide poisoning
  - Ethanol poisoning
- Liver impairment
- Drugs (see below).

Significant lactic acidosis is present if lactate >4mmol/L, with an increased anion gap metabolic acidosis. Conventionally, lactic acidosis due to tissue hypoxia is called type A lactic acidosis, and abnormal lactate metabolism, the under-production or over-utilisation of ATP or other causes of defective gluconeogenesis (drugs!) cause type B lactic acidosis.

D-lactic acidosis is a rare cause of an increased anion gap metabolic acidosis where bacterial overgrowth in intestinal blind loops leads to increased lactate absorption—the proliferating organisms (and not humans) are capable of producing the D-isomer.

Treat the underlying cause—there is *no* role for systemic $NaHCO_3$. So the treatment of type A lactic acidosis involves improving oxygenation: resuscitate shock, restore blood flow and/or improve gas exchange.

Drugs and lactic acidosis

Metformin has long been thought to cause a type B lactic acidosis, particularly in diabetics with renal impairment. There is some doubt about this association, but it is prudent to stop metformin if Cr >150 µmol/L.

Recently, reverse transcriptase inhibitors have also been found to cause an often severe lactic acidosis as a result of mitochondrial injury—in life-threatening cases (lactate >10mmol/L) consider L-carnitine.

Metabolic alkalosis

Metabolic alkalosis is common (as might be expected from its causes), and if severe (pH >7.55), carries a mortality as high as 45%. Either retention of base or loss of acid in the ECF leads to a rising serum bicarbonate and pH. To buffer such changes, patients can hypoventilate to $\uparrow pCO_2$ to as much as 7 kPa ($\times$ 7.5 for kPa → mmHg). For each 1mmol/L rise in serum HCO_3^- above normal, the pCO_2 will rise by $\pm$ 0.08 kPa to buffer the alkalosis (eg, to buffer a serum HCO_3^- of 34 mmol/L, the pCO_2 will need to rise by 0.8 kPa). Causes of a metabolic alkalosis include:

- With low chloride
  - Gastric losses (vomiting, NG suction, self-induced vomiting)
  - Diuretics (thiazide, loop diuretics)
  - Diarrhoea (esp chloride-secreting villous adenoma)
  - Cystic fibrosis
- With low potassium
  - 1° hyperaldosteronism (and less commonly, 2°)
  - Drugs (carbenoloxone, liquorice, laxative *abuse*)
  - Bartter's, Liddle's and Gitelman's syndromes (📖 p.536)
- Other
  - Milk-alkali syndrome (or hypercalcaemia of other causes)
  - Over-zealous bicarbonate therapy
  - Penicillins (cation load → u- HCO_3^- wasting).

Mechanisms for common causes

- Chloride-loss alkaloses:
  - With vomiting of NG losses, the stomach generates replacement gastric HCl, in the process returning HCO_3^- to the ECF.
  - Diuretics block NaCl uptake, with ECF depletion (2° hyperaldosteronism), and $\uparrow$salt delivery to the DCT ($\therefore$ $\uparrow$ exchange of Na^+ for K^+ and H^+). Diuretic-induced $\downarrow K^+$ exacerbates alkalosis further.
- Hypokalaemia and alkalosis:
  - Hyperaldosteronism leads to $\uparrow Na^+$ retention at the expense of K^+ and H^+.
  - $\downarrow K^+$ may increase net acid excretion.
  - The intracellular acidosis found with $\downarrow K^+$ leads to $\uparrow HCO_3^-$ retention in the kidney.

Symptoms and signs

Often due to associated hypovolaemia or hypokalaemia. With severe alkalosis, $\downarrow$cerebral and myocardial blood flow: headaches, confusion, seizures, angina, arrythmias. Compensatory hypoventilation and hypocapnoea may be important in critically ill patients (failure to wean off ventilator).

Investigations
Only consider ABG if evaluating respiratory contribution to a mixed acid–base disorder. U+E ($\downarrow$ K$^+$, $\downarrow$ Cl$^-$). ? $\uparrow$ Ca^{2+}. u-K$^+$, Na$^+$, Cl$^-$.
- Urinary electrolytes:
- u-Cl$^-$ <10mmol/L from gastric losses (► surreptitious vomiting).
- u-Cl$^-$ >30mmol/L if diuretic therapy (abuse), Bartter's, Gitelman's.
- u-K$^+$ >30mmol/L if diuretics, hyperaldosteronism.
- u-K$^+$ <20mmol/L if extra-renal K$^+$ losses.

Diagnosis usually obvious: urinary diuretic/laxative screen, renin and aldosterone if indicated.

Treatment
Depends on the cause:
- Treat $\downarrow$Cl$^-$ alkalosis with *chloride* .
  - If volume deplete: 0.9% saline (NaCl) 3–5L/day IVI.
  - If volume overloaded: KCl rather than NaCl (unless $\uparrow$K$^+$, ?HCl).
- Treat $\downarrow$K$^+$ alkalosis with KCl (📖 p.534).
- Reverse the underlying cause:
  - Stop alkali therapy.
  - Stop diuretics if possible, or add K$^+$-sparing agent, esp. if hyperaldosteronism present (spironolactone)
  - Anti-emetics (e.g. metaclopramide 10 mg IMI/IVI).
  - If NG drainage needed, H$_2$ receptor antagonist or proton-pump inhibitor.
  - Acetazolamide 250–500mg daily will cause Na HCO$_3^-$ wasting.

⚠ Urgent reversal of severe metabolic alkalosis (in ITU)

Indications
- Bicarbonate >45 mmol/L (or pH >7.55) *and*
- Hepatic encephalopathy *or*
- Arrythmias (including digoxin toxicity) *or*
- Confusion, seizures.

Correct K+
IVI hydrochloric acid (HCl) via *central line*: body weight (in kg) × 0.5 (bicarbonate space = 50% body weight) × required $\downarrow$HCO$_3^-$ (mmol/L) = mmol HCl infused at 0.2 mmol/kg/hr.

Example: In a 70kg male, to $\downarrow$HCO$_3^-$ by 10 mmol/L, 0.1M HCl solution (10 × 70 × 0.5 = 350mmol) at 35mmol/h for 10hours to reduce plasma bicarbonate by 10mmol/L. Alternatives include NH$_4$Cl or arginine.HCl. HD or CVVHF also provide rapid correction of severe alkalosis.

Respiratory alkalosis
Always a result of over-ventilation, due to mechanical ventilation, increased central respiratory drive (anxiety, pregnancy, stroke or CNS infection), or hypoxaemia (mild asthma, pulmonary oedema, or emboli). Treatment can be difficult if alkalosis severe.

Mixed grills: acidosis and alkalosis

As a rule of thumb, pH will rise or fall by 0.1 if:
- $[HCO_3^-]$ changes by 6 mmol/L, or
- pCO_2 changes by 1.58 kPA

For example, a fall in $[HCO_3^-]$ from 24 to 12 = pH from 7.4 to 7.2, or a rise in pCO_2 from 5.5 to 7.9 = pH from 7.4 to 7.25.

Normal ranges
- pH   7.38 – 7.42
- pO_2 10 – 13kPa(1 kPa = 7.6 mmHg)
- pCO_2 4.7 – 5.9kPa (mixed venous pCO_2 usually 1kPa higher)
- HCO_3^- 22 – 26mmol/L.

Characteristics of pure acid–base disturbances			
	pH	pCO_2	$[HCO_3^-]$
Metabolic acidosis	↓	ⓧ↓	↓
Metabolic alkalosis	↑	ⓧ↑	↑
Respiratory acidosis	↓	↑	ⓧ↑
Respiratory alkalosis	↑	↓	ⓧ↓

The circled arrows = compensatory mechanism

Mixed acid–base disturbances are not uncommon in hospitalized patients: the key to diagnosis is recognizing when compensation is inappropriate. Using the above table, the following should be expected:
- Metabolic acidosis: pCO_2 falls by $[24 - \text{actual } HCO_3^-] \times 0.17$.
- Metabolic alkalosis: pCO_2 rises by $[\text{actual } HCO_3^- - 24] \times 0.08$.
- Acute respiratory alkalosis: $[HCO_3^-]$ falls to not less than 18mmol/L.
- Acute respiratory acidosis: $[HCO_3^-]$ rises by $[0.75 \times pCO_2 - 5.3] \pm 3$.
- Chronic respiratory alkalosis: $[HCO_3^-]$ falls to not less than 14mmol/L.
- Chronic respiratory acidosis: $[HCO_3^-]$ rises by $[3 \times pCO_2 - 5.3] \pm 4$.

If compensation does not fall roughly within these limits, there is likely to be a mixed component to the disturbance:
1. What is the pH (acidotic or alkalotic)?
2. Is predominant cause metabolic or respiratory?
3. Is compensation appropriate?
4. If not, a mixed acid–base disturbance is present.

The acid–base nomogram

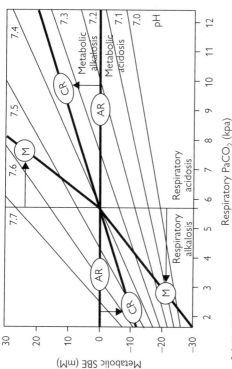

Fig. 9.1 Plot PaCO$_2$ on the x-axis; the left hand scale predicts the base excess/deficit from the intersection with the measured pH. Changes in PaCO$_2$ (i.e. in ventilation) will lead to horizontal shifts, whilst changes in bicarbonate (i.e. administration) will lead to vertical shifts from the original intersection. Metabolic and respiratory changes move the patient along the appropriate axis without altering the other.

Adapted with permission from Schlichtig R, Grogono AW, Severinghans JW (1998) Current status of acid–base quantitation in physiology. *Anesthesiology clinics of North America* **16**: 211–13.

Tubular rarities

Cystinuria

Defective uptake of filtered cystine and other dibasic amino acids from the urine leads to cystine stone formation. Autosomal recessive inheritance of genes encoding tubular amino acid transporter proteins presents in childhood or adolescence with flank pain ± haematuria (calculi).

Urine microscopy shows characteristic hexagonal crystalluria. ↑24h urinary cystine excretion (>2mmol/day, NR <0.15), radio-opaque calculi on plain KUB or USS. Aim to increase oral fluids for UO of >3–4L/day. If u-cystine remains >1mmol/L (cystine is insoluble much above this), add in D-penicillamine 1–2g/day in 4 divided doses. Alternatives include tiopronin up to 400mg daily or captopril. All work by increasing cystine solubility. For managing stones ☐ p.432.

Cystinosis

⚠ *Is not the same disease as cystinuria*

Presents in childhood with growth failure, Fanconi's syndrome, and progressive renal impairment. Eye involvement, hepatomegaly, hypothyroidism, and diabetes, develop as cystine deposits impair organ function. An adolescent variant with normal stature and tubular function but renal impairment offers a better renal prognosis. An autosomal recessively inherited defect in cystine export from intracellular lysosomes leads to accumulation and local injury. Oral cysteamine forms a complex with cystine that can leave lysosomes, ameliorating disease.

1° hyperoxaluria

An autosomal recessive condition presenting in childhood marked by ↑u-oxalate excretion, calcium-oxalate calculi, and nephrocalcinosis. Defective synthesis or targeting of the enzyme AGT, which converts glyoxalate to glycine, leads to compensatory shuttling of glyoxalate to oxalate. Heavy oxalate deposition in the heart, blood vessels, and joints causes significant morbidity. The treatment of choice is combined liver–kidney transplantation, although high-dose pyridoxine offers interim benefit.

Dent's disease

An X-linked inherited defect in the gene encoding CLC-5, a chloride channel responsible for endosomal acidification in the proximal tubule and elsewhere. This leads to impaired endocytosis and uptake of urinary proteins. Presents predominantly in ♂ (♀ may have urinary abnormalities) as Fanconi's syndrome (☐ p.557), hypercalciuria, nephrocalcinosis, and renal impairment. Rickets and osteomalacia is common. Renal transplantation is the treatment of choice for ESRD, and patients generally do well. Older syndromes such as X-linked recessive nephrolithiasis, X-linked recessive hypophosphataemic rickets and idiopathic low-molecular weight proteinuria of Japanese children are now known to be due to the same defect.

Pregnancy and the kidney

Renal physiology in pregnancy

Systemic haemodynamics change early in pregnancy, with changes in renal haemodynamics, tubular function and salt and water homeostasis:
- ↓systemic vascular resistance and ↑peripheral vasodilatation
- ↑cardiac output (by up to 30–40%)
- ↑plasma volume (by up to 30–40%)
- ↓BP and widened pulse pressure (due to vasodilatation).

As early as the 6th week renal plasma flow and GFR increase, under the influence of nitric oxide, vasodilatory prostaglandins, and relaxin. Transglomerular capillary pressure remains the same, with matching dilatation of both afferent and efferent arterioles.

Tubular function

- ↑fractional reabsorption to compensate for ↑GFR.
- Glycosuria occurs, and does not indicate impaired glucose tolerance. Urinalysis should be repeated, and a blood glucose measured if glycosuria is heavy or persistent.
- Proteinuria also occurs (not significant unless >300mg/day). Unlike in non-pregnant women, +ve proteinuria on dipstick testing may be normal. Confirm by 24 hour collection → albumin:creatinine ratios on spot urines less accurate in pregnancy (though a spot urine value of >30 mg albumin/mmol creatinine is highly suggestive).
- Tubular handling of bicarbonate and acid is unchanged, but hyperventilation in pregnancy leads to ↓pCO_2, a mild respiratory alkalosis (↑pH from 7.4 to 7.43). HCO_3^- falls to 18–22mmol/L in compensation.

Salt and water homeostasis

Women gain 9–14kg on average during pregnancy, with up to 8L as ↑total body water. The threshold for arginine vasopressin (AVP) release is lowered: this results in sustained AVP release in the face of plasma dilution, and in a true fall in plasma osmolality of about 10mOsm/kg.
- Serum sodium falls to 132–140mmol/L (Na^+ >140mmol/L may indicate hypernatraemia in pregnancy).
- Rarely, transient diabetes insipidus of pregnancy may develop in the third trimester with marked polyuria, either as pregnancy reveals an incomplete cranial DI in susceptible women, or as a result of increased degradation of AVP. It responds promptly to synthetic DDAVP, an analogue resistant to breakdown.

Anatomical changes
- ↑kidney volume, weight, and size. ↑renal length by 1cm.
- Collecting system dilatation may begin at 8 weeks, and is apparent in 90% of women by 20 weeks gestation. More obvious on right (uterine veins, enlarging uterus, and iliac artery compress right ureter → 'iliac sign' on IVU, with abrupt ureteric cut off at the pelvic brim).
- Collecting system dilatation resolves within 48 hours in 50% of cases, but may still be present at up to 12 weeks post-partum.

▶ Assessments made during pregnancy should be interpreted with caution when comparing to findings pre-pregnancy or post-partum.

Normal values for pregnant women
Creatinine falls from a non-pregnant mean in ♀ of 73µmol/L to:
- 65µmol/L in the first trimester
- 51µmol/L in the second trimester
- 47µmol/L in the third trimester.
Urea falls from preconception mean of 4.6 to 3.1mmol/L in pregnancy.

▶ Cr > 80 or urea of > 5 in pregnant ♀ may indicate renal impairment, and should be evaluated further.

If in doubt, the best measure of renal function is 24hr urinary creatinine clearance: normal range of 125–150mL/min, or 30% above the range for non-pregnant subjects is normal. Formulae that calculate GFR should not be used in pregnancy as they over-estimate actual GFR in pregnancy.

Urate falls in pregnancy: as a rough guide the intrapartum urate should be 0 (gestational age in weeks), i.e. at 26 weeks, urate should be 0.26mmol/L.

UTI in pregnancy

Anatomical, functional, and hormonal changes to the urinary tract make UTI more common in pregnancy. Pyelonephritis is the most common renal complication of pregnancy, occurring in 1–2% of all pregnancies. Preterm labour or low birth-weight infants may be associated with asymptomatic bacteriuria or UTI (co-existing ascending infection causes amnionitis, with ↑inflammatory cytokine synthesis provoking uterine contraction). Untreated UTI may be associated with subsequent develop mental delay in the child, or even an increased risk of fetal death.

Bacteriology

80–90% due to *E.coli*. *Proteus* sp, *Klebsiella* sp or Gram +ve organisms may be implicated. Resistance to first-generation cephalosporins amongst *E.coli* is ± 15% (<1% for cefuroxime). Group B *Streptococcus* (GBS) infection near delivery may lead to vaginal colonization and serious neonatal sepsis. Penicillin prophylaxis should be given during labour if infected with GBS.

Risk factors

Asymptomatic bacteriuria ($>10^5$cfu/mL urine) occurs in 4–7% of women, and in pregnancy is associated with pyelonephritis in 30% of cases if untreated. The absence of bacteriuria at booking is associated with <2% chance of UTI through pregnancy.

Further risk factors for bacteriuria or UTI prior to delivery include:
- UTI before falling pregnant
- UTI in previous pregnancies
- Diabetes mellitus, HIV positivity, or sickle cell disease
- An abnormal urinary tract.

Post-partum UTI is often associated with prolonged labour or delivery by Caesarean section, or labour complicated by pre-eclampsia or placental abruption (and almost always with indwelling urinary catheters).

Diagnosis

- Dysuria, frequency, urgency, or offensive urine suggests UTI. Loin pain, backache, vomiting and fevers are often found with acute pyelonephritis.
- On examination, suprapubic or renal angle tenderness may be found.
- Dipstick for leucocytes or nitrites may suggest a frank UTI, but will often miss asymptomatic bacteriuria. MSU for MC+S.
- If pyelonephritis suspected: blood cultures, FBC, and U+E. Consider USS renal tract. Fetal well-being should be assessed.

Acute pyelonephritis

Pyelonephritis is more common in the second half of pregnancy, and is a significant cause of fetal mortality and maternal morbidity. The increasing size of the uterus may cause ureteral obstruction and impaired urinary flow (particularly on the right), encouraging urinary tract sepsis.

Recurrent UTIs in pregnancy

▶ After more than one UTI (or a single episode in ♀ with an abnormal urinary tract), women should be given prophylactic antibiotics for the duration of the pregnancy.

Post-coital cephalexin 500mg po stat or cephalexin 500mg nocte for one month alternating with nitrofurantoin 100mg nocte have both proved safe and effective: ideally, the choice should reflect sensitivity of the organism cultured. Post-partum investigation for recurrent UTI is recommended (📖 p.426).

Treatment of UTI in pregnancy

Asymptomatic bacteriuria or cystitis
As an out-patient:
- Nitrofurantoin 50mg po qds × 7–10 days or cephradine/cephalexin 500mg po qds × 7–10 days.
- MSU for MC+S monthly to confirm eradication of bacteria.
- Ampicillin 500mg po qds × 7–10 days for group B *Streptococcus* infections.

Pyelonephritis
As an in-patient:
- IV access and rehydration with 0.9% NaCl as required.
- Cefuroxime 750mg IV tds × 3–5 days, then 250mg po tds × 9–11 days.

In select uncomplicated patients with no signs of preterm labour, ceftriaxone 1g IM daily × 2 days as an in-patient, followed by cephalexin 500mg po qds × 10 days after discharge.

Alternative regimens include ampicillin 1g IVI qds + gentamicin 3–5mg/kg per day in 3 divided doses.

Cephalosporins are not known to be harmful to the fetus, and have not been found to cause any physical or mental damage in children with follow-up beyond 18 months. Trimethroprim may be used after the first trimester as an alternative.

⚠ Fluoroquinolones such as ciprofloxacin should be avoided unless resistant organisms are cultured, and cotrimoxazole needs to be used with caution (sulfonamides should not be used in the third trimester).

Acute renal failure in pregnancy

▶ Pre-eclampsia is the most common cause of ARF in pregnancy.
Oliguria is most commonly caused by volume depletion, and responds to rehydration—renal function is usually transiently and mildly impaired. During pregnancy and the puerperium, ARF is now rare in the developed world, though still a significant problem accounting for up to 20% of all ARF in the developing world. Here it usually occurs in early pregnancy, in circumstances where there is no access to safe and sterile terminations.

Septic abortion

Sudden onset (over hours) after any attempted abortion of fever ($\geq 40^\circ$C), rigors, myalgia, vomiting, and diarrhoea (may be bloody). Abdominal pain is common, but vaginal discharge is often absent. Progression to established septic shock with hypotension, tachycardia, peripheral vasodilatation and oliguria is rapid. Organisms include *E.coli* or *Clostridia*.

Investigations

Blood cultures, FBC (haemolysis), G+S, clotting, D-dimers or FDPs (↓Plt and DIC), U+E, calcium and LFT. Perform VE and high vaginal swabs for MC+S. Plain AXR for intra-uterine or intra–abdominal gas. Consider USS to exclude pyometrium.

Management

TPR and BP every 15–30 minutes. FMO$_2$ 2–4L/min. Catheterize and monitor UO. IVI access and resuscitation with colloid and blood pro ducts (e.g. 500mL gelofusin or similar colloid as a rapid infusion—if DIC/bleeding, FFP ± blood).

▶ Benzylpenicillin 1.2–2.4g IVI qds, metronidazole 500mg IVI tds and appropriate Gram negative cover (cefuroxime 1.5g stat followed by 750mg IVI tds or ciprofloxacin 200mg IVI bd adjusted for Cr).

Acute fatty liver of pregnancy

Occurs late in pregnancy or immediately post-partum, and is part of a spectrum of pregnancy-related diseases characterized by endothelial dysfunction and end-organ damage (such as pre-eclampsia). Patients present with nausea, vomiting, and an acute hepatitis with jaundice, encephalopathy, and DIC. ARF due to ATN is common (usually successfully managed conservatively).

Investigations

FBC, clotting, D-dimers, G+S, U+E, LFT, glucose. ↑Urate. Management is largely supportive, and delivery should be expedited if possible.

Cortical necrosis

Once common, esp. after placental abruption. Occurs as a result of sudden and profound renal vasospasm (often with marked hypotension) causing patchy infarction of the renal cortex. Severe oligo-anuric renal failure (persistent anuria often being the first clue), which often progresses to end stage renal failure.

MAG-3 isotope scanning, contrast-enhanced CT scanning or MRI angiography will demonstrate perfusion defects.

Haemolytic uraemic syndrome (📖 p.404)

Used to be known as idiopathic post-partum renal failure—it is very rare, and presents with acute oliguric renal failure progressing rapidly to requiring dialysis in the early puerperium (up until six weeks post-partum) after an otherwise unremarkable pregnancy. Again, endothelial dysfunction with a microangiopathic haemolytic anaemia and coagulopathy is apparent, usually with severe and uncontrolled hypertension. The renal prognosis used to be considered poor, but long-term dialysis is rarely needed, and the prognosis is better than with other forms of HUS.

Hypertension in pregnancy

Hypertension complicates 6–10% of all pregnancies, and is responsible for 15% of all maternal deaths. ↑BP in pregnancy may be due to:

- Pregnancy-induced hypertension.
- Hypertension complicating renal disease.
- Chronic hypertension.
- Transient hypertension.

Classification

- *Pregnancy-induced hypertension* (PIH): ↑BP arising >20 wks gestation.
- *Pre-eclampsia:* is PIH with proteinuria as defined overleaf.
- *Eclampsia:* severe and life-threatening constellation of symptoms and signs characterized by seizures in the presence of PIH progressing to multiple-organ failure.
- *Hypertension complicating renal disease:* occurs in pregnant ♀ with known underlying urinary abnormalities or renal disease.
- *Chronic hypertension:* occurs in ♀ with ↑BP prior to conception, presenting < 20th week.
- *Transient hypertension:* refers to ↑BP in pregnancy that is not found on repeated measurement.

Measuring BP and proteinuria in pregnant women

A variety of classifications exist for diagnosing raised BP in pregnancy: the ISSHP[1] definitions shown opposite seem the most simple. Systolic BP correlates less well with prognosis in pregnancy and hypertension—*but* ↑SBP should still be matched with more regular review of the patient.

Risks to mother and fetus

Mild-to-moderate hypertension (BP 140/90–159/109mmHg) carries little risk, though it may progress to more severe ↑BP (>160/110mmHg), associated with maternal stroke or pre-eclampsia.

☛ *Treatment targets for hypertensive women without pre-eclampsia remain controversial.*

Although there is benefit to the mother in treating high BP, this may come at some cost to the fetus (increased IUGR in particular).

Measuring blood pressure in pregnant women[1]

- Use the bell for auscultation.
- Use a well-maintained sphygmomanometer rather than electronic device (automated devices may underestimate BP).
- Use correct cuff: should encompass 40% of arm circumference.
- Measure with patient sitting after a period of rest with the arm supported at *heart level.*
- Record systolic BP when sounds are first heard *(Korotkoff 1)* and Diastolic at the point of disappearance of sounds *(Korotkoff 5).*

Defining hypertension in pregnancy[1]

Hypertension:

A diastolic BP of ≥ 110mmHg on any one occasion *or*
A diastolic BP of ≥ 90mmHg on 2 consecutive occasions >4 hours apart.

Severe hypertension:

A diastolic BP ≥ 129mmHg on any one occasion *or*
A diastolic BP ≥ 110mmHg on 2 consecutive occasions >4 hours apart.

---

1 International Society for the Study of Hypertension in Pregnancy.

Pregnancy-induced hypertension

Hypertension usually occurring after 20 weeks gestation in ♀ with no previous history of ↑BP. More common in primigravida, and in pregnant ♀ >40 years old. ♀ attending for the first time after 20 weeks and found to have ↑BP should be treated as PIH.

A rise in diastolic BP (DBP) of ≥ 25mmHg above the booking value ('diastolic BP increment'), or even on any value documented during pregnancy is associated with maternal and fetal complications.

Prevention

Prophylactic low-dose aspirin appears to reduce pre-eclampsia (but not PIH) by 15%. Higher risk ♀ who may benefit from aspirin include:
- Primigravida >40 years
- Twin pregnancies
- History of previous pregnancies complicated by PIH or fetal loss
- With raised BP occurring before the 20th week
- Pre-existing renal disease.

✎ Calcium supplementation may also be effective in preventing pre-eclampsia in populations with a low-ish serum calcium. Whether or not all women should be on prophylaxis remains less certain: it is not practice in the UK.

Surveillance

Mild hypertension
↑DBP not > 100mmHg or raised BP arising after 37 weeks gestation.
- Check BP twice weekly
- Urine dipstick twice weekly
- Clinical appraisal of maternal and fetal well-being
- Measure U+E, urate, FBC.

More severe hypertension
Sustained DBP >100mmHg on more than one occasion or a rise in DBP through the pregnancy of >25mmHg or maternal or fetal ill-health suspected (IUGR) or abnormal blood results.
- Check BP three times weekly
- Urine dipstick three times weekly
- Weekly U+E, urate, FBC and LFTs
- Ultrasound for fetal size and liquor volume
- Cardiotocograph (CTG) for fetal well-being.

General principles of management

Bed rest is of no value in mild, non-proteinuric PIH. Although delivery is definitive treatment, non-proteinuric PIH is not an indication for delivery in itself. Drug treatment is not required for non-proteinuric PIH unless:

- DBP >105mmHg on repeated measures
- Hypertension present before 28 weeks gestation

Hypertension <20th week should be referred for specialist investigation and management (including for causes of secondary hypertension). BP lowering is *not* an end in itself—maternal and fetal well-being is a far more important marker of the underlying process.

Prophylaxis for high risk mothers

Aspirin 75mg po daily from week 12—some advocate starting prophylaxis earlier, even as soon as pregnancy is confirmed.

Drug treatment of PIH

PIH (though not pre-eclampsia) is a high cardiac output state with peripheral vasodilatation, so β-blockers are ideal therapy:

- Labetalol 50mg po bd, titrate to 100mg bd or more.
- Atenolol 25mg od titrating up to 50mg od is an alternative (concerns about fetal growth restriction appear unfounded). Advise paediatricians to beware neonatal bradycardia at delivery

  or
- Methyldopa as 250mg po bd, and titrate up to 750mg qds–1g po tds (side-effects are more common than with β-blockade).

Pre-eclampsia and eclampsia

Pre-eclampsia (from the Greek *eclampsus*, or lightning) is a rapidly progressive, life-threatening, pregnancy-specific disease characterized by hypertension, proteinuria and peripheral oedema—it is defined as progressing to eclampsia when seizures occur.

This distinction should be thought of as an arbitrary one—maternal cerebral haemorrhage and may complicate pre-eclampsia prior to seizures. Equally, modest hypertension in the context of pre-eclamptic proteinuria and oedema may progress rapidly to full-blown eclampsia.

Pre-eclampsia remains a leading cause of maternal and fetal morbidity and mortality, complicating about 3–5% of all pregnancies (eclampsia occurs in about 0.05–0.1%). Pre-eclampsia occurs in the presence of a placenta, and its resolution begins with the removal of the placenta. This has informed the obstetric dogma that pre-eclampsia is treated by delivery and delivery alone for more than 50 years.

Pathogenesis

PIH, pre-eclampsia, the HELLP syndrome, acute fatty liver of pregnancy, and HUS in pregnancy are all thought to be diseases manifesting endothelial dysfunction. Pre-eclampsia occurs in a setting of decreased organ perfusion as a result of intense vasoconstriction, affecting almost every organ—the vasculature is highly sensitive to circulating vasopressors (such as AII), reflecting the underlying endothelial abnormality. Decreased intravascular volume as a result of leaky capillaries, and activation of platelets and the coagulation cascade accompany vasoconstriction, exacerbating organ hypoperfusion and leading to formation of microthrombi in small vessels.

In normal pregnancy, endovascular trophoblastic invasion transforms maternal uterine spiral arterioles into dilated low-resistance vessels with little vascular smooth muscle or tone, so providing a blood supply to the fetus. In pre-eclampsia, this response is defective. Endovascular invasion occurs incompletely, without remodelling of spiral arterioles, resulting in abnormal flow in the intervillous space of the placenta. Reduced placental perfusion leads to release of a soluble VEGF receptor (sFlt1) that neutralises circulating VEGF, thus impairing normal vessel function throughout the body[1]. In tandem, increased oxidative stress adds to widespread endothelial damage and intolerance to vasopressors.

1 Maynard SE *et al* (2003). *J Clin Invest* **111**: 649–58.

Diagnosis

Pre-eclampsia refers to new hypertension and proteinuria occuring after 20 weeks gestation in a previously normotensive woman. It may evolve from PIH, or present abruptly. The development of generalised tonic-clonic seizures in this setting is eclampsia.

Criteria for diagnosis

- In ♀ >20 weeks pregnant (who were normotensive < 20 weeks).
- Proteinuria >300 mg/day.
- ↑BP as one of:
  - ↑DBP >15mmHg or ↑SBP > 30 mmHg on early pregnancy.
  - ↑DBP >90mmHg on two occasions 4 hours apart.
  - ↑DBP >110mmHg on a single occasion.

⚠ New dipstick positive proteinuria + ↑BP in *any* pregnant ♀ requires exclusion of pre-eclampsia.

Oedema is present in 60% of normal pregnancies, and is not a sign of pre-eclampsia.

Risk factors for pre-eclampsia

- Nulliparity
- Maternal age >40 years (or ≤18 years)
- Previous pre-eclampsia
- Family history of pre-eclampsia
- Twin pregnancy or fetal hydrops
- Obesity, diabetes mellitus, ↑insulin resistance or ↑testosterone
- Chronic hypertension or underlying renal disease
- Antiphospholipid syndrome, ↑homocysteine or vascular disease.

Affected organs include

- *Circulation* plasma volume, usually increased to 40% above normal in pregnancy, falls as capillary 'leaks' develop. Vasoconstriction and hypoperfusion accompany these changes.
- *Kidney* glomerular endothelial swelling ('endotheliosis') occurs with a fall in renal blood flow (and therefore impaired tubular function with a decreased urate clearance), before proteinuria appears. GFR falls with RBF.
- *Liver* vasoconstriction and hypoperfusion of hepatic vascular bed may contribute to the evolution of HELLP syndrome.
- *Brain* vasoconstriction leads to abnormal electrical activity which may trigger eclamptic fits. There may be associated ischaemia and oedema (often in the parietal and occipital lobes).
- *Coagulation* platelet activation occurs early in the disease, and may become associated with thrombocytopenia. Many clotting factors are elevated beyond the already raised levels seen in normal pregnancy.

Managing pre-eclampsia/eclampsia

⚠ Women with fulminant pre-eclampsia are at high risk—do not leave your patient. Involve obstetric, neonatal and intensivist services early. In all suspected cases, establish the gestational age of the fetus.

- If eclamptic, nurse in *left lateral* with a secure *airway*. Protect airway if depressed level of consciousness.
- O_2 by face-mask at 4–8L/min: monitor O_2 sats.
- *Observations* as TPR ¼ -hourly (more frequently if fitting). Strict intake/output charting.
- Insert an indwelling *urinary catheter* for hourly UO measurement.
- Get *cardiotocograph* trace (CTG) for continuous fetal heart rate (FHR) monitoring. Request fetal ultrasound to confirm gestational age if need be, and umbilical Dopplers to assess placental capacity
- *Investigations*: FBC (↓Plt), film (? haemolysis), clotting, U+E, urate, LDH, LFTs, G+S.
- *IVI access* and give 250–500ml fluid challenge with colloid prior to giving anti-hypertensives. After this, administer 0.9% saline at 85ml/h or as urine output in preceding hour + 30mL.

Delivery

If the pregnancy is near term, delivery should be expedited. If not, and particularly if <34 weeks gestational age, the dilemma is one of balancing maternal health against neonatal outcome. If it is clear that a patient has progressive pre-eclampsia, a decision needs to made on whether or not it is safe for a trial of medical therapy for 24–48 hours after administering corticosteroids to hasten fetal lung maturity. There is rarely a benefit to delaying delivery if placental perfusion is no longer meeting fetal needs, but as the consequences of prematurity are often dire, conservative management of a stable mother is frequently preferred. Maternal complications such as eclampsia, renal, liver, or coagulopathy should be managed by delivery regardless of fetal maturity.

Parameters suggesting a need for delivery

- BP ≥ 210/110 on anti-hypertensives.
- Proteinuria >3g/day.
- Rising urea or creatinine.
- Platelets <100,000/mL.
- Any rise in transaminases.
- Acute changes in fetal well-being: non-reactive non-stress test, abnormal biophysical profile.
- Severe IUGR or abnormal umbilical artery Doppler recording.

Treating hypertension

Avoid sudden ↓BP that may compromise the fetus.

△ The patient is underfilled (reduced plasma volume) and hypertensive!

- If BP >160/110mmHg, MAP >125mmHg or fitting, transfer to HDU. Consider placing an arterial line—treatment is urgent to reduce risk of *intracranial haemorrhage*. Aim for target of 140–150/90–100mmHg.
- *Pre-load* with colloid as above before giving IVI antihypertensives. *Avoid calcium channel antagonists if on MgSO₄ infusion.*
- *Labetalol* 20mg IVI as a slow bolus (over 1min). Double dose every 10min (40mg then 80mg IVI) to a cumulative maximum dose of 300mg. Labetalol 5mg/ml can be infused at 20mg/h, doubling hourly to a maximum of 160mg/h. Avoid in asthmatics.

  or

- Give *hydralazine* 5mg IVI as a slow bolus (at least 5min), and repeat every 20min to cumulative maximum of 20mg. Can be run as an infusion: 100mg in 100ml 0.9% saline at 2mg/h, doubling hourly to a maximum of 20mg/h (2–20mL/h).
- Monitor FHR throughout as hypotension may cause *fetal distress*.

Prophylaxis for and treatment of seizures

At risk mothers should be treated prophylactically, and the underlying pathology reversed—i.e. delivery. Imminent eclampsia is heralded by:
- Apprehension and facial itching
- Headache and visual disturbances ('flashing lights' or blurred vision)
- Epigastric pain
- Hyper-reflexia
- Worsening proteinuria.

- Give 4g *magnesium sulphate* (16mmol MgSO₄) in 100mL 0.9% saline over 10 minutes as a loading dose. Thereafter maintenance infusion of 1g/h (4mmol/h): make up as 24g in 250mL 0.9% saline and infuse at 10mL/h.
- Treatment should continue until 24h after delivery.
- Recurrent seizures may be treated with a further bolus of 2g MgSO₄, or IVI or PR diazepam 5–10mg stat. Uncontrolled seizures should be treated by sedation, paralysis and ventilation on ITU.

Monitor levels: with a target therapeutic range of 1.25–3.25 mmol/L. Toxicity is suggested by central nervous system depression and hypotension. Monitor the following hourly:
- Depressed or absent reflexes (e.g. patellar reflex)
- Respiratory depression (↓RR, or ↓O₂ sats)
- ↓urine output < 30mL/h.

In the absence of serum magnesium levels, maintain at 0.5–1g/h MgSO₄.

Chronic hypertension in pregnancy

Chronic hypertension in pregnancy is ↑BP diagnosed before pregnancy, or before 20 weeks gestation. This group, particularly if newly-diagnosed, will have persistently raised BP beyond 12 weeks post-partum.

Most ♀ with mild essential hypertension (DBP <105mmHg) have uncomplicated pregnancies, but around 10% will develop superimposed pre-eclampsia that is often early in onset and aggressive in nature.

▶ In ♀ with ↑BP <20th week, consider hydatidiform mole.

Prenatal counselling in hypertensive ♀ seeking to conceive

Planned second trimester low-dose aspirin ± calcium supplementation can be discussed. Most importantly, an antihypertensive regime that has the least potential teratogenicity needs to be planned and implemented. ♀ with poorly controlled BP should be advised about contraception (ideally, with an IUCD or condoms, but progesterone-only pills may be an alternative), and the need to achieve ideal control before attempting to fall pregnant.

Antenatal care

As per 'surveillance', 📖 p.574.

⚠ Evolving superimposed pre-eclampsia may be severe in this group, associated with placental abruption, multiple organ failure, and maternal and fetal death. Immediate referral to a specialist centre and close monitoring may be required.

Unplanned conception on anti-hypertensives

Many women worry about potential harm from routine BP medication when discovering themselves unexpectedly pregnant. ACEI inhibitors, associated with fetal renal impairment, IUGR, and fetal death in later trimesters, seem not to be associated with fetal disorders in the first trimester. Nevertheless, they should be stopped as soon as possible.

Optimizing anti-hypertensives before conception

No drug can be thought of as safe. There is little data about the long-term effects of anti-hypertensives on child development. This should always be discussed with pregnant hypertensive women—just as importantly, the greater risk to both her and the pregnancy of untreated hypertension should be emphasized. A treatment algorithm might be:

- *Methyldopa* 250mg po bd, increased to up 1g po tds
  or
- *Nifedipine SR* 30mg od, increased to 60mg bd (sufficient data suggests nifedipine to be safe in pregnancy—amlodipine is likely to be safe as well, but longer experience with nifedipine makes its' use preferable)
  then
- *Labetalol* 50mg po bd, increased to up to 400mg po tds (atenolol 25mg od increasing to 100mg od is an alternative).

Other alternatives include

- *Prazosin* 0.5mg po bd increased to 2–4mg po tds (doxazosin 1mg po bd increased to 8mg po bd is effective, though experience with it is not as extensive as with prazosin)
  or
- *Hydralazine* 50mg po bd, increased to up to 100mg po tds

At the beginning of the second trimester, as prophylaxis against superimposed pre-eclampsia, add in:
- Aspirin 75mg po daily (📖 p.574)

⚠ The following drugs are contra-indicated in pregnancy, or too little experience with them makes their use undesirable: *ACEI inhibitors and angiotensin II receptor antagonists, moxonidine and minoxidil, newer α- and β-blockers.*

Pre-existing renal disease

The ability to conceive falls with ↓GFR, and the danger a pregnancy carries to both mother and fetus rises substantially. Fetal loss, IUGR, and pre-term labour are not uncommon, and irreversible loss of maternal renal function as a result of any pregnancy is a major risk.

↑BP is the single most important predictor of the risk a pregnancy poses to mother and fetus. Such pregnancies should be monitored by a joint obstetric/renal team with specialist neonatal input prior to delivery.

Primary glomerular disease with normal renal function

- The type of glomerular lesion has little impact on fetal outcomes—the presence of *proteinuria* is of far greater importance.
- If nephrotic-range proteinuria (>3g/day, ☐ p.19), ↑perinatal loss (up to 23%) and preterm delivery (35%)—this is double expected if no proteinuria (12–15% perinatal loss and 9–21% preterm labour).
- Rate of spontaneous abortion is not ↑ against the normal population.
- Worsening maternal hypertension occurs in 10–20% of cases, and predicts a worse outcome.
- Relapse of the primary glomerular lesion is rare (► ?pre-eclampsia).
- A permanent deterioration in renal function is unlikely in the absence of renal impairment.

Diabetic nephropathy

Maternal diabetes is usually type 1, but may also be type 2 in young adulthood. Pregnancies may be complicated by prolonged or pre-term labour with large for gestational age babies (40%). Pregnancy does not accelerate the onset of or progression to diabetic nephropathy, but women with overt diabetic nephropathy fare substantially worse.

Non-glomerular disease and normal renal function

Reflux nephropathy is the most common pre-existing renal disease encountered in pregnant women:

- Good outcome if renal function is normal—fetal loss is only about 12%. More frequent and regular MSU for MC+S should be performed, and bacteriuria treated promptly.
- Acute pyelonephritis is more common.
- Children should be screened in infancy (☐ p.430).

Polycystic kidney disease (APKD) has nearly normal outcomes:

- ↑risk of pre-eclampsia.
- If Cr normal but ↑BP up to 45% will develop pre-eclampsia.
- Cyst complications such as cyst haemorrhage or cyst infection in pregnancy may masquerade as obstetric complications.

Women with APKD and a family history of intracranial aneurysms should be screened prior to conception.

Lupus nephritis
- Lupus affects ♀ of child-bearing age—40% will develop renal disease.
- Fertility is normal if GFR normal—cyclophosphamide causes premature ovarian failure in up to 60%, esp. if total dose >10g.
- Progestogen-only pills for contraception if active disease or anti-phospholipid antibodies.
- Wait until off cytotoxic agents, and on <7.5mg prednisolone before trying to conceive (ideally >6 months after full remission achieved).
- If active disease at conception, disease flares during pregnancy are more likely: treatment should be directed in a specialist centre.
- ♀ with antiphospholipid antibodies are at increased risk of spontaneous abortion, and should be managed in specialist centres pre-conception: consider aspirin and LMW heparins from conception—20 weeks if a +ve history of venous thrombo-embolism or fetal loss.
- Fetal outcomes depend on disease control, renal function and the presence of hypertension.
- Active lupus → with increased fetal loss, prematurity and IUGR.

Pre-eclampsia or active lupus nephritis?

	Pre-eclampsia	Lupus nephritis
BP	↑↑	↑↑
Proteinuria	+++	+++
Haematuria	±	+++
Red cell casts	−	++
ALT	↑	Normal
Complement	Normal	↓
dsDNA titres	Normal	↑
Symptoms of lupus	−	++
Response to steroids	−	+

Ante-natal care

Aim to see mother roughly fortnightly until 32nd week, thereafter weekly. Manage as per 'surveillance' 📖 p.574.

- Confirm the underlying diagnosis if possible—if unknown, exclude reflux nephropathy or chronic pyelonephritis
- Check U+E, urate
- Cr clearance and 24 hr proteinuria or albumin:creatinine ratio
- Assess disease activity in systemic diseases like lupus, or in glomerulonephritis (avoid pregnancy while on cytotoxic agents, and until full remission achieved for at least 6 months)
- Plan anti-hypertensives and achieve ideal BP prior to conception—test for pregnancy early, aiming to stop ACE inhibitors/ARB
- Stop smoking, alcohol and caffeine
- Start folate 400 µg od, oral iron and aspirin 75mg od

Outcomes in pregnant ♀ with pre-existing renal disease

Creatinine <125µmol/L
Good maternal renal prognosis, with usually successful pregnancies

Creatinine 125–220µmol/L
Some risk to pregnancy and fetus—real risk to maternal renal function

Creatinine >220µmol/L
Poor fetal outcomes, with high risk of maternal end stage renal failure

Pregnancy in ♀ with CKD (creatinine >125µmol/L)
Fetal risks
- 60% of neonates will be pre-term ± many small for gestational age.
- Fetal mortality is 7% with good neonatal intensive care facilities.
- If maternal Cr >220µmol/L, fetal IUGR present in 57% of cases.

Maternal risks
Significant risk of loss of renal function:
- Cr <125: 16% will experience a transient rise in creatinine.
- Cr 125–175: 40% will have ↑Cr—50% will not recover lost function.
- Cr >175: 65% will have ↑Cr—few regain lost function, and 35% of whom will be dialysis-dependent within one year.
- Superimposed pre-eclampsia occurs in 65%.
- Renal recovery may not be seen until 6 weeks post-partum, if at all.

Diabetics with impaired renal function appear to be at higher risk—pregnancy should be discouraged if significant renal impairment is present.

Disorders of the renal tract in pregnancy

Changes in the anatomy of the renal tract during pregnancy, in particular dilatation of the collecting system (📖 p.567), need to be borne in mind when assessing women with urinary tract symptoms and signs.

Haematuria

In the absence of proteinuria, is usually due to anatomical changes, with bleeding from small venules in dilated collecting systems. On microscopy 2–3rbc/hpf is normal in pregnancy (unlike 1–2 in the non-pregnant population). If Cr normal and no proteinuria, wait until 12 weeks after delivery for further assessment (📖 p.46).

Obstruction

May occur due to mechanical pressure exerted by the uterus (usually on the right ureter, often where the ureter crosses the iliac artery), or pelvic or ureteric stone impaction. Renal stones occur rarely in pregnancy and usually in women known to have nephrolithiasis prior to pregnancy. Collecting system dilatation with stasis, and 2–3 fold increase in urinary calcium excretion may precipitate new stone formation in pregnancy.

Suspect if flank pain, dysuria, and haematuria

- Urine dipstick for haematuria and proteinuria
- Microscopy: red cells (+morphology), casts, pus cells, and organisms
- Urine culture ± stone analysis
- FBC, U+E, calcium, ± PTH (if stones are suspected).

Imaging may include

- Ultrasound
- IVU if obstruction suspected, esp. if with co-existing infection
- (Spiral CT—avoid if possible).

In cases where an IVU is requested

- The radiation exposure is low (0.4–1.5rads)
- Shielding the pelvis further reduces exposure to the fetus
- Limited films should be taken.

Obstruction can be treated by stenting (📖 p.500). Limited experience with external shock wave lithotripsy suggests it to be safe, though best avoided if possible. Consider prophylactic antibiotics through pregnancy.

Pregnancy on dialysis

♀ with ESRD rarely fall pregnant on dialysis: only 0.3–2.2% will conceive. Nevertheless, offer contraception to women who menstruate on dialysis (up to 40%). If pregnancy occurs, and progresses beyond the first trimester, fetal outcomes are often poor, and maternal morbidity is significant.

> **What should women know about pregnancy on dialysis?**
>
> - Between 20–70% of pregnancies will result in a live infant.
> - 13–45% of pregnancies result in spontaneous miscarriage < 20 weeks gestation.
> - Stillbirth, neonatal death, and severe developmental delay are much more common.
> - Most pregnancies (up to 85%) will end in preterm labour and delivery, with a mean gestational age of 32 weeks.
> - Intra-uterine growth retardation and low birth-weight are common.
> - No increase in congenital abnormalities over the normal population.
> - Difficult to control maternal hypertension complicates up to 80% of pregnancies.

Targets for dialysis

No reason for modality switch: HD delivers a higher dialysis dose, but CAPD (esp. APD) offers less rapid metabolic changes and allows steady fluid removal. Residual renal function improves pregnancy outcomes.

Haemodialysis

Aim for urea of ≤ 15mmol/L through daily dialysis for ≥ 20 hours/week. Titrate dialysate K^+, Ca^{2+} and HCO_3^- against serum levels (may require reduction in dialysate HCO_3^- to prevent maternal alkalaemia). Heparin requirements may increase. Avoid hypotension if at all possible—expect 0.5kg/week weight gains from mid-pregnancy onwards.

Peritoneal dialysis

As pregnancy progresses, and intra-abdominal PD fluid volume is less well-tolerated, automated PD becomes necessary with daytime exchanges and CCPD. Peritonitis should be treated vigorously, bearing in mind the potential teratogenicity of some antibiotics.

Diet, calcium and vitamin D

↑protein intake to 1.2–1.4g/kg pre-pregnant weight + 10g per day. For CAPD, take dialysate protein losses taken into account and replace. Daily multivitamin preparation with water soluble vitamins. ↑folate to 1.6mg/day. The placenta produces calcitriol: ↓vitamin D analogue dose. Supplemental K^+ may be required.

Anaemia

Erythropoietin is not teratogenic. Dose requirements in pregnancy will increase by 50–100%. Supplement oral iron. Use low dose IVI iron if necessary.

Labour and delivery

Most units will deliver pregnant dialysis patients early, usually as a result of worsening hypertension, IUGR or both: few pregnancies are permitted to progress beyond 38 weeks.

- Monitoring uterine activity should begin as early as the 26th week, as dialysis may induce contractions.
- Caesarian section is performed for standard obstetric indications.
- PD patients should be drained out for delivery—dialysis can resume 24 hours after delivery with small volume exchanges. Haemodialysis for a fortnight can be used in cases of leakage.
- Assess fluid status carefully: avoid volume overload.
- Infection should be borne in mind, and avoided if possible. Sterile techniques should be used where feasible.
- Neonates should be cared for in specialist units with regular electrolyte assessment.

Renal transplantation and pregnancy

A functioning renal transplant rapidly restores fertility and libido in women with ESRD. About 1 in 50 women of child-bearing age in this group will fall pregnant, and over 14,000 such pregnancies have been reported.

Pre-pregnancy counselling

Many women will not want to fall pregnant: after successful transplantation, barrier contraception with condoms is the safest but not the most effective method (▶ progesterone-only pill). Oral contraceptives may interfere with immunosuppressants or aggravate hypertension. Pelvic infections may complicate IUCD use.

- Review all drugs prior to conception to minimize teratogenicity, with particular attention to anti-hypertensives.
- Inform blood group Rh− women with Rh+ kidneys (they may develop anti-Rh+ antibodies → neonatal haemolysis).
- Live vaccines (such as rubella) are contra-indicated: rubella antibodies should be tested for (ideally, vaccinate before transplantation).
- ± 30% of pregnancies will not progress beyond 12 weeks through miscarriage or termination (similar in general population).
- Beyond this, 95% of pregnancies will succeed. ↑risk of preterm labour and delivery (40–60%), and IUGR (40%).
- No ↑ in congenital abnormalities above general population. Incidence of longer term developmental delay is probably low.
- Successful live births are related to good graft function, the absence of proteinuria, and length of time after transplantation.
- Maternal hypertension will develop or worsen in 30%.
- Transplant function may worsen transiently or even permanently (up to 10% graft loss in the 2 years after delivery), esp. if Cr > 200μmol/L.
- ± 15% of women will experience a decline in GFR with pregnancy.

Ideally

- 2 years post-transplant with stable renal function (<180μmol/L, but <140μmol/L may be a more preferable target) and good patient health.
- Blood pressure control should be good (<135/85mmHg).
- Proteinuria should be less than 500 mg/day.
- No recent transplant rejection episodes.

Potentially teratogenic drugs should have been swopped.

Drugs in transplantation and pregnancy

Ciclosporin: no ↑risk of teratogenicity at therapeutic levels, esp. if dose ≤ 5 mg/kg/day. Monitor levels closely, and adjust dose accordingly. Maternal ↑BP and IUGR may be problems.

Tacrolimus: less evidence available. Transient neonatal hyperkalaemia and renal dysfunction has been reported. Dose adjustment to achieve therapeutic levels often required. Gestational diabetes and preterm labour may be problems.

Azathioprine: widespread experience has not borne out experimental concerns: therapy can be safely continued at low dose (<2mg/kg/day).

Corticosteroids: safe in pregnancy at maintenance doses (<15mg/day). Poor wound healing may complicate delivery (esp. if Caesarean section). Neonates should be monitored to exclude adrenal suppression.

⚠ Breast-feeding is not advocated on maintenance immunosuppression.

The following drugs commonly prescribed in renal transplantation are contra-indicated: MMF, sirolimus, anti-infectives such as ganciclovir, and cotrimoxazole.

Ante-natal care

- Check ciclosporin or tacrolimus levels frequently (weekly).
- U+E, Ca, LFT every two weeks or more.
- FBC 6 weekly.
- Baseline toxoplasmosis, cytomegalovirus, and HSV status.
- Screen for gestational impaired glucose tolerance every trimester.

Labour

- Vaginal delivery is safe, though short labours are preferable.
- Perform all VEs with strict aseptic technique.
- Additional hydrocortisone 100mg IVI or IMI should be administered (or increase oral prednisolone to 15mg od over labour).

Drugs and the kidney

Prescribing in renal impairment

⚠ Always check the recommended dose when prescribing a drug to a patient with renal impairment

Principles

- Most drugs are ultimately excreted by the kidney, though many are broken down in the liver or elsewhere first. Thus renal impairment is likely to affect pharmacokinetics
- In practice, special care is required when using those drugs:
  - With a narrow therapeutic index (i.e. the toxic and therapeutic ranges overlap or are close to each other). (► digoxin, aciclovir).
  - Dose reduction and monitoring of plasma levels may be indicated.
  - In which renal toxicity is a possible effect of the drug, in which case a vicious cycle ensues of worsening renal function, decreased drug clearance, and rising drug levels (► gentamicin, ciclosporin).
- For many drugs, plasma levels are altered by ~ 30% with significant renal impairment (► many antibiotics). Dose reduction may be required, but the wide therapeutic window may make it possible to use the drug safely with simple guidelines for dose reduction (e.g. 'halve the standard dose').

Pharmacokinetics

Renal failure may not just affect the renal clearance of a drug. Other pharmacokinetic changes may also occur:

Absorption

Drugs taken orally are absorbed via the gut. Absorption may be affected by:

- Interactions with other substances in the GI tract (► ciclosporin absorption is affected by grapefruit juice).
- Interactions with other drugs in the GI tract (► phosphate binders).
- Gastric pH may also be important—in renal failure gastric ammonia production may alter gastric pH, decreasing absorption of some drugs (► ferrous sulphate, folic acid).

Protein binding

Changes in albumin concentration affect free drug concentrations of highly protein-bound drugs. In the nephrotic syndrome, hypoalbuminae-mia → ↓drug binding to albumin, and ↑free drug. Accumulation of uraemic metabolites in renal failure, and binding of these compounds to albumin, may also affect protein binding by drugs thus increasing the active fraction of the drug. ► Phenytoin is less protein bound in renal failure, and signs of toxicity may occur at 'therapeutic' levels.

Volume of distribution

Measures the (theoretical) volume occupied by the drug, assuming uni-form concentration in all compartments. Volume of distribution may be affected by renal disease (► digoxin, for which a reduced loading dose may be required).

Clearance

Hepatic clearance: breakdown of the drug to inactive metabolites. Usually occurs either by conjugation (to glucuronide or sulphate) to make a lipid soluble drug more polar (thus increasing renal clearance—see below) or by oxidation/reduction.

Renal clearance:

Smaller molecules (MW<60,000) are filtered by the glomerulus to a greater or lesser extent. Polar molecules are more freely filtered than lipid soluble molecules.

• Tubular reabsorption may be significant, especially of lipid-soluble drugs, as may tubular secretion (acidic drugs tend to be secreted into an alkaline urine and vice versa, eg salicylic acid is better excreted via an alkaline urine). ⚠ In general, as GFR falls, drug elimination by all these mechanisms decreases.

• Most drugs approximate to first order kinetics (the rate of excretion is proportional to the concentration of the drug), and the elimination half life ($t_{1/2}$)is constant. Steady state concentration in these circumstances depends on $t_{1/2}$, which in turn depends on GFR for drugs excreted by the kidney. Thus in renal failure drug levels of renal excreted drugs accumulate unless a dose reduction occurs.

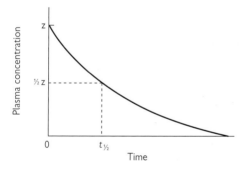

Fig. 11.1 First order kinetics: if the drug is excreted by the kidneys, renal failure will lead to an increase in $t_{1/2}$. Reproduced with permission from Warrell D, Cox T, Firth J, and Benz EJ (eds) (2004) *Oxford Textbook of Medicine*, 4th edn, p.469. Oxford University Press, Oxford.

The septic ESRD patient: drug issues

▶▶ Renal failure is an immunocompromised state. Always consider sepsis in differential diagnosis of any sick patient. The presentation may be atypical and non-specific. Blood cultures (and any other relevant cultures e.g. MSU, sputum, wound site) should always be collected before the first dose of antibiotics in any sick patient.

Choice of antibiotic

- History and examination may reveal the most likely source of sepsis. This should guide the initial choice of antibiotics, but in the sick patient antibiotics should be sufficiently broad range to cover all the most likely and pathogenic organisms. Local antibiotic policies, drawn up in association with the microbiology department, should be adhered to in all but exceptional circumstances.
- Haemodialysis patients: Always consider line sepsis or PTFE sepsis if one of these is present (🕮 p.216).

Empirical therapy in overtly septic HD patients

- Vancomycin 500mg in 100mL 0.9% NaCl IVI over 30min *or* if > 75kg, 1g in 250mL 0.9% NaCl IVI over 60min
- + gentamicin 80mg slow bolus IVI
- Given during the last hour of dialysis or after dialysis.

Levels are likely to remain therapeutic for at *least* 48 hours, and often much longer for vancomycin. Ototoxicity is unusual.

⚠ The effect on residual renal function (an important long-term prognostic feature in ESRD) remains unknown, but consensus remains that the risks of sepsis far outweigh any decline in UO).

▶ *Always* consider removal of any foreign body (line!)
- Peritoneal dialysis patients: always consider peritonitis. Do an exchange and send for culture. Remember that peritonitis in APD patients may be less easily diagnosed (🕮 p.228).
- Transplant patient: consider UTI, chest, atypical infections (esp. CMV, pneumocystis). In the sick patient, give broad spectrum treatment initially until culture results are known (🕮 p.266).

Specific antibiotics

⚠Consult a local or national formulary and/or get expert advice when prescribing any drug for a renal patient.

Penicillins: safe and effective in the non-allergic patient. The highest doses should be avoided in severe renal failure as clearance is reduced e.g. benzylpenicillin, flucloxacillin (give 50% standard dose), piperacillin (4g bd IVI maximum), amoxicillin (500mg po tds maximum)

▶ Neurotoxicity may still occur—watch for confusion, drowsiness

Cephalosporins: usually safe in renal failure as the therapeutic window is wide, but clearance is reduced. Moderate dose reduction is recommended e.g. cefuroxime 750mg IVI bd, cefotaxime 1g bd IVI, ceftazidime 1g daily IVI (500mg if slight)

▶ Neurotoxicity may still occur—watch for confusion, drowsiness.

Quinolones: dose reduction is required e.g. ciprofloxacin 200mg bd IVI or 250mg bd po. If severe sepsis, consider 24–48 hours of full dose prior to dose reduction

Metronidazole: dose should be reduced in severe renal failure e.g. 500mg bd IVI.

Aminoglycosides in renal failure

⚠ Renal excreted, have a narrow therapeutic window, and are nephrotoxic.

A vicious cycle of rising drug levels and worsening renal function can develop. Therefore extreme care is required when prescribing to any patient with renal impairment. Avoid in acute renal failure as ischaemia is synergistic in causing renal injury.

- Freely filtered by the glomerulus (so dosage needs to be adjusted according to GFR), and then partially taken up by tubular cells. Can cause tubular cell injury progressing to frank ATN.
- Standard normograms for calculating dosage regimes must be modified to take GFR into account.
- Peak and trough levels (and renal function) should be measured regularly (after one dose in severe renal impairment). Repeat doses may only be required every few days in severe renal impairment.
- For dialysis patients with no significant residual renal function, gentamicin 80 mg IVI may be given at the end of every dialysis session (check trough levels).
- Resolution of renal dysfunction usually occurs over a few days when the drug is withdrawn unless toxicity is severe. Hyperbilirubinaemia and other nephrotoxins (NSAIDs) prolong recovery time.
- Amikacin, netilmicin and tobramicin have similar pharmokinetics to gentamicin—manage in a similar way.

▶ *Avoid* the recommended 5 mg/kg/day dosing schedule unless eGFR known to be (near) normal

Cardiac drugs in renal failure

⚠ Most big cardiology trials specifically excluded patients with renal impairment.

▶ The indications for using drugs shown to be of real benefit in CCF and IHD (in people with normal renal function) in patients with CKD are therefore unknown and may even be *harmful*.

▶ Ideal dosages in renal impairment are *unknown*

Beta blockers Dose at half the standard dose. Atenolol is renally excreted, and may accumulate causing bradycardia and collapse.

Calcium channel blockers No dose reduction required.

Aspirin May exacerbate the bleeding diathesis of uraemia, but no dose reduction usually recommended.

Clopidogrel Indications and dose in renal failure are unknown. Most clinicians use as for non-renal patients, but caution is required as the risk of bleeding is (probably) increased, and the benefits unproven.

Thrombolytics No dose reduction recommended.

Heparin Unfractionated heparin is usually commenced in standard dosage, titrated against APTT. Low molecular weight heparin has a signifantly increased half life with ↓GFR. Monitoring of activated factor Xa levels is usually recommended but often impractical (it may take too long to get the result for it to be useful). In practice:
• Give as half the standard dose.
• Watch for signs of bleeding.
• Monitor activated factor Xa whenever possible.
• If the risk of bleeding is significant, use unfractionated heparin and measure APTT.

Diuretics As renal failure advances, resistance to diuretics progresses:
• Thiazides used alone are ineffective in advanced renal failure.
• Loop diuretics may require high doses (furosemide 250–500mg/day, bumetanide 5 mg daily).
• Addition of a small dose of thiazide to a loop diuretic may be effective, and beware precipitating over-diuresis (metolazone 2.5–5mg daily, bendroflumethazide 2.5–5 mg daily).
• ⚠ Avoid combinations containing potassium in renal impairment unless monitoring is regular.

ACE inhibitors Recommended for many patients with chronic kidney disease (📖 p.150). A drop in GFR can be expected (up to 20% ↑ in serum Cr) when commencing an ACEI, as can a rise in serum K^+. Always check U+E 1–2 weeks after commencing an ACE inhibitor in any patient with renal impairment. Further falls in eGFR or rises in K^+ may necessitate dose reduction, stopping the drug ± investigation for RAS (📖 p.412).

Spironolactone/eplerenone effectiveness in advanced renal failure is unknown (the big trials excluded patients with a low GFR).

⚠ Risk of hyperkalaemia is significant as GFR falls and needs careful monitoring, esp. if used in combination with ACE inhibitor (📖 p.156).

Digoxin Decreased volume of distribution in renal failure, and thus loading dose should be halved in the dialysis patient. Elimination also depends on GFR, so decreased maintenance dose in renal failure. Monitor by therapeutic effect (e.g. ventricular rate in AF) and by plasma levels.

NSAIDs and the kidney

Mechanism

Non-steroidal anti-inflammatory drugs (NSAIDs) inhibit the enzyme cyclo-oxygenase (COX), part of the major pathway in prostaglandin synthesis. At least 2 COX isoforms have been identified—most NSAIDs inhibit both, while selective COX-2 inhibitors inhibit only COX-2 (purportedly providing fewer GI side effects ♠)

Their potent anti-inflammatory and analgesic properties make these drugs amongst the most prescribed in the world. Adverse effects are comparatively rare, but include:

- Renal toxicity (see below).
- Gastro-intestinal side effects, including peptic ulceration and dyspepsia and small and large bowel toxicity.
- Cardiovascular adverse effects, with increased risk of cardiovascular disease and hypertension (?COX-2 > non-selective ♠).
- Liver toxicity: abnormal LFTs, though liver failure is rare.
- Bronchospasm.
- Anti-platelet effects (decreased production of thromboxane-A2). Beneficial when aspirin is given for ischaemic heart disease, but potentially an adverse effect in those at risk of bleeding.

Renal effects

⚠ NSAIDS should be avoided in anybody with ARF, or at risk of ARF.

- When kidney function is normal, NSAIDs have insignificant effects on renal haemodynamics. When renal blood flow is compromised (renal failure, heart failure, nephrotic syndrome, hypovolaemia, concomitant ACE inhibitor use), then compensatory afferent arteriolar vasodilation by prostaglandins (prostacyclin and prostaglandin E2) plays a key role in maintaining glomerular perfusion.
- Prostaglandins also affect water handling by the kidney, antagonizing the action of ADH. With NSAIDs this diuretic effect is lost. Water retention with hyponatraemia may result.
- COX-2 inhibitors are equally nephrotoxic (though evidence is limited).
- NSAIDs can also cause direct renal toxicity in the form of an acute interstitial nephritis (📖 p.406), or may cause a drug-related nephrotic syndrome—📖 p.394)
- Chronic analgesic nephropathy → CKD may result from prolonged ingestion (usually in combination with other non-NSAID analgesics), though this occurs rarely, and the causative role of NSAIDs remains unproven.

Analgesia in renal failure

Effective analgesia can be difficult to deliver because certain drugs are difficult to use or contra-indicated because of the risk of side effects and toxicity.

▶ Get expert help at an early stage.

Principles in pain control

- Pain should always be treated promptly and appropriately: no patient in hospital should have uncontrolled pain.
- Always give by mouth if possible
- Give regular analgesic medication, and prescribe prn 'top-ups' for breakthrough pain
- Avoid systemic analgesia if possible to minimize toxicity: ideally, use regional pain relief (use of epidurals, nerve blocks, local anaesthetic)
- Use a modified WHO pain control ladder:
  - Start with regular paracetamol 500 mg–1g 4–6 hourly po.
  - Avoid compound analgesics.
  - Consider add-on adjuvant treatments where possible (see below).
  - NSAIDs are contraindicated in renal impairment, but ▶ NSAIDs may be useful in anuric (functionally anephric) dialysis patients for whom further renal injury is unimportant.
  - Add in weak opioid if required, e.g. tramadol 50mg 12 hourly po (alternatively dihydrocodeine-based preparations). *Must* monitor dialysis patients for side effects ☐ p.604).
  - Then add a stronger opiate if needed, e.g. hydromorphone 1.3 mg po 4 hourly, or oxycodone 5mg qds titrating up gradually.
  - If severe pain, consider parenteral diamorphine (or other opiate) starting at low dose (1.25–2.5mg sc, IMI, or IVI). Be careful to review patient and drug chart regularly.
  - Fentanyl patches are usually well tolerated by patients with severe chronic pain. Avoid if opioid naïve (☐ p.604).

Adjuvant therapy

Anticonvulsants

Useful particularly for neuropathic pain. Gabapentin is the best studied, but trials have excluded patients with renal failure. Dose reduction is required depending on GFR with careful monitoring for signs of toxicity. In stage 5 CKD usual dose is 200–300mg alt. day (given after dialysis as partly dialysed out). Toxic effects include fatigue, dizziness, and ataxia. Carbamazepine may be beneficial for trigeminal neuralgia or diabetic neuropathic pain. No dose reduction is usually required in renal failure. Lamotrigine has not been studied in renal failure.

Antidepressants

Tricyclics have analgesic effects at low doses, acting synergistically with opioids. Metabolized in the liver, and accumulation of metabolites in renal failure may lead to side-effects (dry mouth, drowsiness, hypotension). Start with the lowest available dose (e.g. amitryptiline 10mg nocte, increasing to 50mg as required) and titrate up slowly. Avoid higher doses—more side-effects with little additional benefit.

Steroids

May be useful for inflammatory pain and or spinal cord compression. Side effects limit long-term use

Bisphosphonates
May have a role in chronic bone pain (esp. myeloma).

Patient-controlled analgesia (PCA)

A pump provides a continuous IVI infusion of opioid, with the patient able to self-administer a controlled extra bolus dose.

- Although many of the drugs (eg fentanyl) are thought to metabolized and inactivated by the liver, in practice, opiate narcosis remains a real problem.
- With severe renal failure or dialysis dependence, omit the basal infusion and allow the patient to give controlled bolus doses.
- Observations should be frequent and directed to excluding opiate narcosis.

PCA can also be given by the epidural route, when a combination of fentanyl and a local anaesthetic may be useful. As with IVI PCA, avoid basal infusions.

Opioids in renal failure

Opioids act on the endogenous endorphin receptors in the CNS, leading to their narcotic and analgesic effects. As GFR falls, opioid clearance falls, and the dose of opioid should be reduced. Titration is necessary against patient symptoms and side-effects. In general, as with all patients, start with a low dose and titrate upwards.

⚠ The $t_{1/2}$ may be extended up to 10 times (morphine has a $t_{1/2}$ of 3–5 hours with normal renal function, and up to 50 hours in dialysis-dependent patients.

Choice of opioid in renal impairment

Tramadol acts both centrally and peripherally. $t_{1/2}$ is ~ doubled (from 5 hours to 10) in severe renal failure. Max recommended dose in these patients is 50mg bd—watch for side effects.

Codeine should be used with caution—may cause prolonged CNS depression. Dihydrocodeine has potency midway between that of codeine and morphine. As for codeine, use with caution.

Fentanyl and alfentanil tend to be well-tolerated (can be given as trans-dermal patch, but not orally). They are not well dialysed (protein bound, large volume of distribution), so toxicity may be difficult to reverse rapidly. Avoid commencing an opioid-naïve patient on a patch as risk of toxicity.

Hydromorphone appears relatively safe and well-tolerated.

Methadone also appears relatively safe, but should be prescribed by someone with experience of using the drug. With all of these drugs watch for slow accumulation of metabolites and associated toxicity.

Pethidine, morphine, diamorphine and oxycodone may be associated with more side effects (accumulation of metabolites). Diamorphine is metabolized to morphine, and then to morphine-3-glucuronide and morphine-6-glucuronide. These breakdown products are excreted via the kidney—their accumulation (esp. of morphine-6 glucuronide) may lead to the clinical signs of toxicity.

Opiate narcosis in the renal patient

Accumulating opiates and opioid metabolites offer a significant risk to patients with CKD and particularly ARF or ESRD. Patients are often unwell and may even be septic—as such, the side-effects of opiates may lead to clinical deterioration. A particularly common problem in patients stepped down off ITU with recovering (but not recovered) ARF, or ESRD.

Signs:
- Disorientation and confusion → coma
- Nausea and vomiting
- Constipation
- ► Pin-point pupils
- Impaired swallow with risk of aspiration
- Respiratory depression → hypoventilation ± arrest
- Hypotension (and worsening of tissue perfusion).

Be particularly wary in the elderly, as they are susceptible to opioid side-effects, and likely to have unrecognized ↓GFR.

Treatment:
- Sit up and administer face mask O_2.
- If depressed level of consciousness, secure airway.
- IVI naloxone 400–800µg as a bolus. If response (usually the patient 'wakes up'), consider infusion as 10mg in 50mL 0.9% NaCl starting at 0.5mL/min, titrating up or down against response.
- ⚠ Many opiates have a long $t_{\frac{1}{2}}$: expect narcotized patients to deteriorate again until drug removed.
- This may (and often does) require HD.

Poisoning and dialysis

While poisoning (either deliberate or accidental) is common, the need to use dialysis to clear poorly excreted poisons is rare (<1% of all poisonings). Poisonings which lend themselves to extra-corporeal therapies are those in which:

- Toxic effects are severe ± dangerous or potentially irreversible if not treated.
- Elimination is quicker via dialysis, or only possible by dialysis (for example if renal or liver failure is present).
- The poison ± its metabolites can be removed by dialysis.

Characteristics of a drug which is amenable to removal by dialysis are:
- Low molecular weight.
- Relatively small degree of protein binding.
- Low volume of distribution.
- Polar molecule (water soluble).

Dialysis techniques

- The goal is to remove as much of the drug/toxin as possible. Therefore a dialyser with a large surface area, high pump speeds and a long dialysis session (4–6 hours or more) are usually recommended. If renal failure is also present, dialysis disequilibrium (📖 p.121) is a danger and a shorter or more gentle dialysis should be prescribed.
- Haemoperfusion may be helpful for some substances not removed efficiently by dialysis (▶ severe cases of phenytoin or digoxin overdose, or paraquat poisoning: blood is passed over a charcoal or polystyrene resin adsorbent and then returned to the circulation). The offending drug is adsorbed onto the charcoal or resin. Not available except in specialist centres.
- Peritoneal dialysis provides much slower clearance and is not recommended in acute poisoning.

Drugs/toxins for which haemodialysis may provide benefit

Lithium (📖 p.608)	Methanol (📖 p.611)
Salicylate (📖 p.608)	Theophyllines
Ethylene glycol (📖 p.610)	Barbiturates (rare, for severe coma)

Lithium and salicylate poisoning

Lithium

An effective treatment for affective disorders, lithium has a narrow therapeutic window. Blood levels should be measured regularly.

- Toxic effects:
  - Nephrogenic diabetes insipidus (📖 p.523) presenting as polyuria and dysnatraemias—lithium may down-regulate aquaporin production.
  - Goitre—check TSH, though usually remains normal.
  - Acute toxicity causes neuromuscular irritability (tremor, twitching), confusion and drowsiness.
- Lithium excretion mirrors that of Na^+. Freely filtered, lithium is predominantly reabsorbed in the PCT. ~ 20% is excreted in the urine.
- Lithium accumulation may occur whenever the GFR drops (hypovolaemia, NSAID-use, diuretics or ACEI therapy).
- Long-term lithium use may be associated with chronic renal impairment, though evidence of causation is limited.
- With progressive renal impairment, it *may* be necessary to stop the lithium. If GFR is declining slowly, it may be more in a patient's interest to continue the drug if well-controlled.

Treatment of lithium intoxication

- Assess severity—signs of neuro-muscular toxicity, measure lithium level. Measure renal function.
- Fluid resuscitation—correct hypovolaemia. 0.9% NaCl ± 0.45% NaCl (if hypernatraemic) to increase UO and maximize renal excretion.
- Haemodialysis removes lithium effectively. Use high pump speed and large membrane for 4–6 hours. Indications for haemodialysis:
  - Lithium level >3.5mmol/L
  - Lithium level >2mmol/L with severe symptoms ± ↓ GFR.
- Rebound in lithium levels may occur as lithium moves from the intracellular to extracellular space. Recheck lithium levels 6 hours later and give further dialysis if necessary

Salicylates

Aspirin (acetylsalicylic acid) is rapidly converted to salicylic acid after absorption. It is normally highly protein bound (>90%) and broken down by the liver. Only a small fraction is excreted unchanged by the kidney.

In overdose

- 10–20g of aspirin may be fatal in an adult.
- If gastric emptying is delayed → peak levels occur hours after ingestion.
- Direct stimulation of the respiratory centre → over-ventilation and *initial* respiratory alkalosis.
- Cellular injury → ↑anion gap metabolic acidosis.

Symptoms and signs

Correlate poorly with levels (esp. in the elderly), but may include:

- Nausea, vomiting, and diarrhoea
- Tinnitus, vertigo, and blurred vision
- Sweating and hyperthermia
- Pulmonary oedema (increased vascular permeability)
- Confusion and cerebral oedema, esp. if severe acidosis (salicylate crosses the blood–brain barrier more easily if non-ionized).

Once liver conjugation pathways are saturated, the majority of clearance is by the kidney. As salicylates are highly protein-bound (and not filterable), secretion occurs via the PCT anion secretory pathway.

Treatment of salicylate intoxication

Exclude other drug ingestions. Urgent salicylate level:

- Therapeutic level are <300mg/L (2.2mmol/L)
- Moderate toxicity 500–750mg/L (3.6–5.4mmol/L)
- Severe overdose >750mg/L (5.4mmol/L)

U+E ($\uparrow$ or $\downarrow K^+$, $\downarrow HCO_3^-$) and blood gas (early respiratory alkalosis, then $\uparrow$AG metabolic acidosis), lactate, glucose, LFT, FBC, $\uparrow$INR, ECG (?heart block) and CXR (?non-cardiogenic pulmonary oedema).

Monitor in HDU setting. Adminster O_2 if necessary (avoid intubation if possible—if needed (hypoxia), hyperventilate to generate alkalosis.

- Level >500mg/L should prompt aggressive management.
- Gastric lavage up to 12 hours after ingestion (delayed gastric emptying).
- Activated charcoal (50g 4 hourly repeated x 2) may be effective.
- Optimise fluid status. Aim for urine output >100mL/h (fluids below).
- Alkalinize the urine (salicylate is more soluble at $\uparrow$pH). Give $NaHCO_3$ 1.26% IVI until urine pH > 7.5. Maintain u-pH using IVI or oral $NaHCO_3$.
- Give IV glucose if CNS involvement, even if blood levels normal (salicylates cause neuroglycopaenia).
- Correct hypokalaemia if present (allows effective urinary alkalinization).
- Repeat blood gases and salicylate levels 2 hourly until stable.
- Dialysis effectively removes salicylate. Use high pump speeds, and large dialyser for 4–6 hours. Indications are:
  - Blood level >700mg/L (5.1mmol/L).
  - Renal impairment with toxic salicylate level (if GFR >50mL/min, trial of aggressive medical therapy may be appropriate if symptoms are not severe. If levels do not fall, resort to dialysis without delay).
  - Pulmonary oedema (prevents use of bicarbonate).
  - Worsening neurological signs or cerebral oedema.
  - Worsening signs of toxicity despite aggressive medical management.

Recheck blood level 2 hours after dialysis. Repeat dialysis may be required if levels rebound (due to delayed absorption).

Ethylene glycol poisoning

Anti-freeze contains ethylene glycol (EG).

⚠ Ingestion of as little as 50 mL can be fatal.

EG is freely absorbed, and broken down in the liver by alcohol dehydrogenase in an energy-dependent manner to glycolic acid and then on to oxalic acid. Only a fraction of glycolic acid is metabolized to oxalic acid. It is tissue deposition of metabolites which causes renal failure and (long-term) neurological damage.

Symptoms and signs

▶ Patients may or may not confess to ingestion.

Acute symptoms and signs may include:

- Drowsiness, confusion, ataxia (⚠ as with alcohol intoxication).
- Seizures.
- Unexplained ↑AG metabolic acidosis (cause by glycolic acid).
- Pulmonary oedema and respiratory distress in severe cases.
- May present late (after several days) with unexplained renal failure, unexplained neurological signs (cranial nerve palsies, visual symptoms, generalized weakness).

Investigations

Blood gas: ↑AG metabolic acidosis with respiratory compensation (mainly glycolic acid, but lactate accumulation may also contribute to the acidosis).

▶ The degree of acidosis correlates with tissue injury and outcome.

Ethylene glycol level (may be normal if ingestion > 12 hours before): severe toxicity if >500mg/L or 8mmol/L. Check ethanol level if co-ingestion

U+E, salicylate and paracetamol levels (in case of co-ingestion), urine microscopy for oxalate crystals. ↓Ca^{2+} (oxalic acid binds calcium to form crystals), LFT, FBC (↑↑WCC).

▶ ↑Osmolar gap >10mOsm/kg: measured serum osmolality (raised)—calculated osmolality (often normal, as [2 x Na^+] + urea + glucose)

Renal biopsy will show widespread oxalate crystal deposition.

Management

- Gastric lavage if <1 hour since ingestion
- If within 12 hours of ingestion, give *fomepizole*. Competes with EG for alcohol dehydrogenase receptor preventing rapid accumulation of toxic metabolites, with $t_{\frac{1}{2}}$ of 14 hours. Has 8000x greater affinity for enzyme than ethanol. Current recommendations advise:
  - Load at 15mg/kg IVI.
  - Maintenance dose 10mg/kg 12 hourly x 4 doses, then ↑ to 15mg/kg 12 hourly until EG <200mg/L (3.2mmol/L).
  - No need to increase dose during HD (EG and fomepizole both removed).
  - ⚠ Many advocate substantially lower doses (perhaps only 25% of the above schedule).
  - Dose reduce fomepizole after each HD session.

- Ethanol infusion is an alternative (much greater affinity for alcohol dehydrogenase than EG), but less preferred due to intoxication and depressed level of consciousness. Monitor blood ethanol concentration every few hours. Aim for ethanol level of 10–15mmol/L.
- Haemodialysis effectively removes EG and metabolites. Indicated if:
  - Renal failure
  - Plasma level > 500mg/L (8mmol/L)
  - Severe acidosis or neurological signs.
  - ▶ *Always err on the side of early and prolonged HD*
- Adjunct therapies include:
  - NaHCO$_3$ 1.26% IVI infusion for lesser degrees of acidosis (massive doses may be required).
  - Maintain high urine flow rate with IV fluids to minimize risk of oxalate crystal deposition (care needed if renal impairment is present).
  - Thiamine and pyridoxine may be beneficial: prevent conversion of metabolites into oxalate.

▶ Late presentations (no EG detected in blood) do not benefit from the above. Management is supportive. Mortality is high, especially in those who present late.

Methanol poisoning

Contained in de-icing solutions and some varnishes.
⚠ 50mL may be lethal.
Early signs of toxicity include:
- Confusion
- Headache
- Decreased vision
- May lead to coma.

The eye is particularly susceptible. Oedema of the retina may lead to permanent blindness as hypoxia of the optic nerve leads to demyelination. Demyelination of white matter in the brain may also occur. As with ethylene glycol, ↑AG metabolic acidosis with ↑osmolar gap. Diagnosis is confirmed by the history and by measuring blood levels (in early stages). Management is similar to that of ethylene glycol poisoning, with similar indications for fomepizole or ethanol ± haemodialysis. In addition, IVI folic acid may be of benefit.

Appendices

The glomerulus

Structure

Bowman's capsule is a pocket of epithelial cells which are in continuity with the epithelial cells of the PCT. Within Bowman's capsule:

Capillaries: a knot of capillaries lined by endothelial cells. Blood flows in via the afferent arteriole, and out via the efferent arteriole (for a capillary bed to have arterioles on both ends is unique in the circulation). Changes in afferent and efferent arteriolar tone are powerful ways of regulating blood flow and pressure within the glomerulus (🕮 p.616).

The glomerular basement membrane (GBM): Consists of a matrix of type 4 collagen embedded with other connective tissue proteins. Is part of the filtration barrier in the glomerulus (see below). The GBM contains all mesangium and endothelium within in, and all podocytes without.

Epithelial cells or podocytes: attach to the GBM by specially adapted foot processes (hence the name 'podocytes'). Interdigitating podocytes are separated from each other by 'slit diaphragms', the key mechanical and signalling barrier to filtration. Abnormal podocyte function in now considered crucial to proteinuric nephropathies.

Mesangial cells are important regulating cells in the glomerulus. Most are derived from a smooth muscle lineage (and respond to similar stimuli). They are situated adjacent to the endothelium (within the GBM), are active in signalling, recruitment of non-resident cells, and maintenance of vascular tone. Some mesangial cells are derived from macrophages and monocytes, and have phagocytic properties. Mesangial cell proliferation and activation occur in response to immune mediated glomerular injury.

Filtration within the glomerulus

Substances with a molecular weight <5000 Daltons are freely filtered (unless bound to albumin in the plasma). Larger molecules are partially filtered, the filtration fraction depending not just on size but also charge (negatively charged molecules have a lower filtration fraction than similarly sized cationic molecules). Albumin (MW 61000D) is scarcely filtered normally by dint of its size and negative charge.

The glomerular filter comprises 4 levels
• Charged endothelial glycocalyx (charge)
• Endothelial fenestrations (limiting size)
• The glomecular basement membrane
• The inter-podocyte slit diaphragm.

The slit diaphragm offers a mesh of interlocking proteins and lipids important in maintaining the barrier: nephrin, podocin, CD2AP, and podocalyxin all contribute. Podocyte dysfunction impairs both the slit diaphragm and foot process adhesion.

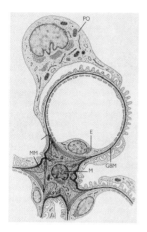

Fig. 12.1A Schematic demonstrating the filtration barrier. The glomerular capillary has a fenestrated endothelium (E). The capillary is surrounded by the GBM, which deviates to cover the mesangial cells (M). The interdigitating foot processes of the podocyte (PO), separated by slit diaphragms cover the GBM and form the final barrier to filtration.

Reproduced with permission from Davison AMA, Cameron JS, Grunfeld J-P *et al* (eds)(2005). *Oxford Textbook of Clinical Nephrology, 3rd edn.* Oxford: Oxford University Press

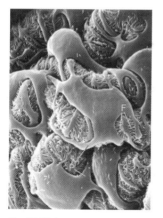

Fig. 12.1B Scanning EM of rat glomerular capillaries. The capillary is covered by branching podocytes. The primary (P) and secondary (F) processes interdigitate, separated by slit diaphragms, and cover the entire surface of the GBM

Reproduced with permission from Davison AMA, Cameron JS, Grunfeld J-P *et al* (eds)(2005). *Oxford Textbook of Clinical Nephrology, 3rd edn.* Oxford: Oxford University Press

Regulation of GFR

GFR depends on:
- Renal blood flow (RBF)
- Glomerular structure (filtration surface area and permeability)
- Trans-glomerular capillary pressure (afferent–efferent tone)
- Plasma oncotic pressure.

Afferent and arteriolar tone

Controls intra-glomerular pressure and flow:
- Increased afferent arteriolar tone (vasoconstriction) leads to *reduced* flow and *reduced* pressure within the glomerulus.
- Increased efferent arteriolar tone (vasoconstriction) leads to *reduced* flow and *increased* pressure within the glomerulus.

Angiotensin II is a potent efferent arteriolar vasoconstrictor (with much weaker vasoconstrictor effects at the afferent arteriole). Thus high local or circulating AII levels raise intraglomerular filtration pressure → maintenance of GFR even if renal blood flow is reduced (hypovolaemia, renal artery stenosis etc.)—this is why ACEI drop trans-glomerular capillary pressures.

Physiological regulation

Glomerulo-tubular balance is the process whereby a change (↑ or ↓) in GFR is compensated for by a corresponding change in absorption by the rest of the nephron (mechanism poorly understood).

Autoregulation preserves glomerular blood flow with variations in systolic BP (local stretch receptors adjust afferent arteriolar tone).

Tubuloglomerular feedback. TGF allows tubular flow sensing to change GFR: Cl^- delivery to the juxta-glomerular apparatus at the macula densa is sensed. ↑Cl^- delivery distally → afferent arteriolar vasoconstriction, thus ↓GFR (mediators include adenosine, thromboxane, NO, and AII). The importance (and beauty) of this mechanism can be appreciated if large quantities of Cl^- (and thus Na^+) are pathologically delivered to the distal tubule (eg non-oliguric ATN). By TGF, ↓renal blood flow ensures ↓GFR, preventing profound diuresis and volume depletion.

Systemic factors. The sympathetic nervous system (noradrenalin, or norepinephrine) effects vasoconstriction of the afferent arteriole. Thus in systemic hypotension (↑sympathetic activity), renal blood flow is reduced (allowing blood to be diverted to the brain and heart). Noradrenalin also stimulates production of renin and AII. AII, with its vasoconstrictive effects at the efferent arteriole, serves to maintain GFR as much as possible in these circumstances. Vasodilatory prostaglandins are also important in these circumstances in maintaining GFR (⚠ hence avoid NSAIDs when renal blood flow is compromised).

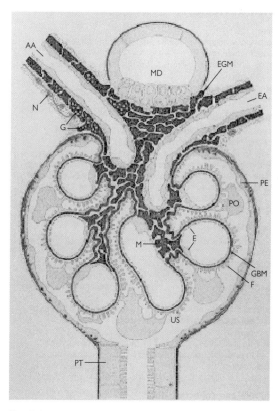

Fig. 12.2 Diagram of a longitudinal section through a glomerulus. Blood enters via the afferent arteriole (AA) and leaves via the efferent arteriole (EA). The capillaries have a fenestrated endothelium (E). The visceral epithelium of Bowman's capsule consists of podocytes (PO), the foot processes (F) of which (with the GBM) cover the capillaries and the mesangium (M). At the vascular pole the visceral epithelium reflects into the parietal epithelium (PE), which itself becomes the proximal tubule (PT) at the urinary pole. US = urinary space.

At the vascular pole the juxta-glomerular apparatus is made up of:
• Extra-glomerular mesangial matrix (EGM) and mesangial cells
• The terminal portion of the AA containing granular cells (G), containing sympathetic nerve terminals (N)
• The efferent arteriole
• The macula densa.

Reproduced with permission from Davison AMA, Cameron JS, Grunfeld J-P et al (eds)(2005). *Oxford Textbook of Clinical Nephrology, 3rd edn.* Oxford: Oxford University Press

Tubular function

The tubules succeed in:
- Reabsorbing the majority of the filtrate (mainly the proximal convoluted tubule (PCT)).
- Regulating salt and water balance (loop, distal tubule (DT) and collecting ducts (CD)).
- Regulating acid/base balance in the body (DT and CD).

The tubule is divided into discrete sections:

Proximal convoluted tubule
- Reabsorbs the bulk of sodium, chloride, bicarbonate, glucose, amino acids, urate and water (see Table 12.1).
- The 'average' PCT is ~14mm long, and offers a large surface area (due to the villous-like arrangement at the apical surface of epithelial cells). The normal kidney contains around 1,000,000 glomeruli, this equates to a potential surface area for reabsorption of >50m^2. The PCT is able to reabsorb up to 65% of the 24,000mmol of Na$^+$ and 160L of water filtered per day.

The loop of Henle
- The loop dives deep into the renal medulla and then back out into the cortex.
- Capillaries serving the loop accompany the loop, enabling a counter-current exchange of urea and electrolytes to exist (🕮 p.622). This helps perpetuate the hypertonic extracellular medium in the medulla, crucial for water homeostasis.
- Divided into thin and thick limbs. The thick (ascending) limb contains cells rich in mitochondria, reflecting the active transport of electrolytes which occurs in these cells.
- The osmotic gradient is maintained by the thick ascending limb, which is impermeable to water but allows urea to diffuse out.
- Filtrate is concentrated in the descending limb by egress of water into the extracellular space and capillaries down an osmotic gradient

Distal tubule and collecting duct
- While only responsible for 5% of solute reabsorption, the DT is the main regulating site for sodium, potassium and bicarbonate reabsorption (🕮 p.626).
- Changes in permeability of the CD allow the formation of a concentrated urine (controlled by ADH).

Table 12.1 Sites of reabsorption of the major ions in the nephron (%)

	Na$^+$	K$^+$	HCO$_3^-$	Ca^{2+}
PCT	65	65	80	70
Loop	25	30	10–15	20
DT and CD	0–10	0–5	0–5	10

The proximal convoluted tubule

Sodium/potassium ATPase
- Plays a prime role in tubular reabsorption.
- Situated on the basolateral membrane (i.e. the capillary side) of the tubular epithelial cell.
- 3 Na^+ ions are pumped out of the cell into the capillary network by an active (ATP requiring) process, in exchange for 2 K^+ ions.
- It maintains a low intracellular Na^+ concentration (20–30mmol/L). The Na^+ concentration gradient between the tubular fluid and the intracellular compartment helps drive reabsorption of Na^+, other solutes and water from the urinary space.
- Intra- and extracellular K^+ concentrations are maintained by specific K^+ channels which allow potassium to be extruded from the cell (down a concentration gradient) in a regulated fashion.

Sodium and chloride
- In the early part of the PCT, most sodium is reabsorbed via specific transporters (Fig. 12.3). Na^+ reabsorption is coupled with absorption of glucose and organic molecules. A further transporter exchanges Na^+ with H^+ ions (see below). The energy for these processes comes from the sodium gradient into the cell, itself generated by Na/K ATPase.
- The gap junctions between the cells are slightly leaky. Chloride (an excess is generated when sodium is absorbed with other anions or molecules) is reabsorbed by this route, as is water.
- Late in the PCT, most of the Na^+ is reabsorbed along with Cl^- (Fig. 12.4). Na^+ and H^+ are exchanged. Cl^- is exchanged for another base e.g. formate, bicarbonate, oxalate. This base is then reabsorbed along with H^+, and thus forms a shuttle, the net result being reabsorption of NaCl. Cl^- leaves the cell in exchange for K^+ or HCO_3^-, or via specific chloride pumps.

Potassium Mostly reabsorbed in conjunction with water via the paracellular space down a concentration gradient.

Bicarbonate Carbonic anhydrase in the PCT cells and on the luminal cell surface allows one HCO_3^- ion to be reabsorbed for every H^+ ion excreted. ▶ *Thus H^+ excretion is equivalent to HCO_3^- reabsorption.* In the PCT H^+ is exchanged for Na^+. HCO_3^- leaves the cell into the interstitium in exchange for Cl^- or in combination with Na^+

Calcium Paracellular reabsorption, down a concentration (and charge gradient).

Phosphate Co-transported into the cell along with Na^+. Inhibited by PTH.

Glucose, amino acids Co-transported into the cell along with Na^+.

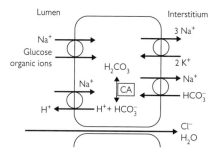

Fig. 12.3 Major pathways of solute reabsorption in the early part of the PCT. Adapted with permission from Greger R (1999) New insights into the molecular mechanism of the action of diuretics. *Nephrol Dial Transplant* **14**: 536–40

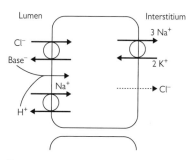

Fig. 12.4 Major pathways of solute reabsorption in the late part of the PCT. Adapted with permission from Greger R (1999) New insights into the molecular mechanism of the action of diuretics. *Nephrol Dial Transplant* **14**: 536–40

The loop of Henle

The counter-current exchange mechanism

- The loop dives deep into the medulla and then back up to the cortex.
- The thick ascending limb of the loop is impermeable to water. Na^+ (with K^+ and 2 Cl^-) is actively pumped from the lumen. The result is to lower the osmolality of the luminal fluid, and raise the osmolality of the interstitium (see Fig. 12.5).
- The medullary blood supply functions as a counter-current—blood flows down into the medulla in the vasa recta and then back up in a hairpin arrangement to the cortex. Counter-current exchange perpetuates the hypertonicity of the interstitium.
- The descending limb of the loop is permeable to water but not to Na^+. Thus water flows down an osmotic gradient into the concentrated milieu of the interstitium. The effect is to concentrate the luminal fluid, so that at the deepest part of the loop the luminal and interstitial osmolality reaches up to 1200mOsm/kg.
- Urea also contributes to the osmolality of the medullary interstitium. Diffusion of urea from concentrated urine into the urea-permeable CD helps generate and maintain the hyperosmolality of the inner medulla.

Concentrating and diluting the urine

Tubular fluid leaving the loop and entering the DT is hypotonic, as a result of active transport of NaCl out of the lumen (~200mOsm/kg, compared with plasma ~285mOsm/kg). Fluid passes down the collecting duct, through the medulla to the renal pelvis. In the absence of ADH, the CD is impermeable to water. Thus the urine remains hypotonic (dilute). ADH makes the CD permeable to water: with ADH the urine can achieve the same osmolality as the inner medulla (~1200mOsm/kg).

ADH

Released by the posterior pituitary in response to rising plasma osmolality and/or significant hypovolaemia. Stimulates thirst, systemic vasoconstriction (V_1 receptors), and in the kidney (via V_2 receptors):

- Conserves water by stimulating water reabsorption in the collecting tubule, thus generating a concentrated urine. The CD becomes permeable to water by the translocation of specific water channels (aquaporins) to the apical membrane.
- Increases permeability of inner CD to urea (via the UT-A1 transporter), thus increasing the osmolal gradient in the inner medulla.

High plasma osmolality → ADH release → binds V_2 receptors → aquaporin 2 translocated → ↑permeability of CD to water → ↑urine osmolality up to that of the inner renal medulla (~1200mOsm/kg)

Low plasma osmolality → ADH release suppressed → no aquaporin 2 translocation → CD impermeable to water → ↓urine osmolality as low as that of tubular fluid entering the cortical CD (~200mosm/kg)

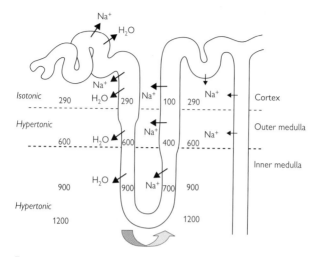

Fig. 12.5 Counter-current multiplication by the loop of Henle The thin descending limb is water permeable. The tubular fluid becomes hypertonic (the interstitium is hypertonic). In the ascending limb NaCl is absorbed (via the NaKCC pump) without water, rendering an osmotic gradient of 200mOsm/kg at any given level. Countercurrent flow in the 2 limbs of the loop multiply this gradient longitudinally. The result is a hypertonic interstitium in the inner medulla (urea also contributes to this hypertonicity—see text).

Thus fluid entering the distal tubule is hypotonic. Further Na reabsorption in the distal tubule can make the fluid still more hypotonic. If ADH is not present the CD is impermeable to water and a dilute urine is passed. If ADH is present the CD becomes permeable to water, and the urine becomes hypertonic as it passes through the medulla. All units are mOsm/kg

Reproduced with permission from Davison AMA, Cameron JS, Grunfeld J-P et al (eds)(2005). *Oxford Textbook of Clinical Nephrology, 3rd edn.* Oxford: Oxford University Press

Solute transport in the loop

The loop:
- Reabsorbs ~30% of filtrate.
- Reabsorbs relatively more NaCl than H$_2$O, thus generating hypotonic fluid in the lumen. Essential for production of a dilute urine.
- Helps generate the counter-current exchange mechanism and hence hypertonicity in the medullary interstitium (📕 p.623), essential for the production of a concentrated urine.

The loop is divided into:
- The descending limb
- The thin ascending limb
- The thick ascending limb.

The descending limb is impermeable to sodium. Water moves into the interstitium down the osmotic gradient (📕 p.623). The result is a high luminal Na$^+$ and Cl$^-$ concentration

Solute transport is passive in the thin ascending limb. Na$^+$ and Cl$^-$ move into the interstitium down a concentration gradient.

In the thick ascending limb, the key transporter is the NKCC co-transporter (see Fig. 12.6):
- NaCl transport without water movement (the thick ascending limb is impermeable to water) allows the loop to generate hypotonic luminal fluid and hypertonic interstitial fluid. This is the fundamental basis of the counter current mechanism.
- The energy for this process is derived from the sodium gradient into the cell and hence ultimately from Na/K ATPase.
- K$^+$ is recycled into the lumen via a specific channel (ROMK channel) ensuring its availability, and generating a net positive luminal charge.
- This positive charge drives reabsorption of cations across the paracellular junction, including Ca^{2+}, Mg^{2+}, NH$_4^+$, and (more) Na$^+$.

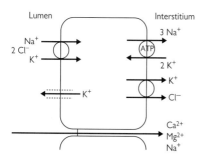

Fig. 12.6 Transport mechanisms in the thick ascending limb of the loop of Henle. The NKCC co-transporter is the key. Potassium can 'leak' back into the lumen via the ROMK channel, rendering the lumen positively charged. This charge gradient facilitates passive reabsorption of Ca^{2+}, Mg^{2+}, and more Na^+ via the paracellular junction.

The distal tubule

The fine-tuning of reabsorption occurs in the distal nephron. The total absorptive capacity of the DCT and CD is not large. Thus mechanisms exist to prevent over-delivery of solute, which would flood the capacity.

The distal tubule is impermeable to passive movement of NaCl (except via specific channels) and water (ADH does not affect water absorption). This allows large concentration gradients to develop when necessary.

Sodium:

~5% of the filtered Na^+ is reabsorbed in the DCT. The NCCT co-transporter is the major route. Some further Na^+ is absorbed by Na^+/H^+ exchange, and some further Cl^- by Cl^-/HCO_3^- exchange (H^+ and HCO_3^- then combine in the lumen to form CO_2 and H_2O—the CO_2 can be reabsorbed and recycled). The energy for the action of the NCCT co-transporter is derived from Na/K ATPase and the resulting gradient aids Na^+ reabsorption into the cell.

Calcium

Absorbed via a specific epithelial Ca^{2+} channel. Reabsorption is partly controlled by PTH and calcitriol.

Thiazide diuretics block the NCCT co-transporter. They also stimulate the pathway for Ca^{2+} absorption (mechanism unknown), thus reducing calcium excretion in the urine.

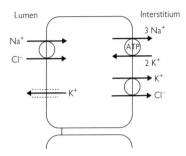

Fig. 12.7 Distal tubular sodium and chloride reabsorption occur predominantly via the NCCT co-transporter.

The collecting duct

The vital role of this segment in control of water absorption is discussed elsewhere (📖 p.622).

2–5% of the total filtered load is reabsorbed. 2 types of cells are important:

Principal cells (~65% of cells)

Sodium: Reabsorption occurs via a specific Na^+ transporter, the epithelial sodium channel (ENaC) (Fig. 12.8). Although only ~5% of filtered Na^+ is reabsorbed by these cells, this is the main site of body Na^+ regulation (aldosterone-mediated). Energy is derived from Na/K ATPase. In contrast to mechanisms of Na^+ reabsorption higher in the nephron, it is not the concentration gradient which drives Na^+ from the lumen into the cell (the luminal Na^+ concentration may be as low as 5mmol/L, significantly lower than the intracellular concentration). The system relies instead on a charge gradient: Na/K ATPase, in pumping of K^+ out of the cell generates a net negative charge within the cell. Na^+ flows down this charge gradient into the cell via ENaC. Tubular fluid becomes negatively charged, allowing Cl^- to move across the paracellular junction.

Control of Na^+ excretion

Aldosterone, after binding its mineralocorticoid receptor, increases the number of open ENaC channels, thus regulating Na absorption (and excretion). Increased intracellular Na concentration is another stimulus (with aldosterone) to increased Na/K ATPase activity.

Atrial natriuretic peptide (ANP) also acts on these channels, with ↑ANP → inactivation of ENaC. ENaC activity may also be affected by *Na^+ delivery* (↓delivery → ↑ENaC activity, reducing Na^+ loss in the urine, thus helping prevent volume depletion). *ADH* may also be important, increasing ENaC activity and numbers. Locally produced *PGE2* also plays a role, decreasing ENaC activity.

Potassium is secreted into the lumen via a specific aldosterone-sensitive K^+ channel, using the favourable charge gradient. High urinary flow rates maintain low intraluminal K^+ concentrations, allowing this channel to operate. Hence hypovolaemia can → hyperkalaemia

Amiloride blocks ENaC, thus reducing Na reabsorption and reducing K^+ excretion. Spironolactone inhibits the effect of aldosterone on its receptor, with similar effects on Na^+ and K^+.

Intercalated cells

Important for acid/base homeostasis. Contain an H^+ ATPase (activity is sensitive to aldosterone) transporting H^+ ions out of the cell into the lumen. Bicarbonate is then returned to the circulation in exchange for Cl^- ions via a co-transporter (see Fig. 12.9). The result is reabsorption of HCO_3^-. Intercalated cells also contain an H^+/K^+ ATPase, allowing some H^+ to be secreted into the lumen in exchange for K^+ absorption into the cell.

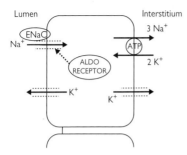

Fig. 12.8 The principal cell in the collecting tubule

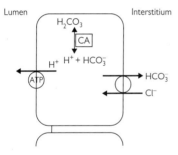

Fig. 12.9 Acid secretion in the intercalated cell in the collecting tubule. Na$^+$/K$^+$ ATPase is an alternative route for secretion of H$^+$ into the lumen (not shown)

Insertion of haemodialysis catheters

Indications

Temporary haemodialysis catheters should be temporary—ideally no line should be in situ for longer than a few days. The risk of infection increases significantly if a line remains in place for longer—switch to a tunneled line if continuing access is required.

Routes of insertion

- The right internal jugular vein is the preferred route. It is superficial, easy to cannulate (in a 'virgin' neck), and joins the SVC in a straight line. The left internal jugular is an alternative, but the guidewire and the line have to curve in order to reach the SVC. The risk of malposition and malfunction (and perforation of the vein) is greater.
- The femoral veins are suitable for short term use and may be the safest and quickest option in an emergency.
- The subclavian route should be avoided: high risk of central venous stenoses, potentially rendering the ipsilateral arm unsuitable for permanent access.

Pre-insertion

- Is the line really needed? Check that dialysis is required, that the patient is not suitable for a tunneled line (📖 p.634) or PD cannula insertion.
- Check FBC and clotting.
- Gain written consent from the patient (verbal and/or family member if in extremis). Consent should be obtained by the operator. Warn about potential complications:
  - Failure to cannulate vein
  - Haematoma ± arterial puncture
  - Pneumo/haemothorax
  - Catheter malfunction
  - Infections.
- Equipment: every renal unit should have a dedicated room for line insertions in a sterile environment containing a 2D ultrasound probe to facilitate vein cannulation. You will need:
  - An assistant.
  - Sterile gown, gloves, drapes, and towels. Iodine or chlorhexidine to clean the skin.
  - Ultrasound probe to guide line insertion (if available).
  - Dressing pack with a supply of syringes, swabs, and needles.
  - Sterile saline for injection.
  - Lignocaine (1 or 2%): 10mL.
  - Line pack (if pre-packed, will contain introducer needle, guidewire and the line itself). Choose a shorter line (e.g. 15cm) for the RIJ route, longer line (e.g. 20cm) for the left side or the larger patient.
  - Heparin (5000units/mL) to lock the line once it is in situ.
- Wash and dry hands as for a surgical procedure, wear sterile gown, mask, and sterile gloves.

- Position the patient slightly head down (for right sided insertion).
- Clean a wide area of skin around the insertion site. Lay out sterile drapes on all sides. Prime both lumens of the line with sterile normal saline solution.

Tips for problematic line insertions

- Stop if your patient is in *pain*. Seek senior assistance. You might be directing the wire or line into trouble.
- Venous blood looks darker than arterial blood and does not fill a syringe with its own pressure: if in doubt, put a 5mL syringe on either hub and see if it fills in a pulsatile fashion. If still in doubt, do a blood gas on the blood. ⚠ Don't take the line out yet (see below).
- Arterial puncture with an 18 gauge needle can usually be controlled by pressure for 5–15min. If the larger introducer needle punctures the artery, it may be safest to abandon the procedure if possible and try again another day. Do not attempt the other side of the neck after significant arterial puncture and haematoma (risk of airway obstruction).
- ⚠ If an artery is accidentally cannulated (i.e. the line is inserted), or if the vein is ruptured and the line tip is found to lie outside the vein, then *leave the line in situ and seek expert help*.
  - Check FBC, clotting and X-match blood.
  - Confirm your concern by aspirating blood (if possible) from both lumens, and if need be check PaO_2. If unable to aspirate, you are in the *wrong* place.
  - Get a CXR.
  - Monitor closely: BP, pulse, and O_2 sats.
  - Find out where the line is: either CT or contrast examination to check where the tip is.
  - Never take the line out: wait until it is known where the distal tip lies, do it under controlled conditions during the day with a vascular/thoracic surgeon aware. If a track has formed around the line, the risks of bleeding into hollow cavities is lower (but not negligible by any means).

Insertion technique
- Establish anatomical landmarks and the planned point of cannulation (see Fig. 12.10).
- Ultrasound guided insertion is now the technique of choice.
- Insert local anaesthetic under the skin. Always attempt to aspirate before injecting lignocaine to avoid inadvertent IV injection.
- Once the needle is in the vein, use the Seldinger technique. Pass the guidewire through the needle (*there should be no resistance*—if there is do not force it but remove the guidewire and check needle position). Remove the needle leaving the guidewire in situ. Use a No 11 scalpel blade to make a nick in the skin. Pass the dilator over the guidewire until it is in the vein. Remove the dilator, keeping the guidewire in position. Without delay pass the line over the guidewire until it is in position. Remove the guidewire.

Vein localization

Ultrasound guided cannulation: most probes have a sterile disposable cover. Follow the manufacturers instructions. After infiltration of local anaesthetic, identify the vein with the probe. The introducer needle can be inserted with real-time guidance.

Blind insertion: the approach can be medial to SCM muscle, between the 2 heads, or lateral to the muscle. Local practice and expertise will dictate the optimal route
- Palpate the carotid artery with one hand (the left for a right sided insertion).
- Insert the needle just lateral to the carotid pulse, aiming at 45° to the skin in the direction of the ipsilateral nipple. Aspirate gently on the syringe as you go until the vein is reached.
- If unsuccessful, withdraw the needle slowly (continuing with attempted aspiration—you may have gone through the vein). Then reinsert, varying the angle of insertion slightly to the medial side. If still unsuccesful, invite a colleague or senior to have a go before you and the patient lose morale.
- Once the vein is identified with a green needle, pass the introducer needle down the same track in the same manner into the vein, palpating the carotid pulse at the same time.

- Check the flows in both lumens. A 20mL syringe should fill easily with minimal aspiration. Flush both lumens with saline (which should also be easy), and then lock with heparin (5000IU/mL). The priming volume will be written on the line (typically 1.3–2.0mL/lumen). Put caps on the lumens, and suture the line in position.
- Arrange a CXR and see it yourself: look for line position (tip should be in SVC) and look carefully to ensure no pneumothorax.

Renal biopsy

Despite improvements in other diagnostic techniques, renal biopsy retains a central role in nephrology.

Indications

- Unexplained acute or chronic kidney disease with normal renal size.
- Histology likely to influence treatment.
- Histology likely to offer prognostic information.
- Information concerning the activity (and reversibility) or chronicity of a known lesion is desirable.

⚠ Renal biopsy is an invasive procedure. An evaluation of the risk-benefit ratio is needed in every case.

Preparation for renal biopsy

- Imaging: confirm 2 normal size, unobstructed kidneys with normal parenchyma.
- BP <140/90.
- Hb >10g/dL.
- Normal clotting and platelet count.
- Send group and save.
- Antiplatelet agents stopped ~5 days prior to procedure.
- Sterile urine.
- Informed consent.
- If renal impairment, the risk of bleeding increases ~2–3 fold. Most units will have their own policy; e.g.
  - If urea ≥20mmol/L or Cr ≥300 give DDAVP 0.4µg/kg IV prior to biopsy (⚠ not if recent or ongoing angina).
  - Some perform a bleeding time and administer DDAVP if >10min.

Contraindications

- Chronic renal failure with small kidneys
- Multiple cysts
- Suspected renal tumour
- Hydronephrosis
- Urinary infection
- Uncontrolled hypertension
- Bleeding tendency
- Uncooperative patient
- Solitary kidney*.

* Not an absolute contraindication

Technique

Renal biopsy is performed percutaneously under local anaesthesia, via a posterior approach. Ultrasound is used to locate the kidneys, determine their size and identify cysts. Either kidney may be biopsied. The lower pole reduces the risk of piercing a major vessel. Real time imaging can be used to guide the needle directly to the kidney, though many favour a non-real time technique once the kidneys have been marked on the surface. CT guidance is a useful alternative when visualization is inadequate with ultrasound; e.g. obesity. The patient is required to hold their breath when the needle enters the kidney. Disposable TruCut® needles or spring-loaded biopsy guns are generally used. If possible, two cores of tissue are obtained to increase diagnostic yield. Routine processing includes light, immunofluorescent and electron microscopy. The patient remains on bed rest with a good fluid intake for 24h* and is advised not to undertake heavy lifting or exercise for 4 weeks.

* Many centres now perform day case biopsies.

Open renal biopsy

Rarely considered if the percutaneous approach carries an unacceptable risk or has been unsuccessful. Allows direct vizualisation of the kidney and easier control of bleeding. More tissue can be obtained. The risk of a GA may exceed that of a percutaneous biopsy.

Trans-jugular renal biopsy

A technique on loan from hepatology. Usually performed by interventional radiologists. The renal capsule is not punctured and the risk of perinephric bleeding is reduced. High success rates have been demonstrated. May be of benefit in obese patients and when a coagulopathy prohibits other approaches.

Complications of renal biopsy

- Pain (usually short-lived).
- Bleeding.
  - Transient microscopic haematuria occurs in virtually all patients.
  - Macroscopic haematuria in ~2%*. Transfusion required in ~1%.
  - Capsular haematoma (pain, drop in Hb) in ~2%. A large haematoma may compress the kidney and cause high renin hypertension.
- Arteriovenous fistula.
  - ~10% on doppler. Rarely symptomatic; may cause persistent haematuria and hypertension.
- Incorrect tissue
  - Usually muscle, fat, liver, spleen.
  - Colonic perforation.
- Death (0.1%).

* Treat with bed rest. Maintain a high urine flow with fluids to prevent obstruction and clot colic. Correct coagulopathy. If severe or persistent, consider arteriography ± embolization and possible surgical intervention.

The role of the renal biopsy

Microscopic haematuria (📖 p.55)

Proteinuria

Non-nephrotic proteinuria (<3.5g/24h)

✦ Many advocate a biopsy at modest levels of proteinuria to ensure potentially treatable lesions; e.g. 1° FSGS and membranous GN are not overlooked. Others argue that the benign prognosis of these conditions when proteinuria is low, make biopsy unnecessary. A fixed 'cut off' level of proteinuria is a compromise (e.g. routine biopsy if >1g/24h). The presence of renal insufficiency weighs in favour of a biopsy.

Nephrotic range proteinuria

Biopsy generally recommended. Two exceptions:
- Minimal change disease in childhood. Here a trial of steroids may be appropriate before biopsy.
- Diabetic nephropathy (✦ 📖 p.438).

Acute nephritic syndrome

The desire to confirm the diagnosis and adapt treatment according to the type and severity of the renal lesion leads most to biopsy, even when the diagnosis is suggested by serological tests (e.g. anti-GBM +ve).

Acute renal failure (📖 p.87)

Chronic renal disease

The most important determinants of the need for biopsy are:
- Renal size. If <9cm:
  - Technically more demanding.
  - Histology likely to show chronic irreversible changes (original insult may not be identifiable).
- Clinical context.
  - May be sufficient for diagnosis; e.g. renovascular disease or diabetic nephropathy.

Preparing renal patients for theatre

Any patient with renal failure is a high risk patient for an operation. Therefore extreme care should be taken when preparing for theatre.

Pre-admission

- Full history. Focus on cardiac and respiratory history, dialysis regime (if appropriate), details about previous anaesthesia. Drug history.
- Can the procedure be done under regional block (most upper arm AVFs can and should)?
- Examination. Listen for murmurs and bruits (carotids), examine peripheral pulses, check lung fields are clear, assess volume status, measure BP (and check BP charts if available). The anaesthetist will prefer a BP of <150/95.
- Investigations. FBC (? anaemia which could be corrected pre-op), U+E ($?\uparrow K^+$), LFT, Ca^{2+}, ECG if any cardiac history (or any patient with ESRD), CXR if breathless or abnormal signs. Echocardiogram if any new murmur or suggestion of poor LV function.
- Liaise with anaesthetist if any doubt about fitness for anaesthesia or if further investigations are necessary.
- Liaise with dialysis unit if the patient is on dialysis. Plan dialysis around the surgery (i.e. day before and day after usually).

On admission

- Repeat full physical examination including BP and volume status assessment.
- If for creation of vascular access, avoid needling ($\triangle$ IV cannulas) the limb targeted for surgery.
- Send bloods pre-op and after last dialysis session. U+E, FBC, clotting, G+S (if surgery carries risk of bleeding). The anaesthetist will prefer a K$^+$ <5.5–6mmol/L.
- Write up drugs to be given pre-op or at induction (e.g. antibiotics).

Post-operative care

- Avoid nephrotoxic drugs if the patient is uric (e.g. NSAIDs, gentamicin), *even if on dialysis.*
- Ensure adequate analgesia is given, but be aware of risks of opioid toxicity (📖 p.605).
- Check volume status and BP. If IV fluids are required, prescribe 1L and then reassess the patient before prescribing more if there is oliguria.
- Measure U+E post-op in any patient with significant renal impairment (depolarizing anaesthetic agents → muscle K$^+$ release and may precipitate dangerous hyperkalaemia in the susceptible patient).
- If AVF or PTFE graft have been formed, check for a thrill over the fistula and avoid any compression or blood tests in that limb.
- Consider ↓ or no heparin if HD is required.

Plasma exchange

A technique in which plasma is separated from the rest of the blood. There are 2 main methods: one by centrifugation (removing plasma by centrifuging the blood) and the other by filtration. Replacement fluid is usually a combination of albumin solution, saline and FFP (hence 'plasma exchange')

Indications

Conditions in which there is a pathological build up of a protein in the plasma should theoretically lend themselves to treatment by plasmapheresis. Those for which the evidence is (relatively) strong are:

- Anti-GBM disease (📖 p.466).
- ANCA-associated vasculitis (certainly if there is associated pulmonary haemorrhage, possibly ☀ if there is severe acute renal failure) (📖 p.460).
- HUS/TTP (📖 p.404).
- Cryoglobulinaemia.
- Hyperviscosity syndrome.

Other conditions which are sometimes treated by plasmapheresis, though for which the evidence is not strong (☀):

- SLE (only for cerebral lupus or if very severe).
- Treatment of antibody-mediated transplant rejection.
- Recurrent FSGS post-transplant.
- Preparation of highly sensitized transplant recipients.
- Myeloma with acute renal failure secondary to cast nephropathy.
- Crescentic IgA nephropathy.
- Non-renal conditions include Guillain–Barré syndrome, myasthaenic crisis, familial hypercholesterolaemia.

Prescription

One plasma volume exchange will lower plasma levels of macromolecules by ≈60%. Exchanges on 5 consecutive days will achieve ≈90% reduction (some rebound occurs as macromolecules are released back into the circulation).

$$\text{Plasma volume} \approx 0.07 \times \text{Wt in kg} \times (1\text{-haematocrit})$$

Replacement fluid should consist of a combination of:

- *Human albumin solution (5%)*: the predominant plasma protein. At least 50% of the replacement fluid should be albumin. More may be indicated if there is hypoalbuminaemia.
- *Normal saline*: Cheaper than albumin, but should make up no more than 50% of the replacement solution (usually 20–40%).
- *Fresh frozen plasma*: may be necessary to replace removed clotting factors, especially if there is a high risk of bleeding. Monitor clotting and adjust FFP appropriately. 2U FFP (more if very high risk) during the last half hour of plasma exchange is an appropriate starting dose. Some conditions (e.g. HUS) require more FFP (📖 p.404).
- *Anticoagulation*: is usually with heparin (usually 2x dose in HD, as heparin is removed during the process). Citrate is an alternative.

Complications

- Hypotension (usually volume related).
- Citrate-induced paraesthesiae (FFP contains citrate). Self-limiting (slow down the rate of infusion).
- Hypocalcaemia: also related to FFP use. Citrate binds calcium, reducing ionized calcium, so a risk when FFP is used. Can be prevented or treated by IV calcium e.g. 10–20mL 10% Ca gluconate during the procedure.
- Clotting abnormalities: patients with high risk of bleeding should receive more FFP and regular monitoring of clotting.
- Infection: risk increased by IV access and associated immunosuppression but not, it appears, from plasmapheresis itself.

(a) **Membrane plasma filtration**

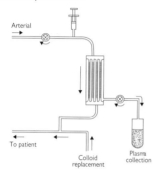

(b) **Centrifugal cell separation**

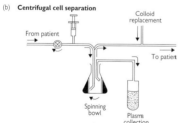

Fig. 12.11 Techniques of plasmapheresis

a) Membrane plasma filtration: blood flow 100–150mL/min. Highly permeable membrane (MW cut off 2000kDa)—most Igs are removed but some larger immune complexes and cryoglobulins may not be well cleared. Cells along with fluid replacement are returned to the patient. b) Centrifugation: plasma is removed by centrifugation using a spinning bowl. Blood is (synchronously or intermittently) returned to the patient along with replacement fluid. No upper limit to the size of protein which can be removed. Can be performed via an antecubital vein.

Reproduced with permission from Levy J, Morgan J, Brown E (2004) *Oxford Handbook of Dialysis*, 2nd edn. Oxford: Oxford University Press.

Clinical practice guidelines

National and international standards (or clinical practice guidelines) outlining the expected level of care for renal patients have been set out by the Renal Association (in the UK), the Kidney Foundation Dialysis Outcomes Quality Initiative (K/DOQI) in the US, and the European Best Practice Guidelines.

These guidelines cover (among other things):
- Pre-dialysis care
- Dialysis prescription and monitoring
- Vascular access preparation and care
- Anaemia management
- Nutrition
- Management of renal bone disease
- Cardiovascular risk factor management
- Management of infection in dialysis patients.

Each of these standards documents makes slightly different recommendations in many of these areas. This is a reflection of the fact that many of the derived standards are the result of expert and consensus opinion rather than good clinical trial evidence.

These standards have informed the advice contained in this book, and in places are quoted directly. The full standards documents can be accessed from the following websites:

Renal Association: *www.renal.org*
K/DOQI: *www.kidney.org/professionals/doqi*
European Best Practice Guidelines: *www.ndt-educational.org/guidelines*

▶ The Kidney Disease: Improving Global Outcomes (KDIGO) initiative was set up in 2003 with the aim of improving international dissemination and cooperation in the development of guidelines (*www.kdigo.org*). Many national and international standards documents can be accessed from this website.

Table 12.2 Guidelines: anaemia management

	UK Renal Association	US K/DOQI
Target Hb (g/dL)	>10	11–12
Frequency of measuring Hb	Monthly for stable HD patients. 3–4 monthly for other stable patients on EPO. More frequently around time of dose adjustments	1–2 weekly at first. 2–4 weekly when stable
Assessing iron status	Ferritin >100mg/L and TSAT >20% (or <10% hypochromic red cells)	Ferritin >100mg/L and TSAT >20%
Frequency of monitoring iron status	At least every 6 months	Monthly if not stable, 3 monthly if stable (3–6 monthly if not on dialysis)
Monitoring of iron status	At least every 6 months	Monthly if not on IV iron, 3 monthly once stable. CKD patients not on EPO: 3–6 monthly

Table 12.3 Guidelines: calcium, phosphate, and PTH management

	UK Renal Association	K/DOQI
Serum phosphate (mmol/L)	<1.8 for non-dialysis patients	Stages 3–4: 0.87–1.49, stage 5 and dialysis: 1.13–1.78
Serum calcium (mmol/L)	2.2–2.6	Stages 3–4: within local normal range, stage 5: 2.10–2.37
Serum aluminium (µmol/L)	Every 3 months (HD and/or if on aluminium containing preparations). DFO test if >2.2	Yearly, and every 3 months if on aluminium containing preparations. DFO test if >2.2
PTH (pmol/L)	<4 × upper limit normal	Stage 3: 3.8–7.7 Stage 4: 1.1–12.1 Stage 5: 16.5–33

Table 12.4 Cardiovascular risk factors

	UK Renal Association	K/DOQI
BP	HD: <140/90 pre-dialysis, <130/80 post-dialysis. PD and transplant recipients: <130/80. CKD patients <130/80 (<125/75 if proteinuria)	<130/80
HbA1c in diabetics	<7%	
Lipids–indications for starting statin therapy	10 year risk coronary disease >30%	Stage 5 CKD: LDL <2.59mmol/L, fasting triglycerides <2.26 mmol/L, non-HDL chol <3.36
Lipids–targets	Total cholesterol <5 mmol/L or 30% reduction from baseline or fasting LDL <3 mmol/L (whichever is the greater)	Non HDL chol <3.36mmol/L

Table 12.5 Nutrition

	UK Renal Association	K/DOQI
Serum albumin (g/L)	If<35g/L (bromocresol green) or <30g/L (bromocresol purple) then investigate. No standard set	>40 g/L (bromocresol green)
Serum bicarbonate (mmol/L)	22–26 (HD), 25–29 (PD)	>22
Screening	BMI, serial weights, albumin, SGA	Serial weights, dietary interviews, nPCR, SGA

Table 12.6 Adequacy, access, and sepsis

	UK Renal Association	K/DOQI
HD		
eKt/V (for thrice weekly dialysis)	>1.2 (or URR > 65%), measured monthly	>1.2 (single pool), measured monthly
Vascular access	>67% patients presenting within 3 months of dialysis start date should commence with a via native AVF	>50% of all new HD patients should have native AVF
	80% of prevalent HD patients should have native AVF	40% of prevalent HD patients should have native AVF
PD		
Weekly Kt/V	>1.7 and/or total weekly Cr clearance >50L/week/ 1.73m^2 (may be higher in APD or high transporters)	Weekly Kt/V >2 and total Cr clear >60L/week/ 1.73m^2 (50L/week/1.73m^2 for low transporters)
Peritonitis rate	<1 in 18 months	
Negative culture rate	<15%	
Initial cure rate	>80%	

Useful websites

Journals

Advances in Renal Replacement Therapy: www2.arrtjournal.org
American Journal of Kidney Diseases www.ajkd.org
American Journal of Nephrology: www.Karger.ch/journals/ajn/ajn_jh.htm
Journal of the American Society of Nephrology (JASN): www.jasn.org
Kidney International (KI): www.blackwell-synergy.com/issuelist.asp?journal=kid
Lancet: http://www.thelancet.com
Nephrology Dialysis Transplantation: www.ndt.oupjournals.org
New England Journal of Medicine: http://www.nejm.org
Transplantation: www.centerspan.org/pubs/transplantation
Peritoneal Dialysis International: www.multi-med.com/pdi

Associations

American Association of Kidney Patients: www.aakp.org
American Nephrology Nurse Association: www.anna.inurse.com
American Society of Nephrology: www.asn-online.com
American Society of Transplantation: www.a-s-t.org
Australia and New Zealand Society of Nephrology: www.nephrology.edu.au
Australian Kidney Foundation: www.kidney.org.au
European Kidney Patients' Federation: www.ceapir.org
European Renal Association: www.era-edta.org
International Society of Nephrology: www.isn-online.org
International Society of Peritoneal Dialysis: www.ispd.org
National Kidney Foundation: www.kidneyorg
Kidney Research UK: www.nkrf.org.uk
UK Renal Association: www.renal.org
UK Renal Registry: www.renalreg.com
USRDS: www.usrds.org
Vascular Access Society: www.vascularaccesssociety.com
World Kidney Fund: www.worldkidneyfund.org

Miscellaneous

Atlas of Diseases of the Kidney: www.kidneyatlas.org
Cybernephrology: www.cybernephrology.org
K/DOQI guidelines: www.kidney.org/professionals/doqi
Kidney disease community: www.ikidney.com
Kidney school: www.kidneyschool.org
Kidney patient guide: www.kidneypatientguide.org.uk
Nephron information centre: nephron.com
Nephroworld: www.nephroworld.com
Nephronline: www.nephronline.com
RenalNet: www.renalnet.org
Renal Web: www.renalweb.com
Travel Dialysis Site: www.dialysisfinder.com

Index